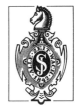

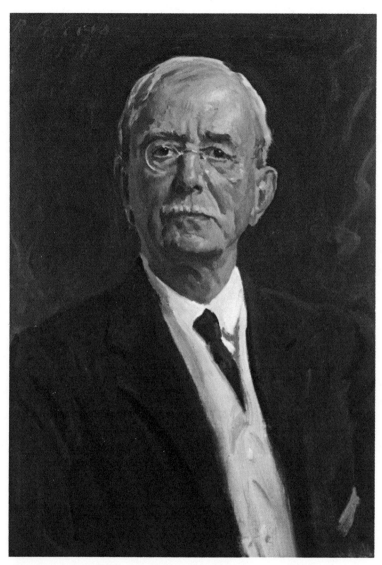

Portrait by R. G. Eves, 1927, in the Sherrington Room,
Woodward Library, University of British Columbia

John C. Eccles   William C. Gibson

Sherrington
His Life and Thought

Springer International 1979

Sir John Eccles

CH-6611 Contra (Locarno) TI. Switzerland

Max-Planck-Institut für biophysikalische Chemie
(Karl-Friedrich-Bonnhoeffer-Institut) D-3400 Göttingen, West-Germany

Professor William C. Gibson

Department of the History of Science and Medicine, Medical School,
University of British Columbia, Vancouver, B. C. V6T 1W5/Canada

ISBN 3-540-09063-0 Springer-Verlag Berlin Heidelberg New York
ISBN 0-387-09063-0 Springer-Verlag New York Heidelberg Berlin

Library of Congress Cataloging in Publication Data. Eccles, John Carew, Sir. Sherrington, his life and thought. Bibliography: p. Includes index. 1. Sherrington, Charles Scott, Sir., 1857–1952. 2. Physiologists-England-Biography. I. Gibson, William Carleton, joint author. II. Sherrington, Charles Scott, Sir., 1857–1952. Sherrington, his life and thought. III. title. QP26.S48E23 591.1'092'4 [B] 78-11359

© by Springer-Verlag Berlin · Heidelberg 1979

Printed in Germany

Offsetprinting and Binding: Appl, Wemding.   2120/3140-543210

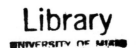

This volume is dedicated to the memory of

Carr and Margaret Sherrington

Preface

So much has been written about the scientific contributions of Sherrington that the man himself, and his thoughts, have been overshadowed. More and more, students of history are calling for creative writing on the whole man, particularly when he is a genius. Those interested in the genesis of ideas want to know the settings for discoveries and the relevant circumstances which ushered in new truths and new insights. The "prepared mind" which Pasteur saw as the only one to be "favoured by fortune" is of immense importance in science, and our account of Sherrington, we hope, will fill a very real gap in this field.

During his life Sherrington actively discouraged any suggestions that a biography be written. For that reason it was not until 1947 that there were any biographical notes by John Fulton, Graham Brown and A. D. Ritchie in a number of the British Medical Journal commemorating his ninetieth birthday, and in addition there was a leading article entitled "The Influence of Sherrington on Clinical Neurology". He left no autobiographical material except the few pages of reminiscences entitled "Marginalia", an essay written in honour of Charles Singer (1953).

In 1952 there were several obituary notices, the most definitive being that of Liddell for the Royal Society. Liddell also wrote charmingly in the Oxford Magazine. Other notices were by Fulton in the *Journal of Neurophysiology* and in the *Lancet*, Denny-Brown in the *American Journal of Psychology*, Creed in the *British Journal of Psychology*, Forbes in the *Journal of Clinical Neurophysiology* and *EEG*, Moruzzi in *Rivista Sperimentale di Frematria* and Eccles in the *British Journal of the Philosophy of Science*. C. S. S. was the subject of a television programme "Medical Explorers" by Gibson for the Canadian Broadcasting Corporation.

In planning the scope of this book we have been mindful of these obituary notices and of the books that have already been written about Sherrington. These publications have contributed notably to the understanding of this many-faceted man of genius. Our aim has been to concentrate on themes that had been but lightly touched upon by previous biographers. We have also the advantage of more than one thousand letters written by Sherrington that have not hitherto been available, and a large number of letters to Sherrington. This voluminous correspondence gives new and valuable insights into Sherrington's activities during his dedicated labours of over fifty years. His diffidence in conversation was overcome, slightly, in his letters, which were so condensed but elegant that the recipient was left with an inexplicable, glowing feeling of awe and affection.

We have passed lightly over the great experimental periods that preceded his Oxford school because there are several admirable and detailed accounts in the biographies of Liddell, Granit and Swazey. In the *Discovery of Reflexes* Liddell has given a most scholarly survey of our knowledge of the nervous system, both experimentally and theoretically, up to the time when Sherrington set about transforming it scientifically. Liddell's Obituary Notice for the Royal Society is a masterpiece of biography that stresses particularly the great contributions of Sherrington to the basic elements of central nervous system physiology. Granit's beautifully written and illustrated biography also concentrates on Sherrington's neurophysiology and then continues on, most valuably, to show how Sherrington's contributions have led to the great discoveries of the last decades, notably in the Nobel Institute for Neurophysiology.

What then will our tasks be? We append a brief outline.

1. Sherrington's dedication to the advancement of science and to the application of science to human welfare. He was a man of affairs exerting an influence of great importance in England and indeed in the world. Sherrington was concerned to analyze the lack of productivity in British medical science in the final years of the nineteenth century, in comparison with that of

France and Germany. He wondered where the compatriots of William Harvey were going wrong, little realizing that he himself was doing for the complicated nervous system what Harvey did for the circulatory system three hundred years before.

2. The preparation of Sherrington for a career of research and teaching. He was well grounded in general biology and basic physiology by professors at Cambridge such as Foster and Gaskell. After teaching human anatomy he studied in Germany with the leading pathologists and bacteriologists of the last century. An undergraduate interest in the nervous system was revived and enlarged when he headed an animal care institute in London and led finally to the chair of physiology at Liverpool. The world-wide network of students and co-workers which he developed there was extended by his appointment to Oxford in 1913. We have chronicled these years in detail.

3. An intimate account of Sherrington the human person and colleague as experienced in the Oxford laboratory of the 1920s and 1930s. We have a narrative to recount from memories and records which may be more appealing than general eulogistic statements. Some of these incidents have their own unique flavour.

4. Sherrington as a builder of theories of the nervous system. This most important scientific contribution has been rather overlooked in favour of the detailed description of experimental results. Yet from 1925 until 1932 Sherrington could be regarded as the great integrator of knowledge of the central nervous system and his theories are still relevant today.

5. From 1933 until his death in 1952 Sherrington was dedicated to the philosophy of the central nervous system. He rightly sensed that it was the greatest problem, both scientific and philosophical, confronting man. He was well fitted for this great task with his comprehensive knowledge both of the nervous system and of the whole field of biology. He brought to this task a wonderfully creative imagination, along with literary, artistic and poetic skills. Furthermore he had the great

advantage of his historical knowledge from classical times. In particular his devotion to Jean Fernel made him a key figure in the project. We feel that the Rede Lecture and the Gifford Lectures give unique insights into Sherrington himself and his sensitive, subtle and imaginative nature. In our opinion they greatly enhance his stature as one of the creative geniuses of our century.

Previous biographers have overlooked the great ethical messages in the last chapter of *Man on His Nature.* Sherrington very strongly expressed his conviction that in the evolutionary process predacity had gradually given place to certain values and that these values were necessary to man's survival – altruism being exalted above all others. His message is both noble and appealing in its urgency.

J.C.E. and W.C.G.

Acknowledgements

The preparation of this highly personalized account of Sherrington's career has involved material and assistance contributed by many wellwishers including his family and contemporaries in the scientific world. The final writing has made possible by an invitation to spend the month of May, 1977, at the Rockefeller Foundation's Villa Serbelloni at Bellagio. There, assisted by our wives, by the Resident Director Dr. William Olson and his wife, and by the scholars in residence and their families, it was possible to compress much of our relevant material into this small volume.

For permission to quote from letters to and from Sir Charles we are indebted to the late Lord Adrian, A. V. Hill, Lady Florey, Mrs. J. F. Fulton and the Yale University Library, the Osler Library and the Wellcome Institute of the History of Medicine, London. The publishers of Sherrington's many works have generously agreed to our use of quotations and illustrations from them. To Christie Stangroom who typed the final manuscript we are deeply indebted. For photographs of portraits we acknowledge the ready co-operation of the H. K. Anderson Library, Cambridge, the National Portrait Gallery, London (Dr. John Hayes and Dr. Malcolm Rogers) and the Biomedical Communications Centre of the University of British Columbia.

To Basil Stuart Stubbs, Anna Leith and Barbara C. Gibson of the University of British Columbia Library System thanks are due for permission to quote from the large holdings of Sherringtonia under their devoted care.

Contents

Chapter 1

The Early Years

Like Leonardo da Vinci, Sherrington began life as a collector of shells and fossils, even venturing into the field of coins dating from the time of Charles I. He grew to young manhood in a home noted for its collection of fine paintings, books and geological specimens. His teachers at the Ipswich Grammar School included a distinguished classical scholar, H. A. Holden, and a gifted young poet, Thomas Ashe, who imbued the sensitive Charles with a desire to read, and especially to write, beautiful poetry. He read widely and, even before matriculating, had studied Johannes Müller's *Elements of Physiology,* given to him by his stepfather, Dr. Caleb Rose.

A bank failure so crippled the family's finances that Charles enrolled at St. Thomas's Hospital Medical School in London in order to permit his brothers William and George to go up to Cambridge ahead of him. On arriving eventually at Cambridge[1], Charles divided his time between his two loves, science and poetry. He sent one of his early poems to Longfellow, who took the trouble to write him a congratulatory letter. Two months later, in March of 1882, Longfellow died in Massachusetts, and Sherrington wrote an appreciation of the poet's work in the *Cambridge Review* which strikes one as incredibly erudite in a student aged twenty-four (Appendix 1). With the limited money available to him, the young Charles bought at Heffer's book shop in Cambridge a first edition of Keats' poems. Also while at Cambridge he purchased in 1887 Nicholas Hawksmoor's personal copy of Bidloo's *Anatomia*[2] published in 1685, a masterpiece of copperplate engraving.

Medical studies at St. Thomas's Hospital in London were interwoven

---

1 Reminiscing years later, Sherrington would chuckle over entrance examinations in which his friend Robert Bridges was reported to have put the Latin piece for translation into Greek and the Greek into Latin.

2 Presented to Dr. F. F. Wesbrook, President of the University of British Columbia in 1915 and now in the rare book collection of the Woodward Biomedical Library.

with his terms at Gonville and Caius College, Cambridge. Three-quarters of
a century later, Sherrington loved to tell the story of being left, one
weekend, in charge of Addenbrooke's Hospital in Cambridge where his
ingeniuity was taxed by a patient determined to jump off the roof. In
London his clinical clerkship in obstetrics was for him unforgettable. His
account in "Marginalia", written at a great age, recalls it vividly (Appendix
2). Both at St. Thomas's Hospital Medical School in London and at Cambridge, Sherrington was an active athlete. In London his delight was in
rugby. At Cambridge, despite his diminutive stature he was active in rowing; his brothers excelled in cricket and one was prominent for years in the
Football Association of Great Britain.

Charles was one of the early devotees of winter sports at Grindelwald.
He described for a much later generation of Cambridge students his
pioneering experiences (Appendix 3).

Despite such diversions Sherrington took a first class in the Cambridge
Natural Science Tripos, Part I, in 1882, and in the following year gained, in
Part II, a 'first class with distinction'. His tutor, the talented Walter Hol-
brook Gaskell[1], wrote to him on 25 November, 1881:

Dear Mr. Sherrington,
You obtained the highest marks in your year for Botany, Human Anatomy and Physiology; and were second in Zoology. You obtained the highest total in your year – that is
261; the next man obtained 253.

As an embryo teacher, Sherrington served, during the following year, as
a "student demonstrator" in anatomy under Sir George Humphry – a man
endowed with revolutionary zeal in the modernizing of the Cambridge
Medical School. His opposite number in physiology was that benign "discoverer of men" Michael Foster. It has been said that Foster discovered and
converted to physiology two mathematicians, W. H. Gaskell and John New-
port Langley. More importantly, he discovered and converted a one-time
classics scholar, Charles Scott Sherrington. Gaskell had part of his training
in the laboratory of Carl Ludwig in Leipzig. Langley founded, and for many
years owned, the *Journal of Physiology*.

Sherrington took his Cambridge medical degree in 1885, having already
published his first scientific paper, with J. N. Langley, on the brain of a dog,
which had been demonstrated by Prof. Goltz at the International Medical
Congress in London. A furious disagreement had broken out on the floor of
the Congress concerning the effect of removing a portion of the brain on the
performance of animals. A committee was set up to make certain anatomi-

---

1 For his appreciation of Gaskell see Appendix 6.

cal studies under Langley's supervision. This research marked the beginning of Sherrington's ensuing 320 scientific publications!

It is worth noting that it was at the same tempestuous meeting that Sherrington first saw in action his hero David Ferrier, to whom he was twenty years later to dedicate his classic *Integrative Action of the Nervous System*. Ferrier demonstrated a monkey which, after surgical removal of part of the brain, exhibited a paralysis on the opposite side of the body. The likeness to the human picture following a 'stroke' was so exact that the great French neurologist Charcot cried out, "C'est une malade!"

For nearly nine months thereafter Sherrington studied in Strasbourg with Professor Goltz, whose dog and whose views had caused so much controversy at the London congress of recent memory. The localization of function in the brain became Sherrington's chief concern while he was in Strasbourg, and it pleased him greatly when, nearly fifty years later, he received an honorary doctorate from that university. Worthy of note also is the warm letter of recommendation which Goltz sent to the University of Liverpool where Sherrington later applied for the chair of physiology. In it Goltz referred to his former pupil as a "good observer" and said that Sherrington was now fulfilling the high expectations which his teacher had long had of him.

In 1885 Sherrington was presented with an opportunity for foreign travel – an addiction which he was only too happy to cultivate. His friend, the newly elected professor of pathology at Cambridge, C. S. Roy[1], had recently solved a problem of infection which was devastating the cattle in Argentina. As Sherrington wrote later, Roy "succeeded in devising a preventive inoculation which alleviated the mischief". The next 'mischief' occurred in Spain in the form of Asiatic cholera, and a Spanish physician was claiming that he had produced a vaccine with which to combat it.

Sherrington was sceptical, however, that a vaccine had been successfully produced in Spain. Thus, with J. Graham Brown, also of Cambridge, Sherrington and Roy set off for the Peninsula. They moved about that land under the auspices of Cambridge University, the Royal Society of London, and the Association for Research in Medicine! In spite of this, however, they were required to pay the commanding army general of the infected area his 'cut' before they could proceed to see cases beyond the quarantine barriers.

---

1 Roy had been the first to hold the 'George Henry Lewes Studentship' in physiology, founded at Cambridge by "George Eliot".

In Toledo an angry mob set upon the trio, and the intervention of the British Consul – a huge Scot who could curse loudly in Spanish – saved their lives. Paving stones were flying through the air by the time he arrived. On their return to England in the autumn, the three decided to send a gift to the Consul and chose a handsome ram's horn into which a snuff-box had been fitted. Alas, the gift was entrusted to C. S. Roy for forwarding. His fatal illness intervened so that the gift never went on its way to Toledo[1].

Parenthetically, it should be made clear that Sherrington did *not* meet in Spain at this time Santiago Ramón y Cajal, as so may biographers have repeatedly stated. Cajal was hundreds of miles away investigating the cholera problem in Zaragossa. He and Sherrington met for the first and only time in London in 1894.

The report presented by Roy, Sherrington and Graham Brown to the Royal Society discredited the claims made for the Spanish vaccine. It confirmed Koch's work on the cholera-spirillum. Sherrington went to Italy the following year to investigate cholera. He also spent time in the Italian art galleries! It was here that his love for rare books developed into an addiction, and many priceless volumes began to find their way to Sherrington's 'secret shelves' in England. Fifty years later he was still pretending that his acquisitions were negligible because, he said of his wife, ". . . dear Ethel would not understand". In fact he became the greatest donor of incunabula to the British Museum in its history[2].

Armed with specimens acquired in these two cholera outbreaks, Sherrington went to Berlin to study with Rudolf Virchow, the professor of pathology who through his great work, *Cellular Pathology,* had applied the 'cell theory' of Schleiden and Schwann to diseased tissues and cancerous growths. Virchow, the son of a country merchant, had scandalized official Berlin by announcing to his students that the King of Prussia had softening of the brain; his paternal ancestor hardening of the brain; and the grandson, no brain at all. After seven years of banishment to Wurzburg, Virchow was invited by unanimous vote of the medical faculty to return to Berlin, to a new institute. It was here that Sherrington went to study pathology, and here began his political education. Virchow, who was elected to the Reichstag before he was old enough to take a seat, was to remain fifty years in that chamber as the implacable enemy of Bismarck. Sherrington used to go to

1 The snuff-box is now at the Woodward Biomedical Library, University of British Columbia.
2 One of his Italian acquisitions, Valla's *Elegantia* (1476) was given in 1938 to the University of British Columbia as a memorial to its first president, Sherrington's colleague of Cambridge days, F. F. Wesbrook.

the Reichstag with Virchow to watch the 'fireworks' as Bismarck would appear from a little cuckoo-clock opening above the assembled lawmakers, shout at them and then withdraw without hearing their deliberations. Between his exposure to Virchow's liberal views and his own memory of the occupation by German troops of Strasbourg, Sherrington became truly anti-Prussian. In the subsequent two world wars he was to become a ready source of help in time of trouble for many refugees from Germany.

Sherrington returned to England to an appointment as lecturer in physiology at St. Thomas's Hospital Medical School and a fellowship at Caius College, Cambridge. He now settled down to his life's work of teaching and research. He kept up a correspondence with Virchow in Berlin on pathological anatomy, only gradually moving towards physiology, or the functions of the body. In 1887 he was studying the spinal cord and medulla of a patient dying after suffering for years with locomotor ataxia. This case study followed that of a patient who succumbed fifty-two days after a cerebral haemorrhage. More studies of brain pathology followed as Sherrington clearly made good use of his opportunities in his busy hospital home overlooking the Thames, whose waters reflect the Houses of Parliament in Westminster.

Already the catholicity of Sherrington's interests was declaring itself, with work on the formation of scar tissue, alternating with that on the nerve cell constituents of the spinal cord of mammals. At the same time he became the Honorary Secretary of the Physiological Society, an office which he held until 1905. He produced with C. S. Roy a work on cerebral circulation which is only today being acclaimed by experts armed with sophisticated techniques.

During his four years at St. Thomas's Hospital Sherrington published more than a dozen papers and began to build the foundation on which modern neurology is based. In 1891 an inspired appointments committee named Sherrington the Physician-Superintendent of the Brown Institution of the University of London located in the Wandsworth Road, Vauxhall. Who was Brown and what did he intend[1]?

Thomas Brown, M. A., LL. B. of Dublin bequeathed to the University of London upon his death in 1854, £ 20000 and the residue of his personal property ". . . for the founding, establishing and upholding of an institution for investigating, studying and without charge, beyond immediate expenses,

---

[1] William LeFanu, Librarian of the Royal College of Surgeons of England, has compiled a synopsis of the founding of the Institution and Sir Graham Wilson is publishing a full history of this unique establishment.

endeavouring to cure maladies, distemper and injuries any Quadrupeds or Birds useful to Man may be found subject to".

This lengthy document goes on to specify that

> ... previous to the Animal Sanatory Institution as aforesaid being opened for the reception of animals and cure of their ailments, a Superintendent or Professor ... shall be appointed by the Chancellor ... the said Professor to have a residence adjacent besides the salary and that he shall give at least five lectures in English and free to the public at some place appointed by the University of London. And I further desire that kindness to the animals committed to his charge shall be a general principle of the Institution.

Brown suggested the appointment of a committee which would control the number and types of diseased or injured animals to be admitted and which would purchase diseased animals or their carcasses for the promotion of science. Failing all this, the funds were to be given to the University of Dublin for chairs of languages!

Sherrington was preceded in this appointment by four distinguished scientists: John Burdon Sanderson, who lectured on inflammation; W. S. Greenfield on anthrax; C. S. Roy on the pathology of the heart and on inoculation against infections (such as his successful solution to the Argentinian cattle disease already mentioned); and the surgeon Victor Horsley, who lectured on the thyroid gland, on infections and on epilepsy.

Since Sherrington was later to have a dispute with the opinionated Horsley, it may be of interest to review briefly Horsley's activities at the Brown Institution. From 1884 to 1891 he published in the *Lancet* very considerable reports of his work, with the result that the Society for the Abolition of Vivisection and certain pamphleteers seized upon this as proof that the bequest was being misused. An appeal was launched to the Charity Commissioners on two occasions and Horsley was cited in a suit in the Chancery Division of the High Court, along with the Chancelllor, Vice-Chancellor and Fellows of the University of London.

In the first sixteen years of its existence the Brown Institution admitted for treatment 45000 animals of all kinds so that the public was relatively satisfied that Thomas Brown's foundation was doing its job. When Horsley left – to run for Parliament and to campaign for anti-alcoholism and dress reform for women – Sherrington proceeded to mobilize the great animal resources of the institution for scientific research. In four years he published another twenty papers, principally on the course of fibres within the nervous system, on the explanation of long-known but not yet understood reflexes, on epilepsy, on the blood and inflammation. Halfway through his superintendency he was elected a Fellow of the Royal Society.

In 1891 Lord Lister, as President of the International Congress of Hygiene and Demography, found himself assisted by two under-secretaries,

Charles Sherrington and Armand Ruffer. These two physicians, interested in infectious diseases and their prevention and cure, were to become the key figures in a diphtheria drama soon to unfold. At the age of ninety, Sherrington gave the following account of the 1894 happenings, written to Sir Percival Hartley of the Royal Society Club on 15 November 1947:

15 Nov. 1947.   12 Grassington Road
                                              Eastbourne.

Dear Senior Treasurer, thank you for kindly writing. Yes, the story was just as you say; except that dear Ruffer's first name was Armand. Poor fellow, he was torpedoed & drowned by the Germans in the 1ˢᵗ World war. He was brother-in-law to Bouchard of Paris, the leading French physician in his line. The story of the horse at The Brown had a dramatic sequel, which perhaps Dr. Drury has not heard; if he has, he will, I hope, forgive my telling it; it may interest you. Ruffer & I had been injecting the horse — our first horse — only a short time. We were badly in the dark as to the dosage to employ, or how quickly to repeat the increasing injections. We had from it a serum partly effective in guinea-pigs. Then, on a Saturday evening, about 7 o'clock, came a bolt from the blue. A wire from my brother-in-law, in Sussex. "George has diphtheria. Can you come?" George, a boy of 7, was the only child. The house, an old Georgian house, 3 miles out of Lewes, set back in a combe under a chalk down. There was no train that night. I did not at first give thought to horse, & when I did, regretfully supposed it could not yet be ripe for use. However I took a cab to find Ruffer. No telephone or taxi in those days — '93 or '94 - Ruffer was dining out; I pursued him & got a word with him. He said "By all means, you can use the horse, but it is not yet ripe for trial." Then by lantern-light at 'The Brown' I bled the horse, into a 2 litre flask duly sterilised & plugged with sterile wool. I left the blood in ice for it to settle. After sterilising smaller flasks, & pipettes & some needle-syringes I drove home, to return at midnight, & decant the serum, &c.

By the Sunday morning train I reached Lewes. Dr. Fawssett of Lewes — he had a brother on the staff at Guy's — was waiting in a dog-cart at the station. I joined him carrying my awkward packet of flasks, &c. He said nothing as I packed them in but, when I had climbed up beside him, he looked down & said, "You can do what you like with the boy. He will not be alive at tea-time." We drove out to the old house; a bright frosty morning. Tragedy was over the place - the servants scared & silent. The boy was very weak; breathing with difficulty; he did not seem to know me. Fawssett & I injected the serum. The syringes were small & we emptied them time & again. The Doctor left. I sat with the boy. Early in the afternoon the boy seemed to me clearly better. At 3 o'clock I sent a messenger to the Doctor to say so. Thenceforward progress was uninterrupted. On Tuesday I returned to London, & sought out Ruffer. His reaction was that we must tell Lister about it. The great Surgeon (not Lord Lister then) had visitors, some Continental Surgeons, to dinner. "You must tell my guests about it." he said, + insisted — so we told them in the drawing-room, at Park Crescent. The boy had a severe paralysis for a time. He grew to be 6ft. or had a commission in the 1st World war.

One of Sherrington's most treasured letters was written to him by Lord Lister on 29 October 1894 from 19 Park Crescent, Portland Place:

Dear Doctor Sherrington,
I cannot but write a line to tell you how much pleasure it has given me to learn that your nephew and also your sister, who took diphtheria from him, are doing well. Believe me, yours very sincerely, Joseph Lister.

A good personal correspondent, Sherrington was also a doughty letter-writer on public issues where misrepresentation of medical science by anti-vivisectionists was involved.

Sherrington's forthright views were clearly stated in his confidential reviews of papers submitted for publication to the Royal Society. Within a year of his election (1893) he was called upon to referee many works in the field of neurology. Taken at random are these statements:

The new matter in the paper is contained in pages 35–47 inclusive ... only a single protocol appears and that is interspersed in the ordinary text somewhat to the obscurement of both ... Considering the slender quantity of new matter added by the communication, the "historical introduction" (going back to Galen and the cartilagenous fishes) is certainly redundant ... I feel strongly that the publication of the paper in the *Philosophical Transactions* would be detrimental to the quality and character of the *Transactions*.

The comment made by Sherrington on H. H. Dale's paper of 1904 "on the islets of Langerhans was: "The paper contains valuable evidence and is written with critical care and very lucidly." Of A. B. Macallum's 1905 paper "on the distribution of chlorides in nerve cells and fibres", his critique was: "This paper is of interest not only from the point of view of the visible structure but of the function of nerve. It contributes to a newly-arisen conception of the working of nerve". Sherrington supported the publication in the *Philosophical Transactions* of F. W. Mott's manuscript on "a complete survey of the cell lamination of the cerebral cortex of the lemur", saying, "The results fill in a gap in our knowledge of the cortex cerebri that has long required to be removed".

Despite his appointment to the Brown Institution Sherrington did not lose interest in St. Thomas's Hospital. He became, in fact, one of the large number who signed a massive deed on 15 December 1892, guaranteeing a sinking fund which was to be raised for the construction of a new teaching building for the medical school. The eminence of his academic colleagues is to be seen from the signatures. Today it is pleasant to record that his favourite subject is taught in a trim brick building beside the Thames, designated as The Sherrington School of Physiology.

The year 1894 saw the publication of one of his finest works in the field of microscopic anatomy. He was able to demonstrate that the "muscle spindles" which his friend Ruffini had shown to resemble little coiled springs between the fibres of muscle, were actually sensory in nature, informing the nervous system of the state of contraction of any skeletal muscle. Professor Denny-Brown has commented on this work, in a personal communication:

> Sherrington was both interested and accomplished in histology . . . His best known contribution is his demonstration of the sensory nature of the annulo-spiral endings in muscle. He told me that he had included a large number of illustrations of the histology, but they were all discarded by Langley who was then the editor of the journal . . . He made a great many preparations of the afferent endings in eye muscle with methylene blue and showed me some drawings of these which were very beautifully done.

Sherrington was responsible for the Royal Society's invitation to Professor Santiago Ramón y Cajal of Madrid to give the Croonian lecture to the Society for the year 1894. To find, especially in far-off Spain, a peasant genius who had for fifteen years been unravelling the secrets of nerve cells under the microscope, was something to celebrate, thought Sherrington. He had read the Spanish and the halting French publications of the Spanish scholar, as few others had done. Cajal had sent reprints of his earliest papers, appearing in *El Diario Catolico* of Zaragossa, to the crowned heads of Europe. In Britain, fortunately, they filtered down to the Royal Society, and thus to Sherrington.

Sherrington had taken on more than he had bargained for in inviting Cajal to be his guest in London. Mrs. Sherrington was to discover that Spaniards stripped their beds each day and hung the bedding out of the window, to the consternation of the neighbours and of the weather prophets in the uncertain climate of London. She also found that Cajal kept his bedroom door locked all day, to protect the little laboratory which he had set up in order to give the final touches to his silver staining of the nervous tissue.

It was difficult to convince Cajal that not all those attending his lecture at the Royal Society's rooms in Burlington House would want to line up for even a rapid look at his preparations under the microscope. Sherrington quietly prepared lantern slides of many of the specimens, but Cajal was at first unwilling to use them. He was, however, so impressed by what he later described as ". . . the hospitality of Ch. Sherrington and his admirable wife, provided with such attention and finesse . . ." that he relented and permitted a few slides to be projected. The fact that Sherrington had provided large flags of Britain and Spain intertwined and a good supply of champagne, impressed his visitor mightily. Michael Foster at the Royal Society dinner remarked that Cajal had transformed the impenetrable forest of the nervous system into a well-kept park! The Spanish Ambassador told his audience that the three most memorable occasions in his life were his first sight of Niagara Falls, his first view of the Coliseum in Rome, and listening to Cajal's lecture to the Royal Society.

The day of Cajal's honorary doctorate at Cambridge provided the best story. Sherrington had to go up the day before for some business and his wife had to put Cajal on the Cambridge train from Liverpool Street on the appointed day. She was anxious to get Cajal ready ahead of time. The cab driver was summoned and given a specially large payment with instructions to put Cajal on the Cambridge train. This he did with enthusiasm because of the large 'bribe', whipping up his horse and arriving in record time. The result was that Cajal was rushed by the cabbie to an earlier train to Cambridge than the agreed one. He arrived in Cambridge forgetful of why he was there with no one on the platform to meet him when we was delivered from the then empty train at Cambridge. He wandered down the street, and passing Emmanuel College, he proceeded to sketch its attractive facade, standing in the middle of the street and blocking traffic. When requested to move he could not understand, and seemed so lost that the police took charge of him.

Meanwhile the correct train had arrived without Cajal, to the consternation of the waiting Sherrington. So he telegraphed his wife asking "Why no Cajal?" She laconically replied by return telegram – there were no telephones in those days – "Cajal consigned by the 11.10 train". But of course this telegraphic exchange took an hour or so and meanwhile the Vice Chancellor's lunch in honour of Cajal, the graduand, had to be held without him. Eventually an enquiry to the police elicited the reply, "We have a fellow along at the station who may be your man". So Cajal was rescued in time for the graduation ceremony but without his lunch!

In his autobiography, *Recuerdos de mi Vida*, Cajal returns again and again to the hospitality of Sherrington and details of the itinerary arranged by him. As he says, Sherrington gave up everything in his daily routine to guide the visitor to the British Museum, the Royal College of Surgeons, three medical schools, the laboratories of Ferrier, Schäfer and Mott, and not least of all, to memorials in Westminster Abbey to Newton and Darwin.

Fifty-five years later the American publisher Henry Schuman was preparing to publish Dorothy Cannon's excellent biography of Ramón y Cajal when it was suggested to him by one of us (W. C. G.) who had worked in Cajal's laboratory in Madrid, that Sherrington, although over ninety years of age, might be willing to write a foreword. What Sherrington provided in a very short time was a seven-page "Memoir of Dr. Cajal" (Appendix 4). This beautifully executed study of a man whom he saw only once in his life – albeit for two concentrated weeks in the Spring of 1894 – tells us much about the author. Sherrington and Cajal, with the help of such scientists as the Belgian van Gehuchten, had pioneered the idea that the basic structural unit of the entire nervous system is a specialized cell with transmission polarized in one direction. Neither of them approved of the way in which Sherrington's colleague of Berlin days – Waldeyer – who had merely popularized their concept as the "neuron theory", was credited with its discovery.

Sherrington has described Cajal's "intense anthropomorphism" in discussing his preparations: "Listening to him I asked myself how far this capacity . . . might not contribute to his success as an investigator. I never met anyone else in whom it was so marked". Our 'poet' concluded his introductory memoir of his much-beloved 'peasant' thus:

> Solicitude for his country's repute deserves explicit mention here; it was perhaps the most powerful driving-force in the make-up of his whole scientific character. It lifted him altogether above all personal vanity. His science was first and foremost an offering to Spain, a spiritual motive which added to the privilege of knowing the man.

(W.C.G.)

Chapter 2
The Liverpool Professor

Sherrington's first appointment to a full professorship came in 1895 when University College, Liverpool, invited him to the chair of physiology – as successor to Francis Gotch, who was leaving for Oxford's Waynflete professorship. Liverpool had some very interesting scholars at that time, including F. J. Cole, lecturer in zoology, destined to become a world authority in comparative zoology as well as a bibliophile, whose great historical collection is today at the University of Reading. Others were Augustus John, the painter, Elton and Raleigh in literature – all on the road to the heights of academia.

Pursuing his research on the organization of the spinal cord, Sherrington was soon invited to give the Croonian lecture before the Royal Society on 1 April 1897. He chose the title "The mammalian spinal cord as an organ of reflex action". Not only was he building up, block by block, the foundation of modern neurology, but also he was tackling the thorny problem of reflex action as opposed to voluntary action, which had bedevilled scholars since the time of Galen, especially Descartes.

Later that year, Professor and Mrs. Sherrington, with Lord Lister, Lord Kelvin and others journeyed to Toronto for meetings of the British Association. Following a week of speeches and dinners, they set out for the Canadian west coast, travelling on the Canadian Pacific Railway, which had been completed only a decade before. They admired the spectacular mountain scenery at Banff, Alberta, where Lord Kelvin made a speech which Sherrington's diary notes as very disappointing. Then down the canyons to Vancouver the party went, wondering how the pioneers had clung to the cliffs and braved the torrents. In Vancouver the party ascended in a "builder's lift" to the top of a "high building" then under construction. Sherrington was sure that a fine view of the mountains of Howe Sound would be afforded them, and gallantly threw open the door at the top of the elevator. The door, as he later loved to recount, led straight into thin air. All gasped and retreated, with Sherrington remarking to Lister, "It's a new country – not everything is finished yet!"

During this interlude the new laboratories for physiology and pathology were being built at Liverpool, the gift of the Reverend S. A. Thompson-Yates. The teaching and research facilities were of world calibre. The opening took place on 8 October 1898, immediately following a ceremony in the great hall of University College, where, before a crowd of 2000 citizens, Professor Rudolf Virchow of Berlin and Lord Lister were given honorary degrees. Lister's address was magnificent, recounting his obligation to great teachers, and making clear the origins of his scientific knowledge which helped him to make surgical procedures safe for mankind.

The hand of Sherrington could be discerned in parts of the speech, especially when Lister discussed operations and demonstrations on animals. The fact that these were done under anaesthesia was underlined several times. Clearly Sherrington was on guard against further outbursts by anti-vivisectionist sympathizers. Two weeks before the opening ceremonies were to take place, Lister had written from a vacation spot in Breconshire to Sherrington:

> My dear Professor Sherrington,
> I am greatly obliged to you for your letter which completely enlightens my ignorance, of which ignorance I have reason to be ashamed.
> I see from the *Lancet* that all the heads of your University and Colleges are to be present at the ceremony of the 8th, and that many distinguished members of our profession besides Virchow are to be there and some men eminent in other ways.
> Your information regarding your benefactor, &c. will be of great help to me in considering what line I ought to take in the remarks I make on the occasion.
> I do not know that anything in my life perplexed me more as to the course I ought to pursue than the Vaccination Bill. But I have been gratified by letters from men whose opinion I respect highly, expressing approval.
> Thanks for your kind care about the robing. Very sincerely yours, Lister.

The eminence of the invited guests meant that Lister's message was conveyed to bishops, parliamentarians, philanthropists and medical practitioners. The press wrote very long reports and editorials on the magnificence of the occasion. They noted that "Professor Richard Caton was an admirable spokesman of the feeling borne towards Lord Lister by the whole world". They also mentioned "those political services by which Herr Virchow has shown that a great man of science can also be a great champion of civil liberty".

In the October 1898 issue of the *Sphinx,* the student magazine of University College, Liverpool, seven pages are given to an unsigned account[1] of the new laboratories, together with Sherrington's views on the relevance of medical science to national and human welfare (Appendix 8).

The celebrations attending the opening of the Thompson-Yates laboratories allowed a burgeoning shipping centre an opportunity to show to the world its international ambitions and to add eventually to the intellectual capital of its people, thanks to local philanthropy. For Sherrington these were stirring and memorable times.

The year 1899 brought fresh opportunity to remind the citizenry of the opportunity and obligations facing them in another international context. On March 9th of that year Sherrington was reported in the *Liverpool Daily Post* thus:

> Professor C. S. Sherrington expressed his conviction of the value of the tropical diseases school not only to Liverpool, but to the whole country. The opportunities afforded by the second seaport in the Empire for the study, sufficiently guarantee the desirability of the foundation of the school here. Years ago Professor Koch had argued the national duty that devolved on England as mistress of India to investigate malaria and cholera. Yet in comparison with the work done by Germany, Italy, and America, England had contributed little to human defense against these diseases, altough the scourge especially touched her own sons. Mr. Chamberlain's advent to the Colonial office had proved a welcome era of medical progress in connection with that department.

A week later the Royal Medical and Chirurgical Society announced the award of its Marshall Hall gold medal to Sherrington ". . . for his services to medicine and surgery by his discoveries regarding the nervous system" over the preceding five years. Marshall Hall (1790–1857) had been an outstanding British physiologist and clinician, whose study of reflexes had opened the way to many new researches. The previous recipients included the eminent contributors to the world of neurology: Hughlings Jackson, Jean Martin Charcot of Paris, David Ferrier and William Gowers. Within a few months Sherrington was singled out by the Royal College of Physicians of London to receive their Baly gold medal ". . . for the person who shall be deemed to have most distinguished himself in the science of physiology, especially during the two years immediately preceding the award". The names of his predecessors in this award make up a veritable *Who's Who* of physiology: Richard Owen, Lionel Beale, William Sharpey, Claude Bernard, Carl Ludwig, Charles Darwin, John Burdon Sanderson, Charles Edouard Brown-Séquard, David Ferrier, Rudolf Heidenhain, Michael Foster, Morris Schiff, W. H. Gaskell and E. A. Schäfer.

While most friends of Sherrington would agree that he was the mildest of men, they would be quite wrong in believing that he could never be tough

---

1 (see p. 14) One of the authors (J. C. E.) has found unmistakable evidence that Sherrington was, in fact, the author, by comparing the wording of parts of the piece with publications elsewhere, signed by C. S. S.

and uncompromising. When unfair treatment was being given one of his friends, whether personal or institutional, he sprang for his pen. Late in 1900 he wrote to *The Times* to defend the National Hospital for Paralyzed and Epileptic in Queen Square London, against virulent and uninformed critics.

In laboratories it is taken for granted that alcohol for use as a chemical starting point or as a preservative should be available at its original cost. In 1901 this was certainly not so, and it is instructive to see Sherrington marshalling support for a proposed change in the regulations. His constant supporter in scientific research was Lord Lister, whose letter to him of 28 May 1901 may be quoted in part:

> The subject on which you have written is certainly a very important one, and I think the Council of the Royal Society might quite well approach the Chancellor of the Exchequer on the matter, perhaps in conjunction with delegates from other scientific bodies, provided we had a clear workable scheme to put before him for providing the much needed relief for scientific workers and teachers without risk of alcohol being diverted to other objects.

The summer of 1901 marked the arrival in Liverpool of an American brain surgeon who was to enjoy Sherrington's close friendship for the rest of his life. Harvey Cushing, trained at Yale, Harvard and Johns Hopkins, had completed a year of study in the best European clinics and, presumably at the suggestion of William Osler, his hero in Baltimore, had come to visit Sherrington en route home. He assisted with the professor's work on the electrical stimulation of the cerebral cortex in the higher primates and put to good use his skill as an artist. His maps of the cortex, sometimes in colour, were some of the finest ever printed. Although he could stay only one month with Sherrington, Cushing alluded to these early studies in many later addresses and publications. In addition he found Sherrington just as "exophthalmic with bibliomania" as he was himself. Later in this volume, we shall enlarge on this friendship.

One year later another American arrived, fresh from an apprenticeship with Professor E. A. Schäfer in Edinburgh. Robert Sessions Woodworth, who was to become the doyen of American psychologists, worked with Sherrington from 1902 to 1903 and only reluctantly returned to Columbia University, so entranced was he with Sherrington's developing views on the physiological basis of psychology. He was to learn at Liverpool that first class physiologists could be interested in the very real problems of psychology. Sherrington was an early advocate of physiological psychology in the curriculum of all teachers' colleges. When Woodworth began to write textbooks in this field, Sherrington found a life-long exponent of his views.

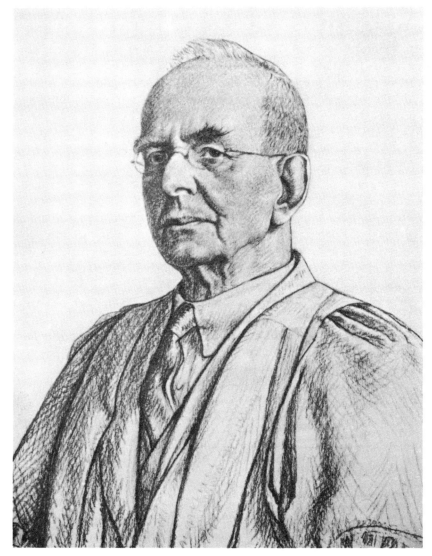

Fig. 1. C. S. Sherrington by Francis Dodd (Liverpool period) 1901

To the Liverpool Teachers' Guild and the British Child Study Association Sherrington was lecturing on *suggestion* including "Sources of suggestion acting on children in school life", "Individual differences in suggestibility", and "Suggestibility as an element of child character". To the Liverpool
Medical Institution he was lecturing on "The circle of Willis" and on "The

Listerian system". To the King Alfred School in Hampstead he read a paper on "Physiology for teachers", and he travelled to his old home in Ipswich to speak before the Parents' National Education Union on "Fatigue in children".

Before the Pathological Society of London, Sherrington was discussing localization of function on the surface of the brain. To Liverpool teachers he was speaking on "The horizon of the senses". The Royal Society had already published his paper "Experiments on the value of vascular and visceral factors for the genesis of Emotion". Ventures into such fields must have caused near apoplexy in the more traditional physiologists of that era, but Sherrington always had an intense interest in people – as individuals, not in some imaginary herd or mass.

To lay groups, Sherrington was keeping up his public information lectures – first on "The health requirements of children" and then through a series on "Fatigue of body and mind, its causes and consequences". The announcement of these speeches at Warrington noted "all the lectures will be illustrated by limelight views".

Sherrington's desire to travel was gratified in 1903 when he was invited to join William Osler, the Professor of Medicine at Johns Hopkins University in celebrating the union of Trinity College's medical school (where Osler began the study of medicine) with that of the University of Toronto. The ceremonies also included the opening of a new laboratory building for the pre-clinical sciences. It was in this building that Banting and Best eighteen years later discovered insulin.

On the afternoon of 1 October Sherrington addressed the large gathering on Medical Science (Appendix 5). In the evening Osler, by now a Canadian legend, filled the University gymnasium with enthusiastic students, faculty and members of the public, as he gave possibly the finest address of his career, "The master word in medicine". Both speakers received honorary doctorates, along with William Welch of Hopkins, W. W. Keen of Philadelphia, Russell Chittenden of Yale and H. P. Bowditch of Harvard. Sherrington was introduced to the vivid autumn colors of the Muskoka area of Ontario by his friend Professor A. B. Macallum. For the rest of his life he spoke nostalgically and wrote about Canada and its varied scenery spread over an immense area. His holiday time was shortened by an urgent invitation from Rush Medical College in Chicago to speak to its medical faculty. Sherrington was awarded their honorary doctorate on October 5. Meanwhile the President and Fellows of Yale University were selecting a scholar to give the annual series of Silliman Memorial Lectures, on "the wisdom and goodness of God as manifested in the natural and moral world". Happily they chose Sherrington. His "Integrative action of the nervous system", which embodied his 1904 Silliman Lectures, has become a classic. As has earlier been remarked, it did for the nervous system what William Harvey's *De Motu Cordis* did for the circulatory system.

Undoubtedly Harvey Cushing's interest in Sherrington's research had weighed heavily with the Yale committee and when, in 1904, Sherrington arrived in New Haven, Cushing wrote from Baltimore to make sure that his teacher from Liverpool would visit Osler's new faculty there. The Yale invitation meant that Sherrington had to work over the text and his illustrations for months. It was as if he had been asked to write a Magna Carta for the nervous system, based on his own discoveries. With characteristic generosity, however, Sherrington cited more than three hundred workers in the field. So impressive were his lectures that a letter signed by Philadelphia's neurological leaders Frazier, Reichert, Stille and Spiller, invited him to give two lectures there before he returned home. Sherrington's concluding statement in *The Integrative Action* reads:

> The cerebrum ... comes ... to be the organ *par excellence* for the readjustment and the perfecting of the nervous reactions of the animal as a whole, so as to improve and extend their suitability to, and advantage over, the environment. These adjustments, though not transmitted to the offspring, yet in higher animals form the most potent internal condition for enabling the species to maintain and increase in sum its dominance over the environment in which it is immersed. A certain measure of such dominance is its ancentral heritage; on this is based its innate right to success in the competition for existence. But the factors and the elements of that competition change in detail as the history of the earth proceeds. The creature has to be partially readjusted if it is to hold its own in the struggle. Only by continual modification of its ancestral powers to suit the present can it fulfil that which its destiny, if it is to succeed, requires from it as its life's purpose, namely, the extension of its dominance over its environment. For this conquest its cerebrum is its best weapon. It is then around the cerebrum, its physiological and psychological attributes, that the main interest of biology must ultimately turn.

The *Yale Alumni Weekly* for 18 May 1904, commented:

> The attitude of the lecturer towards his task was essentially different from that of the man of the platform in the ordinary course of lectures on literature or law. In such courses the recognized purpose is instruction. Professor Sherrington on the contrary, adopted the methods traditional in such an institution as the Croonian Lecture of the Royal Society. Not to instruct but to suggest questions was his purpose.
> The effect of this treatment upon the various members of the audience was strikingly paradoxical. This is well illustrated by the comments of one of these gentlemen who, though neither a physicist nor a physiologist, attended some of the lectures of Professor Thomson last year and as many of Professor Sherrington's. Of the former he remarked, "I understood all the words; but I sat there for an hour, and I did not know a thing the man had said; and I thought that was fine". Of Professor Sherrington's lecture on Scratch Reflex, he remarked, "I understood the whole of it. Everyone knows how a dog scratches himself when a flea bites him".

The review, signed by Yandell Henderson, concluded:

> The Silliman Lectures for this year have formed a fitting sequel to those of a year ago. Together they promise that in future this course will serve as a torch to keep alight the fires of scientific investigation in the university amid the obscuring elements of mere teaching, athletic interests, college tradition, and those currents which tend to the production of citizens rather than to the development of scholars.

The *Alumni Weekly* noted also that Professor Chittenden gave a dinner for the Sherringtons at the Graduates Club, where in addition to Yale faculty there were many outside guests. Among these were Professors Bowditch and Porter of Harvard, Professors Reichert and Abbott of the University of Pennsylvania, Professors Lusk and Kunham of the Bellevue Medical School and Professor Lee of the College of Physicians and Surgeons of New York. At an official university dinner the outsiders included Dr. Cannon of Harvard, Dr. Thorndike of Columbia and Dr. Yerkes of Boston. The menu was couched in Sherringtonian terminology.

The people of New Haven could not understand why the Sherringtons would go for fifteen mile walks in the country! To be given a testimonial dinner by the medical students was indeed a unique experience for any visiting professor. The visit was a breath of fresh air for Yale University.

Echoes could be heard in the contemporary press and in every scientific journal in the biomedical field. The echo that meant more to Sherrington than many others, however, was that from a pupil – Robert Sessions Woodworth, writing later with George Trumbull in their volume *Elements of Physiological Psychology:*

> Probably the greatest authority on reflex action in general is Sherrington, and in what follows reliance will be placed chiefly on his numerous special studies, and especially on his philosophical presentation of the whole matter in his book with the title *Integrative Action of the Nervous System.*

Thirty years later – even sixty years later, such echoes persisted. In the dark days of November 1939, Dr. F. M. R. Walshe, F. R. C. P., editor of the British journal *Brain,* wrote to Sherrington concerning a volume of his selected writings: "I look to it to turn my mind sometimes from the grim world that surrounds us all now, and to renew in its pages some of the delight that I found when Bayliss first gave me my copy of *The Integrative Action* some thirty years ago when I was a student. Such as my work has been since, what I got from the book has been the best part". Similarly, in 1947, Dr. Hugh Clegg, F. R. C. P., editor of the *British Medical Journal* wrote to Sherrington: "I still remember the thrill with which as a student at Trinity College, Cambridge, working for the Natural Science Tripos, I bought your *Integrative Action of the Nervous System* when it was first published". In 1967, Professor Jerzy Konorski of Warsaw, who in his student days had never been exposed to Sherrington, wrote in his own volume, *Integrative Action of the Brain:* "These simple and seemingly primitive reflexes require for their elicitation very fine and elaborate stimulus-patterns which must fit them as exactly as a key fits a lock, to use Sherrington's ingenious comparison".

An interesting insight into Sherrington's character is given in an 'exchange' with the *British Medical Journal* which, on 9 March 1907, printed a five-page review by F. W. Mott, of *The Integrative Action.* On 16 March Sherrington wrote to the journal concerning Mott's "extremely generous" review, protesting that he was being given credit for work actually done by Mott! From that Sherrington went on to thank the British Medical Association for financial help over the years in carrying on his work, and in fact he said that he spoke for many other medical researchers so helped. Sherrington used the opportunity to call attention to the pittance of £ 4000 per year given by the Imperial Government to the Royal Society of London to support research in the whole of the British Empire in all fields. He asserted:

> But what is £ 4000 as a sum with which to cover so vast a field of needs in the whole expanse of natural knowledge throughout the confines of the most extended, most populous, and most complex empire of the modern world! The sum is about the same in amount as – sad to say – the average yearly takings of a public-house in a poor quarter of this city; and of this sum only about a tenth part can . . . be allotted to research bearing on medicine . . . I may be forgiven if I express my conviction that among all the varied purposes served by the Association and its organization, none are of higher usefulness, not only to our own profession but to the community at large, than that which is expressed by the foundation and distribution of this [B. M. A.] fund.

While concentrating on his teaching, research and publications Sherrington still found time to address the summer meeting of the Psychological Society held in Cambridge, on "reaction times" from the physiological standpoint. The programme included a paper on vision by W. R. Rivers and one by Sherrington's associate of earlier days at Cambridge, William McDougall on "The bearing of modern experimental work on the problem of the unity of the mind". In Paris the *Journal des Débats* gave half a page to the Cambridge meeting, in a full exposition of Sherrington's work. As president of the Liverpool branch of the British Child Study Centre, Sherrington gave a public lecture on "Growth". Clearly his public service continued despite his heavy scientific obligations.

Following the success of the Silliman lectures, the University of Toronto invited Sherrington, the rising star, to fill its vacant chair of physiology. They sought a man of international reputation and they made their offer so generous that he was sorely tempted. Liverpool University liked the kudos which he brought but they were niggardly in their support[1]. He had, for example, no secretarial help, though his wife filled in nobly. Thus, on a Friday night, Sherrington wrote and mailed an acceptance of the Toronto offer. He could not sleep all night and went to the Liverpool postmaster on Saturday and received permission to go through all the trans-Atlantic mail in search of the letter. He finally found it and was allowed to retrieve it, so that Toronto lost a good candidate.

It was not long, however, before the remarkable president of Columbia University in New York, known to generations as Nicholas "Miraculous" Butler, wrote an expansive letter to Sherrington offering him the professorship of physiology which was about to be vacated by the veteran John G. Curtis. The selection committee included Dr. George S. Huntington, of Huntington's chorea fame, and Dr. Christian Herter, Professor of Therapeutics. The president mentioned, very wisely, that Sherrington would find his old pupil Woodworth in the Department of Psychology, along with Cattell and Thorndike. Coming from Johns Hopkins University to take the chair of pathology was a pupil of Osler and Welch, W. G. Mac-Callum.

It was all in vain, however, and Sherrington chose to stay in the United Kingdom rather than to endure the stress of life in a very large city. His laboratory was by now clearly on the beaten track, and almost weekly, the trans-Atlantic steamships docking in Liverpool brought laboratory visitors and research students. These in turn brought an increased correspondence, all dealt with personally and by hand. It has been said that Florence Nightingale wrote thousands of letters. She would be hard pressed to compete with Sherrington. To one correspondent alone we have found nearly two hundred letters. The total number of letters to correspondents in Sherrington's ninety-five years must be in the tens of thousands.

From the date of the Silliman Lectures in 1904 to his appointment to the chair at Oxford late in 1913, Sherrington published seventy-seven papers. Most of these concerned his research on reflexes, the reciprocal innervation of antagonistic muscles and the localization of various functions in the brain. There was, however, in addition, a wide spectrum of other subjects such as the effects of chloroform on the heart – a study sponsored by the

1 The medical dean at Liverpool, an anatomist, in order to increase the curricular time allotted to his subject, tried to reduce physiology's time by one-half and pathology's by one-third. Sir John Burdon Sanderson came forcefully to the rescue and William Osler wrote, "I would get rid of all lectures in anatomy. It seems to me they are the most superfluous things given in medical schools".

British Medical Association and the British Government. For the Board of Trade Committee on Sight Tests Sherrington served and helped to write the report. With William McDougall he reported to the British Associaton on mental and muscular fatigue. To the same association he reported with S. M. Copeman on body metabolism in cancer. With his pupils he published on tetanus, vision, strychnine, the cranial nerves, the importance of longer hours of sleep at public schools, training for teachers of hygiene and the scientific education of the medical student. In the historical field he gave a public lecture on "Old pages from the story of physiology". He agreed to give the Croonian Lecture for 1913 to his colleagues at the Royal College of Physicians on "Principles Evident in the Co-ordination of Muscular Acts".

Sherrington's medical correspondents varied from Oliver Lodge to Walter B. Cannon of Harvard. Lodge wrote:

> I find it difficult to decide whether George Bernard Shaw married for money. You see he is a man who would prefer what is called "sense" to beauty, but I think it was inevitable he should stultify himself in so far as he has done so. He is the opposite of Morris, being clever and not great. Still he did some good work before he got the idea that he was a Puritan, since which he has ceased to matter; in my opinion his last book is poison rather than rubbish. However, I believe he is doing good work as a borough-councilor (St. Pancras).

Cannon, on the other hand, wrote:

> Two new examples of your beautiful work came yesterday morning in the two notes from the Royal Society *Proceedings*. I promptly took to the country, accompanied by the reprint, and filled myself with refreshment by reading it. There is a rare pleasure that one has in feeling one's insight into the mists of the nervous system physiology grow deeper and clearer, as it does with every paper that comes from your laboratory.

The Liverpool phase of Sherrington's life was to come unexpectedly to a close in 1913 with the death in Oxford of Francis Gotch, Waynflete Professor of Physiology. The electors to that chair were summoned by Sir William Osler, Regius Professor of Medicine, and unanimously recommended Sherrington for the post without considering any other candidates. He took up his new work in January 1914.

(W.C.G.)

Chapter 3

Oxford 1914–1920

At age fifty-six most men are not seeking a new post, a new challenge, nor anything more than a new set of joints, limbs, eyes and possibly ears. Not so Charles Sherrington. In 1913 he entered upon the busiest period of his career, at the very cross-roads of the academic world. Cecil Rhodes's dictum that nowhere could he find an Oxford man at the top of the scientific tree, was about to be disproven.

Alan Gregg, the 'wise man' of the Rockefeller Foundation for so many years, has recorded a conversation with Sherrington during this remarkable epoch. On asking what Sherrington thought was the real function of Oxford University in the world, Gregg received this reply:

> After some hundreds of years of experience we think that we have learned here in Oxford how to teach what is known. But now with the undeniable upsurge of scientific research, we cannot continue to rely on the mere fact that we have learned how to teach what is known. We must learn how to teach *the best attitude* to what is *not yet* known. This also may take centuries to acquire but we cannot escape this new challenge, nor do we want to.

It is precisely this attitude which Sherrington communicated to the students who came to work with him in his new setting. At the beginning and at the end of his twenty-two years among the spires, the bicycles and the bookshops of Oxford, he was telling students in his quiet, highly personalized way, "The more intelligent the question you put to Mother Nature, the more intelligible will be her reply". To those rushing through merely for a medical qualification, this was considered, probably, as an aberration. But from those who understood came many future leaders of the scientific and educational world in medicine.

The Rhodes Scholars from the Commonwealth and from the United States came in increasing numbers to work with Sherrington. On arriving in Oxford he found Wilder Penfield, born in the far west of America, a Princeton graduate, who was to spend a lifetime advancing and broadening his teacher's concepts of the functions of the various areas of the human brain.

In the same group were Wilburt Davison, who built Duke University Medical School in North Carolina, and Emil Holman, who created a school of surgery at Stanford University in California. John Fulton carried the Sherrington torch to Yale. Three Nobel Prize winners were among Sherrington's Oxford students – Florey, Eccles and Granit. These are but the highlights of the influence of one professor in that ancient seat of learning.

What was Sherrington's day-to-day life in Oxford? The first thing to say is that his life became intertwined with that of his long-time friend, Sir William Osler, who presided over the medical faculty. Both had been students of the great Berlin pathologist, Rudolf Virchow. Both were admirers of Canada – Osler by birth and Sherrington by repeated contact. Both were bibliophiles and medical historians. Their families in Oxford were the closest of friends. From the beginning, therefore, Sherrington felt at home in the new setting. Gradually and patiently he began, in his quiet way, to energize what had been too long a sleepy, if not moribund part of the university. When, soon after his arrival, he felt that the students were being given less than a fair opportunity to study the rapidly developing field of pharmacology, he prevailed upon the Rhodes Trust to provide a readership in that subject.

When the first World War broke out he soon found his physiology classes decimated. Only three physically unfit men and three women remained, together with the three American Rhodes Scholars already mentioned. Penfield, in the Oxford vacations, crossed the Channel to work in the American volunteer hospitals set up in France and was seriously injured when the *Sussex* was torpedoed. Sir William Osler heard that he had been landed at Southampton and took him to his home, "The Open Arms", at 13 Norham Gardens, until his recovery from a shattered leg was complete.

Davison was sent by Osler to be "in charge of all bedpans in Bulgaria" as he used to phrase it, during the investigation of the difference between typhoid and parathyphoid fevers. Since at Oxford there are only three terms of eight weeks each, one has time for far-reaching vacation experiences. Wherever a student was going for these non-resident periods, Sherrington was anxious to provide introductions. Sherrington was not surprised, at the end of hostilities, to receive a letter dated 21 August 1919, from Davison, by now back at Johns Hopkins Hospital in Baltimore saying, "I have been here since my release from the Army in March. I am an instructor in Pediatrics and am doing the bacteriology for the Children's department. Most of the latter consists in research on the etiology of Infantile Diarrhoea". The impact of the commencement of war upon Oxford is well illustrated by the letter of 5 December 1914 from Sherrington to E. A. Schäfer:

You may like to hear how Oxford is; from all colleges most of the students are gone – to the Army. In the death-roll of every college there are, I believe, some undergraduate names already. Magdalen has only 24 men instead of its normal 160. New College has no less than 226 undergraduates in the two services. In the laboratory we had 74 students last term and have 18 this, and most of these in khaki. The laboratory fees as estimated for 1915 will amount to £ 230 whereas £ 810 has been the average annual fee-total for the past ten years. But everyone is keen to spare no effort or sacrifice to help the country and its cause. Most of the Colleges have taken in soldiers into their vacant quarters. We had 70 sleeping in the Dining Hall for some time – the last occasion was for Cromwell's troopers.

At the end of term in June 1915, Sherrington cycled off to Birmingham whence he wrote to a correspondent: "I am a munition worker at Vicker's works here until next Monday, when I return to Oxford. The hours are very long, 7:30 a. m. to 8:30 p. m. with only 1 hour off, and Sats. and Sundays until 6:00 p. m. This particular 'shop' turns out now 28000 three-inch shrapnell a week".

To Schäfer whose son Tom was reported "missing in action" Sherrington wrote: "I cannot say how deeply we hope time will bring news of Tom. We all know of instances where much longer has elapsed, but each week nevertheless aggravates the misgiving". Of his own son, Carr, he added: "He rejoins the Battalion on Tuesday next at Weston-super-Mare for further divisional training – some 40000 men there now, we hear. He is well and likes his brother officers very much – ³/₄ Oxford and Bucks Light Infantry. He will be 19 next March".

When March 1916 came, Sherrington was in the thick of an academic fight, brought on by the war, as he told Schäfer: "I am busied with rather a heavy struggle here just now to get women admitted to our medical school. The chief opposition so far has been from inside the Medical School itself, but Osler is heartily sympathetic and most helpful".

In reviewing papers submitted by London specialists with a view to publication Sherrington could be very cutting. But when in 1916 a young Dutch worker submitted a paper, he wrote: "I have read it, and its English is very bad, but I don't mind the trouble of rewriting the text". He then told Schäfer: "I hope Jack is well; no doubt on service . . . What with pottering about trying to be of some use as a swab diagnoser, etc. at the hospitals here, the long vac. has slipped by before one is aware. Oddly I went to Sheffield for one night and there was a Zeppelin raid there – in consequence a rather heavy loss of life".

"Pottering about" was not quite what Sherrington had been doing. In 1915 he had landed a bombshell at the War Office in the form of a report on his personal experience and study of fatigue in war factories. What he did not put in his report, but what gave him a feeling of pride for the rest of his life, were the remarks of the foreman when he left the Birmingham munitions factory: "Sherrington, I don't know why you want to leave us in the middle of a war. You have been very helpful in talking French to those Belgians in the plant, and if you ever need a reference you can use my name".

The war as seen by his friend W. B. Cannon of Harvard is well described in letters of early 1916. Alexander Forbes wrote from Boston concerning a joint paper on acoustic reflexes: "I feel rather ashamed to have allowed my name to take first place in authorship when you conceived the idea, made the first observation and wrote the paper. But knowing your ways I decided it would be futile to attempt an 'after you' controversy across 3000 miles of water".

It was not long before Forbes was telling Sherrington:

> I am growing impatient under our persistent official neutrality and 'friendly relations' with Germany. It bothers my conscience to sit here in peace while your men are dying for the freedom of which we call ourselves the foremost bulwark (or perhaps 'Exponent' might be more just)... Last night a professor of music said to me that he couldn't stand it any longer, that he felt he must go to France to help. He said he must for his own self respect.

W. W. Keen, the Philadelphia surgeon echoed this view after reading Sherrington's letter to Forbes in the October 1916 *Atlantic Monthly.*

Soon after this Forbes put his own considerable talents to work for the Allies. One of Sherrington's favorite stories twenty years later concerned Forbes's eventual status as an 'Admiral'. He was arrested for driving wildly in Boston clad only in his pyjamas, while trying to overtake a suburban train, two of whose passengers he had to 'intercept'.

Sherrington was consulted endlessly on wartime matters. He wrote bluntly in reply to an enquiry from Harrison at the Royal Society: "The appropriate place for the Newton relics just now is in the cellar". At Oxford he "fumed and fussed" according to Cox, his laboratory assistant, over some fine steel microtome blades which he had sent early in 1914 to the Sartorius factory in Germany for re-sharpening. The blades did not come back and throughout the war years Sherrington would pace about the histology laboratory saying, "Those poor boys, those poor boys, being killed with that steel I sent over there. Why did I ever send those knives to be sharpened?" At the end of the war the blades arrived back with a note: "Due to unforeseen circumstances delivery of these blades has been delayed."

Though Sir Charles might be in Hull or London, his wife kept the hospitality fires alight at 9 Chadlington Road, Oxford. The Rhodes Scholars were always finding their way back to that haven as they did to the "Open Arms", the Osler residence in nearby Norham Gardens. Sherrington "just happened" to locate a London research fellowship for Wilder Penfield after he had left Oxford. This athletic young American used to cycle from London to Oxford every week-end during his year's further study in post-war London. His classmate and erstwhile wrestling partner, C. F. Krige, a South African Rhodes Scholar, had earlier come back to Oxford to follow the ward rounds of Sir William Osler at the Radcliffe Infirmary.

Krige's interesting volume, *A Doctor's Autobiography,* gives an account of war-time human experiments at Oxford only three centuries removed from those of Wren's day. He writes:

> Physiology as taught at Oxford under Sir Charles Sherrington was an outstanding course. With a limited number of students working in pairs we could make our own graphic records . . . This was the time when four of us became human guinea pigs by being injected with the experimental 'combined T. A. B.' vaccine as produced by Professor Dreyer and Dr. Ainlie Walker at Oxford. The other three were Cluver, Penfield and Holman. The release of this vaccine had become urgent as men were dying like flies at Gallipoli from paratyphoid A and B infections. Army headquarters would not allow the vaccine to be used until officially tested, and this would have meant months of delay. We suffered no ill effects and expedited the use of the vaccine on the troops.

To his close friend of Cambridge days, Frank Wesbrook, President of the University of British Columbia at Vancouver, C. S. S. sent his cherished copy of Bidloo's *Anatomia* (1685). In a clear hand he inscribed in it the story of the court proceedings which followed the publication by William Cowper, a London surgeon, of the Bidloo plates to which he had supplied an English text. Bidloo was awarded damages of one shilling. In addition Sherrington wrote the history of Nicholas Hawksmoor, the domestic clerk of Christopher Wren and architect of many London churches and Oxford colleges, who had been the first owner of the book in 1693. Finally, many of Sherrington's friends who visited his laboratory in 1915 were asked to place their signatures in the volume, as a surprise and as encouragement to Wesbrook who was trying to build a new university in the face of the World War. The names included William Osler, John McCrae, author of *In Flanders Fields,* Walter Raleigh, Frederick Gowland Hopkins of vitamin fame and Professor Arthur Thomson, the Oxford anatomist. Years later Sherrington would laugh as he confided that he had dispatched the book at a time when the submarine menace was thought to be least. Records later showed that it was the worst possible time but, as he said, "The book arrived safely, did it not?"

Wesbrook replied that he and his colleagues were overwhelmed at such generosity, especially from one so preoccupied with the war, adding:

> Out of this little college with about 290 students of whom 150 are men, 57 students and ex-students have gone to the front . . . The mortality has been very high amongst our men but every bit of news from the front helps to stimulate recruiting . . . Whenever opportun-

ity is offered for enlistment, it is oversubscribed three or four times almost instantaneously . . . If you can give me any news of McDougall I shall be glad to receive it . . . I have not given up the hope of inducing him to come to us.

In addition to McDougall in psychology, Wesbrook and Sherrington were hopeful that Julian Huxley in biology and William Bragg in physics could be 'captured' for the "second Cambridge" which Wesbrook was trying to build in Vancouver. Sherrington told Wesbrook that Bragg was a "good bet" and likely to be heard from in the future! From Caius College, Cambridge, W. B. Hardy wrote: "Many thanks for opportunity of seeing Wesbrook's letters . . . a remarkable testimony to Canadian spirit".

Forbes wrote that his paper with Alan Gregg had been published, but lost no time in getting back to his chief interest, American participation in the war: "I watch the papers eagerly for indications of the collapse of Germany". He published in an American periodical some possibly classified material which A. V. Hill had communicated to him from London, and it took all of Sherrington's diplomacy to reassure Hill that no questions would be asked in the House of Commons.

Meanwhile Sherrington's wife was writing to Sir William and Lady Osler to say that Carr had been awarded the Military Cross for "bravery, courage and endurance", but that the corporal who had supported him throughout with machine gun fire had died of wounds sustained. She hoped that the Oslers had good news of their son Revere, but this was not to be. He received a terrible head wound, and although cared for by their devoted Harvey Cushing, died in France – a death which literally broke Sir William's heart. As Sherrington's laboratory man said so wisely, commenting upon the change which came over the Regius Professor, "It's Mr. Revere, sir, and Sir William won't ever recover".

With the American declaration of war, letters from Forbes at Harvard and Frederic S. Lee at Columbia University became ecstatic. Forbes was immersed in wireless work but was keen to join A. V. Hill in England on anti-aircraft gun research. Apart from a busy trans-Atlantic correspondence Sherrington had many matters to deal with in Britain. Horace Darwin was collecting a memorial fund for the Cambridge genius Keith Lucas, who was killed while serving as a test pilot. William Bayliss, the London physiologist, was writing to say that the Women's Medical School of the University of London had taken in a class of 110 students. From Scotland, Mrs. Nellie Watt wrote at least a letter a week asking Sherrington to get her psychologist husband out of a prisoner-of-war camp in Germany because he had a heart ailment. Pavlov's pupil, Beritoff, wanted a paper published. And so it went.

Amidst all these demands on his time by others Sherrington could still enjoy his search for rare books. His friend Walter Morley Fletcher, Cambridge muscle researcher *par excellence* and fellow bibliophile, was wearing himself out trying to get Britain's new Medical Research Council on an even keel. Sherrington relates, of this period:

> Walter had given his own fine copy of the rare book 'Tractatus quinque' by John Mayow, most generously to Osler – to Osler's intense delight. He had done so because, visiting Osler, he had noticed that the copy of the book in his library was a poor one. Osler a little later told me of this. I happened to have a good copy like Walter's so sent him mine to make good his loss. Thus everyone was pleased, when I got the following letter from Walter:

> My dear Sherrington:
> I came back tired this evening and found your parcel here, and your delightful surprise has cheered and wholly revived me. I can't tell you how grateful I am for your kindly idea of sending me the Mayow. I am only nervous lest you have not a second copy yourself – for the Oxford Professor of Physiology *must* have one. But I shall always be very proud to have a copy of yours – and one I see that you must have bought almost as an undergraduate. Believe me too when I say that much as I value the book and shall always value it, I value almost immeasurably more your kind letter that came with it, and the friendship which you let me claim. I wish I could deserve either – but you hearten me wonderfully to make an effort not to deserve them so little. I thank you most warmly.

Sherrington was still trying to keep up his research on the cortex of the brain. He told Schäfer: "I confess this paper grew rather weary work to me . . . Yes, I quite agree, 'figures' as a verb is bad American . . . 'Schema' too is rather jargon . . . If I had written these last week I should put it down to the influence of the series of Americans who have been going through here – including Cannon, Cushing and Crile, on their way to France . . . As I write there are nine aeroplanes in the sky at one time".

Six months before the war was over Sherrington was trying to find a post in England for the displaced Russian histologist Maximov, who had written to Osler in search of a haven. On the same day he was consoling his brother physiologist Schäfer who had just lost his second son in the war: "I did not write to you about your recent loss; it is almost too sad to speak of. I mean the personal aspect of it. But we feel such sympathy I cannot refrain from mentioning it now. Jack had such character, and the work he had done and was doing was so fine a line of duty; it must touch your pride in him as well as your sorrow".

Before and throughout the war Sherrington had been working to develop a new type of laboratory guide for students in physiology. When it appeared in 1919 as *Mammalian Physiology; a Course of Practical Exercises,* he wrote to Schäfer:

> A danger ahead of physiology itself in this coming time of reconstruction is, I think, lest the medical profession jib at the time spent on some of the older muscle and nerve amphibian exercises; e. g. paradoxical contraction – controversy long turned to fossil; the students themselves consider some of these things out-of-date and respectfully try a boycott . . . I have finished my small practical book and a copy will reach you. I hope it has not many mistakes, but a rather novel venture is bound to have some.

According to some foreign reviewers the book had one unforgivable mistake – the illustrations were all by Englishmen! In fact, most of the illustrations of laboratory recordings were the very tracings achieved by such American students in Sherrington's classes as Penfield, Davison and Holman. We shall deal further with the mammalian physiology class in Chapter 4. Lord Bryce had little suspected such a practical response to his note of 21 December 1915 to Sherrington: "All success to your efforts at Oxford to create and draw Americans to post-graduate courses".

Sherrington could look back over a period of four years of unremitting war with little inner satisfaction. His research had been sacrificed but he counted this as little compared with the human sacrifice around him. His most poignant poetry was written in the war years as we shall see later in this volume.

Early in the war he had signed a declaration, "Why Britain Fights" which was distributed to scientists and others around the world. From his friend Ruffini in Bologna he had a warm letter of support. From von Uexkull in Germany he had the following message: "Dear Sherrington: In these serious times the Reply to German Professors as published in *The Times* of Oct. 21, 1918 was a real joy to us all. We never laughed so heartily. The only thing I regret was to find your earnest name connected to this nonsense".

In 1919, Sherrington had to listen to a counter-blast, this one from T. D. Acland, who wrote on 4 March of that year demanding the removal from the Physiological Society of all German professors: "The Huns are not a civilized nation; they made war like barbarians and have conducted it like brutes, and no self-respecting Society in this country ought to include any of them on its roll of Honorary Members until they have shown by their actions that they are ashamed of themselves".

We can only conjecture what Sherrington replied to this, for on March 12, Acland returned to the attack: "I am very sorry to gather from what you say that there are so many unpatriotic Englishmen. How anybody can have anything to do with a Hun passes my comprehension . . . I thought better of physiologists".

In happier correspondence John George Adami, the pathologist trained at McGill and Cambridge, wrote on June 3rd, 1919, thanking Sherrington for a note congratulating him on his elevation to the Vice-Chancellorship at Liverpool University: "This post at Liverpool appealed to me largely as a link between Canada and England . . . We are at the opening of a new social era . . . and I believe the provincial universities are the fitting places to train the new leaders".

Once the faithful correspondent Alexander Forbes returned from overseas to his Boston laboratory he had new experiences to relate to C. S. S.:

> Stanley Cobb and I had the good fortune to take an electrocardiogram and an electromyogram of an elephant a few days ago. The circus people sent two of them and some other side-shows to amuse the children at the Children's Hospital next door; and I induced the keeper to let one of them stand under my windows while we ran wires out and did the trick. He was well trained and co-operated with us perfectly, contracting his trunk muscle for the electromyogram when told to; altogether the best experimental animal I have worked with.

In December, 1919, Sir William Osler died – a terrible blow to Oxford, but especially to the Sherrington household. The British Medical Journal soon carried Sherrington's tribute, reading in part:

> To my own thinking, among the characteristics which endeared Osler to his friends none was perhaps more striking than the combination of an intense affection for the past . . . with an enthusiastic receptivity for the new . . . To run his eye backward and forward along the historic continuity of medicine seemed with him a daily and hourly habit . . . there was never a greater believer in the young generation than Osler, or a more generous encourager of it.

But Sherrington little suspected that his highest office was waiting for him, 'round the corner'.

(W.C.G.)

Chapter 4

The Years of the Presidency
of the Royal Society, 1920–1925

In 1920 Sherrington assumed the presidency of the Royal Society – that ancient body chartered by Charles II in 1662, and successor to the Invisible College of Christopher Wren's day. On October 28 Sherrington received a letter from the retiring president, J. J. Thomson, the distinguished physicist and Master of Trinity College, Cambridge:

Dear Professor Sherrington:

I am writing at the unanimous request of the Society Council to ask you to allow yourself to be nominated at the Anniversary Meeting for the office of President.

I think that some explanation is required that this request has not been forwarded to you earlier. What has happened is this. When the question of the vacancy in the Presidency was considered by the Council, they were of the opinion that the next man of science to be offered the Presidency should be a biologist and were unanimous that you should be that biologist; it seemed however, to the Council that at the present time there were special reasons why Mr. Arthur Balfour[1] should be asked to take the office, and the nomination was offered to him. Unfortunately he has been away from England for some time and it was only yesterday that a reply was received saying that he was grieved to say that the proposal was impractical.

The Council then, as I have said, decided unanimously to ask you to undertake the office at once instead of after a short interval. I hope you will see your way to accept as I am sure the proposal will receive the approval of every member of the Society and that you will receive a most cordial welcome from all your colleagues who are engaged in the work of the Society.

Sherrington must have wondered at the evident haste, but he accepted the challenge and for five years guided the Royal Society through some uncharted seas as the post-war development of science proceeded. He told Schäfer: "The nomination was quite unexpected by me. I shall want all the indulgence of my friends in trying to occupy the office, and very much of its proper distinction must go unfulfilled in my tenure". In a footnote to Schäfer he said: "If you call your letter to me poorly legible, what of mine – it is like a spider's trail".

---

1 Chancellor of Cambridge University, former Prime Minister, leading British delegate to the Peace Conference, and an eminent philosopher.

Sherrington was in the chair when the Royal Society had its anniversary dinner on November 30th, the distinguished guests including a number of ambassadors, maharajas, the Prime Wardens of the Fishmongers' and Goldsmiths' Companies, the editor of *The Times,* vice-chancellors of universities and the respective presidents of the Royal Colleges of Physicians and Surgeons.

Lord Sumner in proposing the toast to the Society was reported by *The Times* as saying that ". . . they had before them the greatest of conquests, and that was the conquest of the public mind. The public mind was at present devoted to an orgy of waste. The whole world was devoted to waste. The natural resources of the universe, so far as they were within the reach of man, were being squandered as fast as they could be". Sir Charles used to blink when confronted with some amazing new prophecy, and presumably he blinked repeatedly during this toast. Two years later the toast was given by Mr. Justice Darling, *The Times* reporting "laughter" following each paragraph. When Sherrington came to reply, however, he insisted, in the presence of the Archbishop of Canterbury, that Science and the Church had a number of ". . . ties strong enough to draw them together, as at the present time. The bond between them was social service, something towards the benefit of the whole community. There was another tie between them. They both set truth as an ideal, as worth the devotion of a lifetime".

Letters of congratulation began to pour in upon the diffident little man. The great physiologist William Bayliss wrote: "It is with much pleasure that I write to tell you that the Physiological Society at its meeting yesterday decided to send unanimous congratulations on the honour to physiology and to its distinguished exponent by making him President of the Royal Society".

From William Bateson, father of the term 'genetics' came an unusual note:

> When some 35 years ago I drank your tea in the Lambeth Road it did not happen to strike me that we might one day be congratulating each other on quite this scale! Thank you for what you have said. I am proud of my work-a-day honour. [Royal Medal] But here's to you in your glory! We have now a President in whom we can all feel satisfaction and pride, who will show the world that a man of science is not necessarily innocent of all the graces and all the arts. We shall look to you to bring the Royal Society back a little nearer to its proper place. Advisory Office to Govt. is not good enough. May you find Newton's chair stuffed with good things!

One of Sherrington's first projects in January of 1921 was to assemble a committee with the help of Lord Bryce to help "Russian Emigré Savants", telling the members: "Need for moving seems to be rather urgent".

In the summer of 1921 Sherrington was given the honorary degree of Doctor of Science by the Victoria University of Manchester. The citation, read by Professor A. V. Hill, was both illuminating and entertaining, and it was made very clear that Manchester had decided to honour Sherrington even before his elevation to the Presidency of the Royal Society.

Sherrington was probably relieved that there was no student demonstration in Manchester comparable to that at Cambridge when Pavlov received an honorary degree. There the students had lowered on strings from the gallery a model of a dog bearing endless tubes and wires! Pavlov felt it to be a great compliment.

The summer of 1921 was also a time for touring the battlefields of France. As Lady Sherrington recounted to Harvey Cushing in a letter from Amiens:

Yesterday Charlie and I walked over a great part of the Somme battlefield, taking train to ruined Albert and then walking to Thiepval and Pozieres, more especially choosing the former, because there it was 5 years ago next Sunday that dear old Carr gained his Military Cross for holding a trench so long – 48 hours, going in 160 [men] and only 18 left, 17 besides himself when relieved.

Then she wrote to Harvey Cushing of Oxford happenings:

I went to see Grace Osler just before [coming away]. She was feeling the heat greatly, and could not understand Charlie and my rejoicing in this summer . . . or real heat and sunshine continuously which we really do enjoy though I fear England has suffered badly in many places from want of water, especially in the country. We have no arrangements for such a continued drought . . . We are greatly interested in William's [Osler] life. No one but yourself could more fully have loved and fully understood him. Oh, how greatly he is missed and loved still[1].

Since Cambridge days Sherrington had been closely in touch with William McDougall, the medically trained psychologist who, with other graduates in medicine such as Rivers, James and Lange greatly influenced the development of the subject in North America. Now Sherrington was to learn of McDougall's determination to leave Britain permanently:

I feel that I must make some personal explanation to you in justification of my nefarious conduct. I tried to set out my reasons pretty fully to [Walter Morley] Fletcher in telling him that I am frankly feeling the difficulties of the job of trying to do anything for English psychological medicine by direct action. I am afraid I would spend my remaining years in fruitless efforts.

Sherrington had little time for depressed dons, however, and relished the creative minds of the Royal Society. He was sometimes three half-days and an evening per week in London and had, in addition, to receive visitors from North America, the continent and even from Siam. One of his greatest satisfactions came from his friendship with Sir Alfred Yarrow, F. R. S., the

1 Cushing's two-volume *Life of Sir William Osler* won the Pulitzer Prize in 1925.

shipbuilder, whose gift of £ 100,000 to the Royal Society was a great stimulant to research in Britain. He wrote to Sherrington: "I should prefer that the money be used to aid scientific workers by adequate payment and by the supply of apparatus or other facilities, rather than to erect costly buildings, because large sums of money are sometimes spent on buildings without adequate endowment, and the investigators are embarrassed by financial anxieties".

Sir Alfred wisely added: "Care must, of course, be taken that a gift from the Fund shall in no case lessen any Government grant . . . I recognize conditions alter so materially from time to time that, in order to secure the greatest possible benefit from such a Fund, it must be administered with unfettered discretion by the best people from time to time available". A year later yet another Yarrow professorship was created thanks to Sir Alfred's munificent gift to the Society.

While these developments in research support were taking place, Sherrington was keeping up his world-wide correspondence. His friend A. B. Macallum, the biochemist, had been in China, setting up departments of physiology, pharmacology and biochemistry at the new Peking Union Medical College, financed by the Rockefeller Foundation. He had some penetrating things to say:

> I would have gladly accepted a permanent appointment out there were I twenty or thirty years younger . . . China is also intensely interesting, as much so as the world of another planet . . . Though life is cheap it is injoyed by the Chinese as I believe it is nowhere else and under conditions which we of the west would not tolerate . . . In Japan things were not so interesting . . . the system of teaching copied almost wholly from the German universities . . . Japan has 4,800,000 trained soldiers. She could land 500,000 men in China in a week, another 2,000,000 in a month, and her armies could not be dislodged.

At the end of each year since 1901 Sherrington had exchanged Christmas greetings with Harvey Cushing, the acknowledged master-surgeon of the brain. Thus, on 22 December 1921, Sherrington wrote to him at Harvard:

> Life is up to the chin in things that call for their doing – and that makes our miss of Osler all the sharper. Years will intensify still more the memory of that strength he had to bind those of his time together, no matter across what distances . . . I am glad Penfield has a good appointment and opening . . . he deserves it, and so does she. Malloch[1] blows in from time to time always on a cheery note.
> I dined with Chas. Ballance[2] in London the other evening – dear old Ferrier was there – told me he is reading Thucidides in the original to enjoy a few months stay in Sicily the

---

1 Archibald Malloch, M. D., who was cataloguing, with Reginald Hill and Osler's nephew, Dr. W. W. Francis, the incomparable collection at Norham Gardens before its journey to McGill University in Montereal, as The Osler Library.

2 Ballance wrote from 106 Harley Street to Sherrington in 1922: "It was Ferrier, not any surgeon, who was the originator and founder of modern cerebral surgery".

more. I got an interesting account out of him of his original brain expts, that started the modern physiology of the cortex. He was so modest about all that first-rate work, done in a little private room in a Yorkshire Asylum, by himself with very little to guide or help him; and the results so clearly and simply set forth in those early papers by him . . . Christmas Eve, all go en famille to carol singing at Magdalen till midnight "and then to bedde" as Pepys used to write.

What Sherrington wrote about Ferrier's early work could be written about Sherrington's young colleague of Liverpool days, Alfred Campbell, an Australian graduate of Edinburgh. As director of the pathological laboratory at Rainhill Asylum he often observed the mapping of the cerebral cortex by Sherrington and Grunbaum. From 1900 to 1903 he cut transparently thin serial sections of the preserved brains of twenty-five higher apes turned over to him by Sherrington for study. He stained, alternately, sections for fibres and for cells – a colossal undertaking. Sherrington arranged for a grant from the Royal Society to aid in the publication of Campbell's great atlas by the Cambridge University Press. It is a classic, impossible to purchase today, for as the gifted Lorente de Nó, Cajal's pupil, has said: "The only good architectonic pictures are those of Campbell . . . the only cytoarchitectonist who has described facts and only facts".

Echoes of Osler returned again and again in Oxford, and in the spring of 1922 Lady Sherrington wrote to Cushing in Boston:

No, Grace Osler and you were and are very kind and flattering re C. S. S. holding the Regius Professorship of Medicine, but honestly, I fear its many more social duties would have worried C. greatly, especially by taking him even more away from research work, always his first great love, and we both think our *earned* income too small for the much that – as you know – has to be done. Sir W. and Lady Osler were so wonderful in their really loving kindness and hospitable home offered to so many[1].

Since Sherrington was in constant personal touch with his close associates in Britain his correspondence was, in large measure, directed to his many overseas pupils and colleagues. Jacques Loeb, one of his visitors in Liverpool days, wanted Sherrington to visit him at the Rockefeller Institute in New York after opening the new Biology Building at McGill. Considerable correspondence developed concerning Banting and Best's spectacular success in producing insulin for the treatment of diabetes. Gowland Hopkins, the vitamin researcher at the Sir William Dunn Laboratory of Biochemistry at Cambridge wrote to Sherrington concerning the honorary doctorate about to be conferred on him by Oxford. He told Sherrington:

I know that the high honour I am to receive from Oxford must have come to me largely because of the friendship that you personally extend to me . . . It is really true however, to

---

1 For Sherrington's *Osler at Oxford* written for the hundredth anniversary of Osler's birth 1949, see Appendix 7.

> say that I have been feeling some actual discomfort due to doubts of my adequacy . . . I
> have always looked upon on honorary degree from Oxford . . . as an honour *in excelsis* . . .
> There is nothing in the world . . . that I could have wished for so much.

Sherrington must have felt that talent and industry were rewarded when this pioneer in the metabolism of muscle and former insurance clerk turned forensic laboratory chemist – a butterfly pigment researcher who discovered that accessory food factors were necessary for life – stepped forward to receive from Oxford's Chancellor its highest award.

As if the Presidency of the Royal Society were not enough for one man, Sherrington was prevailed upon to be president of the British Association in 1923. It met in Hull and Sherrington's address was widely reported (Appendix 8). Among other things he stressed the value of Banting and Best's discovery of insulin. The press dealt generously with his discussion of the nervous system – taking fewer liberties with the text than had *Punch* when Sherrington had last addressed the British Association on this subject in 1904. At that meeting in Cambridge *Punch* pretended to have a special correspondent who reported Sherrington as having delivered an address on "The physiological interaction of capillary splanchnics", saying in part, "The reflex arcs of the pianistic system converge in their course so as to impinge on kinks" possessed by various groups. The main principle established was ". . . the intercombustion of trypsinogenous splanchnics about their common afferent root-neurone". It was noted that one professor spoke in Magyar, and that Tibetans showed "luxuriant capillary Splanchnics!"

Correspondence ranged from a formal note by Albert Einstein, elated with his admission as a Foreign Member to the Royal Society, to doggerel from John Sampson, on a trying colleague of the Liverpool years:

> He lived in other people's ways
> To get himself a shove;
> A man who it was wise to praise
> And difficult to love.

Sampson, the University Librarian at Liverpool, noted impishly that he had just been staying with a real poet, Robert Bridges, the Poet Laureate, at Oxford. Concerning Liverpool he noted that ". . . our little University is as live and pleasant a place . . . as ever".

Reviewing Sherrington's busy life in 1922, we find him writing to congratulate his Cambridge colleague H. K. Anderson, now Master of Caius College, on his knighthood in the Birthday Honours list. On 6 June, Anderson wrote to C. S. S.:

> You are always too appreciative of the feeble efforts of others, and too blind to your own
> great achievements. That is the only fault that your friends and admirers can find in you

... It is the pride of my life to have the friendship of a scientific man to whom all the physiologists of England, and I believe in the world, look up as their leader, in all that is good and unselfish.

When, in 1926, Anderson was host to a group from the Commonwealth Universities' Conference at Cambridge, he referred to Wesbrook's work as a Caius man, trying to build a university in wartime at Vancouver. He became so emotional about Wesbrook's contributions that he broke down and had to leave the dinner. Such too were Sherrington's feelings about "dear Frank Wesbrook" as he always called him.

For Sherrington and for Oxford, 1921 was to be a banner year in the number and quality of Rhodes Scholars arriving. At Magdalen College he had John Fulton from Harvard and Howard Florey from Adelaide, South Australia. At Merton, succeeding Penfield, was Marshall Fulton from New England. This situation recalled Cecil Rhodes' six wills, in the first few of which he was giving one scholarship to each of "the thirteen colonies". When it was pointed out to him that there were forty-eight states, he did some arithmetic and soon saw that to give one per state would be enough to outnumber the rest of the world's Rhodes Scholars. He finally settled for a lesser number, thirty-two in fact, but the American influence was to remain strong at Oxford. In later years, of course, the Oxford influence in the United States and Canada became, reciprocally, very strong and was one of the keystones in the Anglo-American alliance in the second World War.

Meanwhile the correspondence kept mounting up, with Léon Fredericq of Liege writing, as he said, "du fond du coeur", and Zieman, Rector of the University of Amsterdam, thanking Sherrington and the Royal Society for conferring the Rutherford Medal on him, and commenting: "I was much impressed by the long after dinner speeches, and admired the great energy the English speakers had at their disposal, after the fatigues of the day. This refers especially to yourself". Eddington, president of the Royal Astronomical Society wanted Sherrington to attend their centenary dinner, and excused him from having to prepare a speech. Sherrington was asked to give an address at the presentation to the British Museum of the portrait of the evolutionist Alfred Russel Wallace, O. M., F. R. S., Darwin's contemporary. The debate between Huxley and the Bishop of Oxford in 1860 was probably forgotten as the Archbishop of Canterbury accepted the portrait on behalf of the trustees, but one can be sure that Sherrington smiled gently.

Sherrington's interest in the discovery of insulin at Toronto kept recurring often during 1923. His peppery correspondent, Oliver Lodge wrote: "I shall never forget your early and instructive remarks to me about Insulin and its Canadian discoverer, before the subject got into the papers and became known . . . We rejoice in your high scientific position and, if I may say so, at the modesty and dignity with which you sustain it".

As early as 4 January 1923, Professor H. J. Hamburger, a longtime friend from Groningen, wrote to Sherrington to say an attempt was being made in Holland to produce insulin. In the meantime he wondered if Sherrington could send some from Britain for a very sick patient. One month later J. J. R. Macleod, Professor of Physiology at Toronto, received a cable from Sherrington announcing his election to the Royal Society. Macleod replied: "I wish particularly to thank you for the kindness which prompted you to send me the news by cable. Nothing in the way of honours could possibly please me more than to be an F. R. S." Sherrington probably reflected on the fact that it was his pupil during his Liverpool period, Professor Fred Miller, now of the University of Western Ontario, who had sent Banting to Macleod in Toronto to discuss his proposed research on insulin.

At the Royal Society Sherrington was watching carefully the weaknesses which might be developing in the committees charged with study and recommendations to the government in special fields. He recommended, for the Sectional Committee on Physiology and Medicine, Henry Head, the neurologist and outstanding student of speech and of its loss – aphasia. On eight distinct grounds, not least of which was Head's research as a medical student in Prague on the Hering-Breuer reflex, Sherrington thought the Council should appoint him. (Head, as a student, is reputed to have introduced the game of soccer to the Czechs, but he was never sure, after seeing international matches thereafter, whether his had been a friendly act or not.) Sherrington in early 1923 was encouraging Head to publish his long-awaited book on aphasia, to which Head replied:

> Your letter gave me the greatest pleasure and heartened me up for future efforts; for the work has been long and arduous and sometimes I have almost lost courage, especially when I think of how much pleasant travel I have deprived my wife on account of the necessity of taking our holidays in a place where I can write. Poor thing! She wishes la petite aphasie as her French friends call it, would be less sluggish in making its entry into this world.

Lady Sherrington could echo such sentiments! She wisely refused to go with Sherrington to meetings where there was little diversion for wives, even in Paris where her French blood would have made her feel at home. She told Harvey Cushing that for a Royal Wedding they had given up their

> . . .twice sixteen inches of space allowed in the Abbey seats to others more anxious to view the ceremony. Alas I am still loving all unconventional and outdoor things as well as I did

in the old days in Cheshire . . . and indeed live mostly out of doors on a push bike still!!! Also am immensely enjoying watching Rugger intercollegiate matches this week, the Toggers (on the river) when such real healthy delights can be edged in somehow between more serious entertaining and work. Charlie is tonight being entertained by the Fellows of the Royal resident in Oxford – 30, I think.

No place, alas, for Lady Sherrington at a men's dinner given at the home of Lord Mildmay of Flete on 1 May 1924, in Berkeley Square, who wrote to Sherrington: "I am earnestly hoping that you may be able to join us. I am asking the Editor of *The Times,* Admiral Sir Roger Keyes, Field Marshal Massingberd, the President of the Royal Academy, Sir Robert Horne, Lord Bryce, Hailsham, Winston Churchill and the American Ambassador". It was shortly after this dinner that John Jacob Astor, owner of *The Times,* asked Sherrington to give him "a few minutes" in London to discuss the future of his family's paper.

To Sir Humphry Rolleston, President of the Royal College of Physicians, Sherrington wrote that despite his many meetings he felt that he could manage four per year for the Council of the College. From the famous Warden Spooner[1] of New College, Oxford, he received a note: "It is very kind in one so distinguished as you are to think about and remember my very humble self – I am grateful". What Sherrington did not tell the Warden in reply was that his favorite pun-cum-Spoonerism was "mooning in the spoonlight". Carr Sherrington, his son, loved to tell of his father's childish delight at the invented variety. Wilder Penfield enjoyed telling Wykhamists the story of Spooner inviting each Fellow as he met him in New College gardens to come for sherry before dinner to meet a new don. When the astonished don was thus addressed by the absent-minded Spooner, he replied, "But sir, I *am* the new don". "Good," said the Warden, "come anyway."

Professor James Jeans, F. R. S., was always very helpful to Sherrington in dealing expeditiously with Royal Society business. When Sherrington stepped down from the Presidency in 1925, after five eventful years, and Rutherford took over, Jeans sent Sherrington a graceful message saying how pleasant all members of the Council had found the work with Sherrington. One note passed by Jeans to Sherrington at a Council meeting to hear a submission, has survived. In it, Sherrington is advised: "This man is a terrible bore. I should feel inclined to cut the discussion short and not ask him to reply".

Sherrington's final year in the Presidency of the Royal Society had seemed a race between his correspondence and his survival. Friends as well

---

1 The Reverend Doctor Spooner was a stout supporter of the natural sciences at Oxford.

as people of whom he had never heard rained on him personal letters, requests, congratulatory messages, and sometimes, thanks. Sir Otto Beit, proud of his Fellowship in the Society, admitted that it was ". . . something I should like to have one day as an acknowledgement of my interest in science – but I never dreamt that it would come true". Gowland Hopkins told Sherrington: "I am not sure whether you yourself recognize how consistently throughout the years you have afforded me kindness and appreciation". Santiago Ramón y Cajal wrote concerning Wilder Penfield's projected visit to work in his institute in Madrid. Then he wrote again to "Mi antiguo y buen amigo" to say that Dr. Raoul May of Paris was translating his two-volume work, *Degeneration and Regeneration in the Nervous System.* Louisa Garrett Anderson, on behalf of the London (Royal Free Hospital) School of Medicine for Women thanked him for his presence at their Service of Thanksgiving.

From the War Office Sir William Leishman, a fellow pathologist and contributor in the campaign against typhoid, thanked Sherrington for "securing" his election to the Athenaeum – something never admitted unless one is a Lieutenant-General in charge of Army Medical Services. Sir Arthur Schuster wanted to thank Sherrington for sending him the key to the new gates of the National Physical Laboratory. Raymond Dodge sent a group of reprints from the Division of Anthropology and Psychology of the National Research Council in Washington, D. C. "with deep appreciation" for Sherrington's introduction of workers in vision to the "final common path". William Bateson in acknowledging "a pocket Rossetti which shall ease off many a journey" commented in passing that he had learned while in Russia that Sherrington had been made a foreign correspondent of the Leningrad Society of Naturalists. "This took place a year or two ago, I believe, but a similar notice in my case only arrived long afterwards."

Thus Sherrington concluded his immense work at the Royal Society. What he most wanted was to return to his researches with a new generation of students, and he wanted time for sustained correspondence with his old ones.

(W.C.G.)

Chapter 5

The Last Decade at Oxford 1925–1935

A. Oxford Hospitality

Number 9 Chadlington Road was the delightful home of the Sherringtons at Oxford. It was in a road of fine homes and gardens and conveniently within walking distance to the Physiological Laboratory through the magnificently treed University Parks. The daily walks to and fro gave C. S. S. exercise and refreshment as so felicitously described in many poems.

On arriving at the Laboratory in October 1925 I gave Sir Charles a letter of introduction by Professor W. A. Osborne, his old friend and the Professor of Physiology at Melbourne University, where I had been his student. To my delight there was immediately an invitation to afternoon tea next Sunday at 4 p. m. Robert Aitken had already been a year at Oxford and knew the ropes, Denny Brown and I being the novices. It was my first experience of the English hospitality that I learned to appreciate so much. The rules were of charming simplicity. There would be no further invitations, but every Sunday afternoon in term time at 4 p. m. the door was open and you entered without knocking and went to the drawing room to seek company. There could be up to twenty guests, mostly students like ourselves from overseas, and some young ladies also mostly from overseas. Lady Sherrie was a delightful hostess and Sir Charles came down from his study upstairs to join in entertaining the company with fascinating stories of his experiences enriched by so much remembered detail of people and places. Then came the time to move into the dining room for tea (Indian or China) which was served by Lady Sherrie to us all seated around the fine dining table that was replete with good things to eat. Of course there were maids to help and the conversation sparkled. About 5:30 was the usual time of departure. As I walked home that first evening through the Parks with Robert and Denny I realized that I had entered into a new world – a world of culture and style that I had never known before.

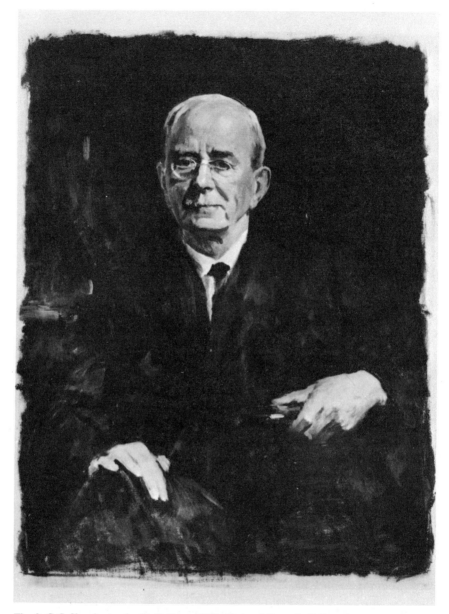

Fig. 2. C. S. Sherrington by R. G. Eves, 1927. National Portrait Gallery, London

It was an education to be in a drawing room with walls lined by books, being particularly rich in poetry and art. Sir Charles would often select a book and read some lines of poetry that were particularly apt for the conversation. He had an amazing memory for all the riches stored in his books.

I became a devotee of those lovely Sunday afternoons. Sometimes, when most had gone, one got the word from Lady Sherrie to stay for an informal evening meal. Occasionally in summer, when the weather was good, there was tennis on their lawn court, and I can remember Sir Charles playing quite a good doubles game. Some of us had the pleasure of dinner-theatre parties that Lady Sherrie arranged. Sir Charles never came, Lady Sherrie saying that he had no interest in theatrical presentations or in music. But she took great enjoyment and we had many delightful evenings in her company, beginning with dinner usually at the Northgate Restaurant.

I have enduring memories of Sir Charles as a raconteur. It seemed to happen regularly that, when in the middle of the main course at some dinner party, he would start on a long story sparkling with many detours. Though a joy to listen to, it was unfortunate for the hostess because he would forget to eat for as long as a quarter of an hour. He would be so deeply engaged in his fascinating story long after all of us had finished the course that he had scarcely begun. I remember an occasion where he had a piece of roast potato on his fork half way to his mouth for what seemed to be an interminable time. The hostess and indeed the whole company had their eyes glued to this potato, but to no effect! His plate was cleared in the end, almost untouched, so that the next course could follow. So rapt was he in his memories that he did not seem even to notice what was happening. He seemed on these occasions more like an ethereal or bird-like spirit that had no need of material sustenance.

B. Sherrington's Lectures at Oxford

When I arrived in Oxford in 1925, Sherrington was in his sixty-eighth year. I had hoped to commence research, but was persuaded by Magdalen College to become an undergraduate and read Physiology and Biochemistry in the Faculty of Natural Sciences. For me Sherrington's lectures were the star feature of the course. I was a skilled note-taker and my lecture note books give an authentic record of Sherrington's lectures[1], both of the lecture itself

---

1 Now in the Sherrington Room, Woodward Library, University of British Columbia.

and of all the illustrations. As I turn the pages of my notebook I can confirm my impression that at that time Sherrington was a good lecturer. He did not have the flow of eloquence of C. G. Douglas, but he presented the physiology of the nervous system as the fascinating story of its theoretical and experimental investigation from Descartes right up to his latest work with Liddell on the myotatic reflexes. Of course there were the detours so characteristic of his rich memories and experiences, but they did not detract from the main story that he was developing. They merely served to embellish it. I attended his lecture course for the two years of my undergraduate career and much appreciated it. My opinion was shared by the other students. The attendance was good throughout the whole course.

In 1952 Liddell wrote a good posthumous appraisal:

> As a lecturer, Sherrington was not rewarding to everyone because, especially in advanced lectures, his mind often seemed to work in three planes – the subject immediately in hand, though presented with great care, then at uncertain intervals came an elevated and rather distant diversion to contemplate possible plans for research on the subject, interwoven again with an even more elevated discourse on its place in the whole of learning. To the few who could follow these altering elevations of theme, the lectures gave a wealth of information and inspiration, and were also, as were his writings, an example of artistry in the choice of words.

I give these accounts because in the existing biographies it is stated that Sherrington was a poor lecturer, tending to confuse students rather than to instruct them. I think this was true in his later years – from 1930 onwards. I did not then attend any lectures, but we tutors encouraged our students to attend. They did for the first few, but thereafter, sad to relate, the numbers rapidly dwindled to zero! The students reported that they could not even hear most of the lecture, which was delivered to the blackboard on which illustrative diagrams were being drawn. It was before the age of neck microphones and the acoustics of the lecture room were appalling. No doubt also the detours were more obtrusive than before. It was embarassing for us to realize this breakdown of communication at a time when Sherrington had so much to give. We could only guess what Sherrie felt about this failure, because not one of us would dare to enquire. But I believe it strengthened his resolve to retire at a time when we were all urging him to stay on. We needed his leadership, and the reality of our need was all too obvious when he left.

C. The Mammalian Laboratory Class

In his later years at Liverpool Sherrington had been concerned with the obsolescence of the traditional physiological practical courses for medical students. He incorporated some experimental work on cats in the Liverpool classes. Taking advantage of this early experience, he was at Oxford able to develop a systematic experimental course in Mammalian Physiology that became world famous. During the war there were few students, so there was excellent opportunity to work with them in evolving the course. The tracings of blood pressure, of secretion and movements were recorded on a smoked drum kymograph, and the best specimens were carefully fixed by varnish and framed with the names of the students responsible. As soon as the war was over, it was possible to produce a printed laboratory manual giving the experimental procedures and the physiological interpretations with the chosen illustrations of the pioneer investigators. The book *Mammalian Physiology: A Course of Practical Exercises* published in 1919 was the text for this quite unique practical course. Nowhere else in the world was there anything like it.

For two years I was a student taking this course in the Final Honours School, then for ten subsequent years I was a demonstrator. In order to comply with the Home Office regulations on animal experimentation, the animals during an initial anaesthesia were either decapitated or decerebrated by the Sherrington guillotine. The students could hardly realize the intensive preparation that preceded by one hour the commencement of the class at 10 a. m. on each Thursday. Up to twenty cats were prepared in that hour. One of us demonstrators carried out the surgical procedures, and the whole technical staff under the stern eye of George Cox were mobilized in the anaesthetization and subsequent care of the preparations with attention to haemostasis, respiration and temperature control. It was rather like the feverish preparation before some dramatic performance. But when the curtain went up at 10 a. m. the prepared cats were awaiting the students. There were two students to a cat, so they had excellent technical training in the canulation of arteries and veins, in intravenous injections and in nerve dissection and stimulation. Throughout the three hour session the several demonstrators were checking the students' dissections, and their relevant physiological knowledge. During the class the best experiments were displayed and at the end of the class the smoked kymograph tracings were preserved in varnish for illustration by the students in their practical notebooks.

In 1952 Liddell wrote about Sherrington and these classes:

> His enthusiasm and zest in the conduct of that class were the key to its success. His urgent emphasis on correct procedure, his scorn of slovenly work (which could be surprisingly emphatic), and his excited interest in good results kept every member on his toes. Having the advantage for close work of short-sight, Sherrington would slip off his pince-nez the better to get a nearer view of the work in hand and aid some floundering student, to emerge at last triumphant, and gropingly retrieve his glasses.

The Thursday mammalian class was the great dramatic event of the week, and so it remained during the whole of Sherrington's Oxford period. A revised edition of the book with Liddell as co-author was published in 1929. Comparable mammalian classes soon were initiated in many medical schools throughout the world. In recent decades the trouble has been the prohibitive cost of cats, which were so cheap in the Oxford days – certainly less than ten shillings.

D. Research

In the 1920s and into the 1930s Sherrington's laboratory would have been generally regarded as the leading laboratory of the world in the field of central nervous system physiology. This exalted status derived of course from the greatness of Sherrington. Yet it was amazingly modest, ill-organized and ill-equipped by present day standards. Even when biochemistry moved into its new laboratories in 1927 the physiology facilities were poor. Denny-Brown had inherited the sole well-equipped room from John Fulton in 1925. It had the only electrical recording system, a string galvanometer, and it had the other standard equipment of a falling plate camera, optical myographs and stimulating equipment built up of various key arrangements for single and repetitive stimulation using induction coils. In October 1927 I had been accepted as a D. Phil. student with Sir Charles as my supervisor and due to his support I had in December 1927 been appointed as a Junior Research Fellow of Exeter College; yet I had no laboratory in which to work and had never carried out a scientific experiment! Five of us research associates were quartered in the old mammalian laboratory with no office equipment other than a table, a chair and the partial privacy given by a folding screen: Granit, Denny-Brown, Olmsted, Marcu and myself. This was as far as Cox's patronage would go. George Cox had been Sir Charles' factotum for over thirty years. Otherwise we had to fend for ourselves. Fortunately Creed asked me to join him on a research problem. This gave me my chance because he moved into vision research and I inherited his very modestly equipped research room in 1928.

That was most valuable for me because in January 1928 Ragnar Granit came from Helsingfors to work in Sherrington's laboratory, and Sherrington thought that we could work together, a choice for which we are eternally grateful. In those primitive days research problems were not easy to formulate or to implement when your total equipment was an optical myograph, a plate camera and sundry induction coils. Our chosen problem was to do for the crossed extensor reflex what Sherrington, Cooper and Denny-Brown had done for the ipsilateral flexor reflex. It was on the theme that dominated the research projects of the Oxford School at that time, namely the interaction of reflexes. Before dealing with these developments, two early experiences of my research with Sherrington may help to give some feeling for the dramatic atmosphere at that time.

i. The Motor Unit

Throughout the 1920s the investigations on reflexes by Sherrington and his associates – Liddell, Sassa, Creed, Cooper and Denny-Brown were discussed in terms of motor units. These units were defined as the axon or nerve fibre arising from a motoneurone in the spinal cord and the assemblage of muscle fibres innervated by it. He had already recognized in the 1890s that there was no peripheral inhibitory mechanism such as occurs with crustacean muscle. Once the message was discharged by the motoneurone it inevitably resulted in a contraction of the innervated muscle fibres. Investigations by Fulton and others had revealed that it was only rarely that two motoneurones innervated the same muscle fibre. Thus for practical purposes the territory of muscle fibres innervated by one motoneurone could be regarded as the private preserve of that neurone, always contracting at its bidding. Hence arose the Sherringtonian concept of the motor unit, which was the natural unitary constituent of all muscle contractions. Thus, interaction of reflexes was interpreted quantitatively in terms of the activation of motor units.

In 1928 Sir Charles was enquiring more sharply about this unitary constitution of all movements. It was necessary to know the average amount of the contraction delivered by motor units of different muscles, both for single twitch responses and for the steady muscle contractions evoked by repetitive stimulation – the motor tetanus as it was called. For this purpose he required merely a count of the motor fibres to a muscle and the tensions developed in its isometric twitch and tetanic responses. He had shown in the 1890s that the nerve to a muscle contains a large proportion of sensory fibres from the receptor organs in the muscle. It was essential to eliminate these from the muscle nerve and then the number of motor units would be given simply by counting the fibres in a histological preparation of the transverse section of the nerve.

Thus the plan of the experiment was firstly a complicated aseptic operation in which the spinal canal was exposed with the sensory ganglia on the dorsal spinal roots. These ganglia had to be excised from the roots supplying the muscles to be investigated, but the underlying ventral roots containing the motor nerve fibres had to be left intact. This is a delicate operation requiring surgical skill of a high order, but Sherrington was a master of such technique. After allowing the time of about 2 weeks for complete degeneration of the sensory fibres so that they would not be counted, I assisted in the mechanical recordings of the various muscle contractions. Then the muscle nerves were excised for histological staining by osmic acid. This Sherrington did with consummate skill so as to avoid shrinkage of the fibres. He did the dehydration in a succession of alcohols all through the night, taking home the nerves carefully 'splinted' on filter paper for the treatments during the night in his bathroom.

The resulting histological preparations were unrivalled, as can be appreciated by reference to the published paper. These superb transverse sections were given to me for counting. Never before had completely deafferented motor nerves been examined histologically. The first glance was a revelation. Instead of the expected population of nerve fibres of fairly uniform large size, there were distinctly two populations with almost no transitional fibres. Immediately I did a count for plotting a size spectrum and confirmed this surprising discovery. When Sir Charles arrived, I already had the story clearly displayed. It posed two related questions: how to account for this duality of size? and how to enumerate the motor nerve fibres for evaluating the average contractions of the motor units? In retrospect our decisions on these questions seem inexplicable. We produced a developmental theory to account for the sizes of the fibres, postulating that the small fibres came from motoneurones whose axons had arrived at the muscle too late to secure an appropriate ration of muscle fibres for innervation, hence they lived on in an undeveloped state. We divided the muscle contractions by the total number of muscle fibres, small and large, and hence recognized that we had underestimated the tensions given by the average large motor unit. Later by graded stimulation of the motor nerve it was shown that the small motor fibres did not add in any detectable amount to the contraction produced by the large fibres.

In part we missed the significance of the small fibres because Sir Charles

was engaged on a study which well illustrates his perfectionism in histological investigations. Implicit in the use of the counting procedure to provide
an enumeration of the motoneurones supplying a muscle was the assumption that the motor axon did not branch on the way to the muscle. To test
this the nerve to a muscle – usually gastrocnemius – was dissected out as far
proximally as possible as it lay embedded in the sciatic nerve. This long
nerve (up to 5 cm long) was sectioned and counted at different distances
proximally from the muscle. The numbers decreased considerably as one
followed the nerve proximally. So, clearly, the individual nerve fibres did
branch, and counts close to the muscle would overestimate the number of
gastrocnemius motoneurones. It was, however, reassuring that this branching was negligible in the most proximal segment that could be dissected.
Counts at that level were used for the calculation of the mean contraction
tension of the motor units.

However, Sir Charles was not content with this arithmetical demonstration of branching. It was too indirect. So he set about the laborious task of
teasing deafferented motor nerves in order to see an actual branching of
fibres. During the summer of 1929 he was teasing nerves day after day. I
have never known him so happy and absorbed as he was in this mechanical
task with the rewards every now and then of a beautifully displayed branching – it was like pure gold! Meanwhile I was working in the same room (his
study) doing the measurements that gave the plots of fibre size against
number. It was at the time of the International Physiological Congress at
Boston and he sent from the laboratory a cable to Professor Cannon con-
veying greetings and best wishes to which he insisted on appending my
completely unknown name.

The correct explanation of the size duality of motor nerve fibres was
given by Granit's pupil Leksell many years later (1945). He showed that the
small motor fibres innervated the muscle spindles. The large fibres were in
the alpha class of nerve fibres and came from alpha motoneurones, while
the small ones were in the gamma class and came from gamma
motoneurones whose unique function was to innervate the highly
specialized receptor organs in muscle that are called muscle spindles. As
stated above, our failure to give the correct explanation of the clear duality
of motor fibres is all the more inexplicable when it is recognized that Sherrington had identified the motor innervation of muscle spindles in the 1890s
and had in his Linacre Lecture of 1924 specifically raised the question of
the function of the motor innervation of muscle spindles. I have never
discovered if Sherrington ever realized our mistake. He would have been
most intrigued by Leksell's discovery and the experimental follow-up by

Granit and his school. I tried to tell him of this in 1952 when I saw him again after my fifteen years sojourn in the Antipodes. But it was too late. His interests had by then moved on to the philosophical problem of brain and mind. I could not arouse his attention to these scientific problems that had been so central to his earlier life. One is reminded of the line: "There is a tide in the affairs of men . . .".

ii. The Angle

In the 1920s optical myography was perfected. It was the technical procedure of which we at Oxford were most proud. The aim was to have the most faithful recording of the tension exerted by a muscle contraction. For that purpose contracting muscle had to be allowed the smallest possible shortening so that the contraction energy would not be dissipated in the internal friction deriving from the muscle viscosity. Sir Charles set great store by the myographic technique, as well he might, because it was the procedure whereby he obtained all the quantitative investigations in the 1920s. A string galvanometer was not installed until late in 1929.

With the mirror myographs so ably constructed by the instrument maker O'Neill, the torsion of the steel rod was greatly amplified by an optical beam that was reflected from a mirror on the rod and photographed by a moving plate camera. In that way beautiful photographs could be taken of a unitary muscle contraction, the muscle twitch. John Fulton had systematically studied muscle twitches in the early 1920s, and had reported extraordinary features by his refined analysis. It was of particular interest that at the summit of contraction there was a steady maintenance of tension that abruptly terminated in a rapid relaxation, the sharp transition being named the 'angle'. The sharpness of the angle was in fact used as a criterion of the faithfulness with which the myograph recorded the muscle contraction.

I, too, believed in the angle, so much so that I planned an investigation designed to throw light on the nature of the relevant mechanical events in the muscle, namely its viscosity and elasticity. For this purpose of vibratory analysis the bearing of the torsion rod was redesigned from support by a V-shaped slot to an axial knife-edge supported on a flat steel base. To our amazement the angle had disappeared, the muscle twitch showing a smooth rise to a summit and a smooth decline therefrom. Within the few minutes required for transposition it was possible to show that the same muscle on the old torsion myograph gave twitches with good angles. Superposition of the two myographic pictures gave the explanation of the discrepancy. The

V-shaped support of the torsion rod provided a frictional resistance to its rotation. The resulting distortion appeared as three features: a delay on the rising phase of the recorded myogram; a lowered summit at a maintained plateau; a sharp onset (the angle) of the falling phase that was delayed until the frictional resistance could be overcome. It was so obvious that the old myographs were gravely defective in design, yet it had not been recognized because, ironically, we believed that the excellence of their recording was guaranteed by the sharpness of the angles in their myograms!

I immediately informed Sir Charles of this embarrassing discovery. He had of course believed the authenticity of the angle, as had all members of the Oxford School. He carefully inspected the myograms and the myographs, and was greatly disturbed – as also was I – at the impending blow to the prestige of the Oxford laboratory. However, next day he had fully recovered his equanimity. He confessed that he had gone home to read right through the publications of his researches using the optical myographs. His verbatim comment was: "Aren't I lucky? I found that I had not mentioned the word 'angle' once".

Nevertheless he recognized that a report of the faulty myograph design should be made to the Physiological Society. It was duly made at the St. Thomas's Hospital meeting in December 1929. He presented our conjoint communication and I followed by a communication giving a comparison of the twitch myograms of the same muscles with the friction and the frictionless myographs. Many years later there was a piquant aftermath. Lord Adrian wrote to me in 1952 saying how much he appreciated the way in which I had renounced my hypotheses of electrical transmission at excitatory and inhibitory synapses. He went on to remark that he was reminded of the charming manner in which many years before Sherrington had admitted the errors arising from the faulty myograph design. "But Jack," he wrote, "this was long before your time!"

iii. Synaptic Mechanisms

We can now return to the principal activity of the Oxford laboratory at that time, namely the attempt to discover the nature of synaptic action, both excitatory and inhibitory. The available techniques prevented such procedures as unitary analysis with microelectrode recording, but we could hope to gain evidence about the time course of synaptic action by studying the interaction of the central events produced by two afferent volleys set up in peripheral nerves that converged on the same spinal cord centres. For example we used the two nerves to gastrocnemius muscle as afferents and recorded the reflex response of a flexor muscle of the same limb. When either volley alone evoked no response, two at a short interval apart were effective (facilitation). Sir Charles and I studied the time course of this facilitation by varying the stimulus interval and plotting the size of the facilitated response against the stimulus interval. Unfortunately the choice of the flexor reflex entailed the complication of an interneurone in the spinal reflex path, but it was the best we could do when our recording was restricted to muscle contractions. Nevertheless the facilitatory curves in their simplest form did give the right answer of about 15 ms for the duration of synaptic excitatory action. More complex forms could plausibly be attributed to the interneuronal complication.

I was very excited by these discoveries and proceeded late in 1929 to write them up for publication. I can remember that I invited Sir Charles to dinner at Exeter College and after dinner I read to him some of the manuscript that was to be our conjoint paper. He was helpfully critical as usual, and made good suggestions on word usage. In fact at that time he gave me a copy of *Roget's Thesaurus* which is inscribed: "My joke, C. S. S.". The paper was duly published in the *Journal of Physiology:* "Reflex summation in the ipsilateral spinal flexion reflex". As we sent it in to press Sir Charles shyly told me that it was the first of his published papers that he had not written himself. I was dumbfounded!

An amusing incident occurred when Sir Charles and I were to demonstrate reflex facilitation at the Oxford meeting of the Physiological Society in 1929. The preparation was set up in good time, but developed for an unknown reason an irregular twitching of the flexor muscle whose twitch contractions were to display the facilitation. Such twitchings would confuse the whole demonstration. Careful examination showed that the twitching was not due to any local injury of the muscle, but was genuinely a reflex, perhaps arising from some area of cut skin. Then Sir Charles discovered that this reflex twitching could be inhibited by steady squeezing of the cat's tail. So we worked out our strategy for the demonstration. We would not confuse the onlookers by telling them what we were doing. Sir Charles would sit so that he could unobtrusively hold the tail of the cat in his hand, and, as soon as the demonstration of the reflex facilitation was to be given, he squeezed it, so providing the quiet background for the display of the reflex facilitation. During the hour-long demonstration to wave after wave of observers we kept up our strategy, never revealing it. So our demonstration was saved, and we felt the shared happiness of co-conspirators!

Determining the time course of synaptic inhibitory action provided a tougher challenge. Sir Charles entered into the planning with enthusiasm. He had always been emotionally attached to synaptic inhibition. Inhibition in the central nervous system was really his scientific discovery in the 1890s. Before that, there were only a few crude anecdotal accounts. His attachment was amply demonstrated when in 1932 he gave his Nobel lecture with the title "Inhibition as a coordinative factor".

The research strategy was to have a steady background contraction of the quadriceps muscle that could easily be provided either by our equipment for giving a steady stretch of the muscle in our decerebrate preparation or by a crossed extensor reflex. A central inhibitory action would be exhibited as a brief relaxation of this steady reflex. To our delight we found out that we could demonstrate facilitation of this relaxation, particularly with the crossed extensor reflex. We could choose two nerve volleys that alone gave a slight inhibitory relaxation, but together were much more effective. But the facilitation differed from that for excitation in that the facilitated inhibitory relaxation was usually greatest when the two volleys were 10–30 ms apart. It declined to zero with further lengthening of the stimulus interval. We thought we had evidence on the time course of central inhibition; but more of that anon.

I have vivid remembrances of the heroic experimental procedures required in those days to carry out some simple tests. The device for giving two stimuli at chosen intervals was an enormous pendulum that from a 'remote' era had been fixed on the wall of a room adjacent to our research room and the only communication was by a small window. The whole area had been McDougall's laboratory with the walls blackened presumably for his visual experiments. After assisting with the experimental preparation Granit's task was to lift up the massive pendulum, which was held by a magnetic release. Then he set the two break keys to the required interval, which was accurate to 0.1 ms. Meanwhile in the research room the muscle stretch had gone on, then the falling plate of the camera was released, tripping on the way the electrical circuit of the pendulum magnet. Down came the great pendulum weighing many kilograms with a swing of about 2 m breaking the contacts of the two circuit keys and so activating the induction cells that provided the nerve stimulation. After all this commotion in the adjoining room Granit's face would appear in the little window to hear of the results and to be given the instruction for the next stimulus interval. All of that work for just one point on the curve, and so on through the day! It was well that Granit was a great strong Swede.

Unfortunately after all this experimenting we were confronted by Denny-Brown's criticism and we had to accept it, which we did with gratitude. It was simply that we had overlooked the complication ensuing from the time required for the onset of a muscle relaxation. Even though a single stimulus gave no relaxation of a crossed extensor reflex, it could still have silenced the motoneuronal discharge for a time (say 20 ms) too brief to allow for a relaxation. Thus in our experiments two stimuli individually ineffective could give a relaxation because they lenghtened the silencing of the muscle long enough for relaxation to ensue. This accounts for the optimal interval at 10–30 ms. If there had been any inhibitory facilitation in our experiments, it had been inextricably complicated by this relaxation phenomenon. We now recognized the danger of relying exclusively on mechanical recording. If we had had electrical recording from the muscle, we would not have been misled. Thus our so-laborious experiments were abandoned and remained unpublished. I was very sorry because Ragnar Granit was soon to leave and this was his only opportunity to publish a paper with Sir Charles. A year or so later Sir Charles and I did manage to redesign our inhibitory experiments and obtain some evidence on the time course of synaptic inhibitory action on flexor reflexes.

There was one good aftermath. Sir Charles and I recognized the necessity for electrical as well as mechanical recording. So our research room soon had a string galvanometer. Together we learnt the technique of electrical recording from muscle, one of us near the end of his experimental life, the other at the beginning. The string galvanometer was the first step and was good for many studies on the effects of firing impulses back into neurones from their axons that normally carry these messages in the reverse direction – from neurone to muscle. This physiological trick was introduced by Denny-Brown as a procedure for analysing the responses of nerve cells, and we exploited it in that last hectic year before Sir Charles gave up active experimental work. The experiments were complicated and one hesitated to break off once they were running well. So in this arduous life during the years 1929, 1930 and even into 1931 our experiments went on all day with no lunch break. Then usually at about 4 p. m. we went down town for an enormous afternoon tea before returning for a final session. Lady Sherrie was rightly concerned at this strenuous existence – often with two such experiments in a week, and early in 1931 the last physiological experiments were done, Sir Charles then being in his seventy-fourth year. Thereafter he returned to one of his first loves – neurohistology.

I give two quotations from an excellent posthumous account (Liddell, 1952):

> In physical build Sherrington was small and wiry, and as with Harvey, his eye was "full of spirit". He spent long hours in the laboratory over arduous experiments, often in a stuffy

dark-room, and even when no longer young, he would work away without appearing to become tired or indeed aware of anything at all except the purpose of the moment, the revealing of new knowledge. Gifted insight kept him poised steadily in his course of progress. It had been said of him, and truly, that he knew what questions to ask of Nature, and how to ask them. He knew too when he had the right answer. Now, years after, when more refined methods are available, there is much coming to proof that he had foreseen or surmised by clear hard thinking and deduction.

As head of a laboratory, 'Sherrie' was ever genial and sympathetic with a standard of criticism whose topmost height was barely seen by others. His own example set a standard of achievement, and of modesty. The work that mattered most came first, and that was research. There was so much to do, so much to think about. He knew where and how he could achieve supreme results. Except at the intenser moments on the "sacred days" of long experiments any young researcher, hot on a trail, was greated on equal terms, for a talk on things physiological which could be both questioning and informative. Then might rapidly appear on any handy scrap of paper delightful rough drawings to show a plan for future battle. Thus were ideas poured out.

iv. Memories

From these years there remain memories of striking incidents. One morning Sir Charles arrived with an inspired look on his face. He recounted vividly how he had seen a cat walking solemnly on a stone wall that was interrupted by an open gate. The cat paused, inspected the gap, then leaped exactly to the right distance, landed with ease and grace and resumed its solemn progression. A very ordinary happening, yet to Sherrington on that morning it was replete with problems for future research. How had the visual image of the gap been transmuted by 'judgement' into the exactly organized motor mechanism of the leap? How had the strength of the muscle contractions been calculated so that the leap was exactly right for the gap? How had the motor machinery been organized so that there was this elegant landing on the far side of the gap? How after the landing was it arranged that the stately walk was resumed? Of course these questions were largely for the future, but some, such as the landing mechanism, could in part be answered. After almost fifty years we can make partial attempts at some of the questions. In Granit's recent book on *'Motor Control'* there are partial answers based upon our present knowledge of the neural machinery of the spinal cord and its control. And there are glimpses of answers in the unfinished studies of cerebro-cerebellar circuitry and of cerebro-basal ganglia circuitry, as well as in the studies of the cerebro-spinal and the cerebello-spinal pathways. But the satisfactory answers to Sherrington's questions on that morning will be long in coming.

The electrophysiological research continued in the last years of Sherrington's Oxford period. Amplifiers appeared with firstly a Matthews oscillograph and then cathode ray oscilloscopes and two shielded rooms were constructed. By present standards it was simple. The stimulus timing was provided by the Lucas spring pendulum, a much simpler device than the massive gravity pendulum. Sir Charles regularly visited the laboratories and took a professional interest in the new experimental procedures and the scientific results. Some years later when I was in Sydney and sent him pictures of the research room there and of the contraction of an innervated strip of soleus muscle he was to write, "I could almost see the sluggish contraction and hear the Keith Lucas hammer fall".

This strictly scientific story has left out delightful concomitants of our life together in the laboratory. As is usual many experimental procedures were routine, and this gave opportunity for listening to Sir Charles as he drew on his accumulated wisdom. He had an expert knowledge of Italian painting, and believed that in the Renaissance some of the painters' studios were like scientific laboratories today. He illustrated this idea by Verocchio's studio in Florence, where there was study of anatomy by dissection, a study of perspective and geometry, a study of pigments and media, a study of colour and shadow. Furthermore there was continual discussion and criticism. And so a youth of fourteen goes there as an apprentice and emerges six years later as Leonardo da Vinci. I was so enthused by our art discussions that I spent four weeks wandering in the hill towns of Tuscany and Umbria during Easter vacation of 1930. Penfield has said that Sherrington's memory was superior to that of anyone he had known. It was remarkable not only in the wealth of the store but in its quality, and in the aptness of his remembrances according to circumstances. So good was his sequential memory system that it would often sidetrack him from the matter in hand. One had to be patient – and we were. You could always anticipate an exciting adventure back into his life.

Besides art his other great love was poetry, and above all Shakespeare and Keats. I can remember his frequent quotations from Keats during our daily work. He greatly enjoyed Middleton Murry's book *Keats and Shakespeare,* which appeared about 1930, and we were regaled with the story day by day as he read through it every evening. Then he gave me a copy, and recently I reread it, along with Keats, when I was confined in a hospital. I was almost unconscious of those unhappy surroundings because I was reliving the days of my Oxford life with Sir Charles. Another great joy for him was Robert Bridges' wonderful epic – *The Testament of Beauty.* We were all reading it as soon as it appeared and quoted it to one another. It seems to have been lost sight of in these more violent and uncultured times. I recently reread it and found it still had the same enchantment. I think Sir

Charles would have felt this age as less attractive culturally than the nineteenth century and the earlier decades of this century.

E. Sherrington's Contribution to Theories of Nervous Function, 1924–1934

On our chosen theme, as given by the subtitle of this book, the theoretical and imaginative writings of Sherrington are of particular interest, not the conventional reports of laboratory experiments. In this work we are endeavouring to paint a picture of him as the creator of so many of the fundamental concepts of modern neurology, though of course he was also a skilled experimentalist. He was much in demand as a lecturer in the early 1920s, but of particular importance for our theme is the Linacre Lecture delivered at St. John's College, Cambridge on 6 May 1924. It was entitled "Problems of muscular receptivity", and has undeservedly been almost forgotten.

After a general introduction to the manner in which muscles are at the service of the nerve centres, he gives a characteristic philosophical aside:

> The skeletal muscles are the motor machinery for all the life of the animal which the older physiologists were wont to call the 'life of external relation'. Of the importance of that life of external relation the moralist has written that even in man the crown of life is an action, not a thought. Should we demur to this distinction, we can still endorse the old adage that to move things is all mankind can do, and that for such the sole executant is muscle, whether in whispering a syllable or in felling a forest.

Yet he goes on to say that muscles are not purely passive at the service of a nervous system informed by receptors providing signals about the external world. That this is so

> ... is shown by their possession of receptors of their own. On their own behalf they send messages into the central exchanges. This must mean they have some voice in their own conditions of service, perhaps ring themselves up and ring themselves off. Let us attempt to penetrate into the significance of their 'receptivity'.

This introduces the theme of the lecture with the further pregnant sentence:

> Following the functional scheme of all receptors, we may be sure that the central reactions provoked by the receptors of muscle will be divisible into, on one hand, the purely reflex and on the other hand, those which subserve mental experience.

The lecture is mainly concerned with the purely reflex function of muscle receptors and is excellently illustrated by his studies with Liddell on postural or stretch reflexes. The influence of higher centres on the spinal reflex mechanism is illuminated by a wealth of knowledge. He concludes:

> The two reactional aspects, the sensual and the purely reflex, of muscular receptivity reveal therefore two sides of, broadly taken, one singly-purposed function addressed to a single problem, in brief, the taxis of execution, the management – from rough adjustment onward into minutely refined *finesse* – of the acts of our skeletal muscles.

This statement provides the theme for investigations right up to the present time. It was prophetic. "Its content of unanswered questions is legion."

However, later in the lecture he ventures into the perplexing field of the functions of the various histological types of muscle receptors that he had recognized in the 1890s.

> In perception of postures and movements there seem traceable, as underlying data, degrees of muscle-tension. Some muscle receptors may be length-recorders, others tension-recorders; one would suppose the Golgi tendon-organs among these latter. As to the 'muscle-spindles', the muscle fibres they enfold, though differing within the spindle from those outside, yet receive motor-terminals; one would suppose active contraction to supply their stimulus. Through them and through other receptive endings which clasp muscular fibres, the active contraction of the muscle might be expected to evoke reflex reactions, and to furnish a contraction datum for perception of active postures and movements.

These statements were highly speculative in 1924, but in their essentials they have been corroborated. They provided a challenge and a programme for research that have been among the great achievements of neurobiology during the subsequent decades. As mentioned in the section on the motor unit, this reference to the motor innervation of muscle spindles was unaccountably overlooked when we discovered some five years later the two classes of motor nerve fibres, large and small.

When I arrived in Oxford in the autumn of 1925 there was much discussion about Sherrington's recently published theoretical paper in the *Proceedings of the Royal Society* (Sherrington, 1925). It was rather coyly entitled "Remarks on some aspects of reflex inhibition". It seems that the intention was to present an alternative theory of inhibition to the interference theory that had been so ably developed by Lucas, Forbes and Adrian. Their theory had the attraction that it was based on scientific studies of nerve fibres and nerve-muscle junctions during repetitive stimulation, but it also had the weakness of an analogy that was based on a very improbable central design.

Sherrington had realized that this interference theory was unable to account for all the gradations that he had observed in reflex responses under the interactions of excitation and inhibition. In order to present this theory of inhibition he had first to give an account of the synaptic mechanisms of excitatory pathways from afferent nerves to motoneurones to muscles. In the spinal cord there was a simple arrangement of branching of the three afferent fibres and their convergence on the three motoneurones to muscles in a simple explanatory diagram.

The term (motor unit) was coined for the anatomical arrangement of the axon of the motoneurone and the muscle fibres that it innervated. There has been earlier reference to this very useful term, which implied an all-or-nothing unit of muscle contraction.

The key feature of the new theory was the postulate that at the synapse the incoming afferent impulse ended, its excitatory action being effected by an intermediary process of the recipient neurone. This intermediary process had a longer duration than the impulse and was capable of summation with similar intermediary processes produced by impulses incident on other synapses of that neurone. Summation to a critical level resulted in the discharge of an impulse by the motoneurone. Thus was born the concept of the central excitatory state (c.e.s.), which was to dominate the thinking and the experiments of the Oxford School from that time onwards and which is still with us in an updated form. On the basis of this simple theory it was possible to account for a great many experimental findings. Amongst those listed were gradation of reflex discharge with increase in stimulation of an afferent nerve, and the after-discharge with its increase under similar circumstances. The reflex responses evoked by repetitive afferent nerve stimulation were accounted for in all their variety.

The schema for inhibitory synaptic mechanisms was developed on similar lines. An important postulate was that inhibition was not just a neutralization or diminution of the excitatory processes, but that it existed independently as a central inhibitory state (c.i.s.), capable of giving a state more depressed than the unexcited state. On the basis of this hypothesis of two complementary synaptic processes it was possible to account for all the experimental findings of Sherrington and his school on the interaction of excitation and inhibition; for example, that inhibition could be effective on a later excitation. Because of the duration of a unitary inhibition, repetitive stimulation of an inhibitory afferent could give a steady inhibitory action. It was proposed that there were two classes of synapses; but, because the synaptic knobs showed no differentiation, it was assumed that excitatory and inhibitory synapses differed in respect of the postsynaptic membrane. In almost all of its features this hypothesis of synaptic action is in general agreement with the very sophisticated synaptic mechanisms as understood today. There was even a suggestion of humoral synaptic transmission. The rival interference theory did not survive.

This frankly speculative paper was not received enthusiastically. Most scientists erroneously believe that science should be concerned only with experimentally discovered facts. I arrived in Oxford some months later and heard the derisory comment from my turor, "The old man has delivered himself of a bunch of speculations!" As I read and reread this paper I recognized that the theories there enunciated provided the guidelines for years of experiment. It was a great illuminating experience and in my collaboration with Sir Charles the experiments were designed to discover more and more about c.e.s. and c.i.s., in particular the time course of these postulated states when set up by a single afferent volley. My D. Phil. thesis of 1929 with Sir Charles as my supervisor was built upon these fundamental concepts of 1925. Long after the demise of the Oxford School these ideas were current in other laboratories, for example in the Rockefeller Institute with Lloyd. But the final justification for these speculations of Sherrington's came in 1951 in New Zealand when intracellular recording from motoneurones revealed that these two states did indeed exist as depolarization and hyperpolarization respectively of the neuronal membrane with a unitary duration of 10–20 ms, very much as originally proposed by Sherrington (Brock, Coombs and Eccles, 1952).

The next important general contribution by Sherrington was the Ferrier Lecture (Sherrington, 1929), "Some functional problems attaching to convergence". Here were displayed the fruits of the quantitative studies of the motor unit constitution of muscle. Central to it were considerations of the numbers of motoneurones in the motoneurone pool (as it was called) supplying a muscle and of the contraction tension developed by the average motor unit. The interaction of reflexes could be quantitatively considered in terms of the numbers of motor units concerned in occlusion or facilitation. These operations were illustrated in attractive diagrams of motoneurone pools (Fig. 3). They are reproduced here in order to display the vivid pictorial thinking of Sherrington in explanation of experimental findings. When the two afferents excite many neurones in common, their interaction results in a reflex contraction less than the arithmetical sum of the constituents. The reflexes are said to be occluded. When on the contrary there is a large overlap in the subliminally excited neurones (the subliminal fringe, as it was called) the interaction gave facilitation, there being a larger reflex contraction than the sum of the constituents. The concepts of c.e.s. and c.i.s. were valuable in accounting for the experimental findings, and already our earliest studies on the duration of the c.e.s. (16–40 ms) were displayed in plotted curves.

A valuable part of this lecture concerned the interactions of excitatory and inhibitory actions – or c. e. s. and c. i. s. in the new terminology. Old observations on the interaction were reconsidered. The general story emerged that in the confluence there was a conflict of exctatory and inhibitory actions (the so-called algebraic summation), each of which could

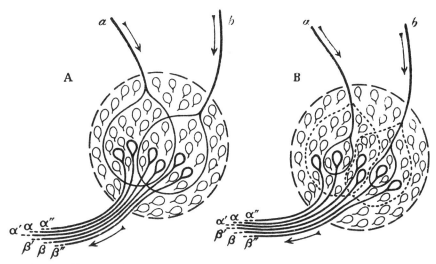

Fig. 3. *From Sherrington's Ferrier Lecture, 1929*
A Two excitatory afferents, a and b, with their fields of supraliminal effect in the motoneurone pool of a muscle. *a* activates by itself 4 units (α', α, α'' and β'); *b* by itself 4 (β', β, β'' and α'). Concurrently they activate not 8 but 6, i. e., give contraction deficit by occlusion of contraction in α' and β'. **B** Weaker stimulation of a and b restricting their supraliminal fields of effect in the pool as shown by the continuous-line limit. a by itself activates 1 unit; b similarly; concurrently they activate 4 units (α' α, β' and β) owing to summation of subliminal effect in the overlap of the subliminal fields outlined by dots. (Subliminal fields of effect are not indicated in diagram **A**)

be graded, and the observed reflex was the outcome of this conflict. For example weakening of a reflex by fatigue makes it more susceptible to inhibition. Under special conditions a steady state of neuronal excitation can be secured by a balance of the intensities of excitation and inhibition. One of the sections has the surprisingly modern title: "The discharging nerve cell in the hands of central excitation and inhibition". Already the analytical investigations of Adrian and Bronk on the one hand and of Denny-Brown on the other had refined our thinking by making it possible to consider the frequency of firing of the individual motoneurones. It had actually been shown by Denny-Brown that inhibition could slow the rate of discharge of a neurone to a steady value. New insights were thus given into the subtle interactions of nerve cells in the spinal cord.

The conclusion is worth quoting in extenso:

> ... though trains of impulses are the sole reactions which enter and leave the central nervous system, nervous impulses are not the sole reactions functioning within that system. States of excitement which can sum together, and states of inhibition which can sum together, and states which represent the algebraical summation of these two, are among

the central reactions. The motoneurone lies at a focus of interplay of these reactions and its motor-unit gives their net upshot, always expressed in terms of motor impulses and contraction. The central reactions can be much longer lasting than the nerve impulse of nerve trunks. Further, these central states and reactions are, as compared with the processes of nerve-trunk conductions, relatively very sensitive to physiological conditions, and are delicately responsive to fatigue, blood supply, drugs etc. The specific cell units, the neurones, far from behaving merely as passive recipients and transmitters of impulses, modify as well as transmit what they receive. They can develop rhythm of their own, and their rate of discharge can rise and fall with intensity of central excitation and inhibition respectively.

Two years later (Sherrington, 1931), in the Hughlings Jackson Lecture, he developed further the theme of the motor units as is indicated by the title "Quantitative management of contraction in lowest level coordination". The numbers and contraction values of motor units were given for a representative selection of muscles. In a motoneurone pool reflexly excited at a steady level there could be four levels of excitation: maximal, subtetanic, subthreshold and zero. With the maximal the discharge rate is so rapid that the muscle contracts with maximum tension. With the subtetanic the frequency of discharge is so low that the motor unit gives a tremulous contraction of low tension. Using this basic criterion the effects of stronger or weaker excitation of the motoneurone pool were readily explicable by a movement respectively upwards or downwards in the array of levels. A great wealth of observations was shown to be readily interpretable on the basis of the levels of excitation. As finally stated in Sherrington's inimitable style:

> . . ., the motor centre – old but expressive term – is not a mere passive relay on the path out to its muscle, not merely a place of passive assembly of impulses converging upon the muscle. The motor centre grades the excitation of the individual motor unit, causing its faster or its slower firing. The motor centre is a central instrument which adjusts *actively* the contraction-strength of its reflexes; it works on the basis of the 'central excitatory state'. Driven and fed by centripetal impulses, it deals with them on the summation basis. It is in short a 'summation-mechanism'. It operates on the individual motoneurone by excitation-summation; in that way it can exert a whole scale of degrees of excitement upon one and the same individual motor unit, firing it faster and so obtaining nearer full tetanic value of contraction, or slower with greater defect from full tetanic contraction. It also shows changes in extensity with variation in the number of motoneurones. Yet, since central impulses in order to excite a motor unit must be summated, the central mechanism is ultimately wholly a summation apparatus. One secret of its co-ordinative power lies in its power of summating, with almost negligible time-lag, shifting fringes and mobile shades of excitation that meet and overlap upon it. These join and disjoin, expand and shrink as afferent channels leading from various sources come into or drop out of action; and each and every time the central apparatus subjects them to or releases them from its summation.

No doubt such imaginative concepts recommended themselves very strongly to the assembled neurologists gathered to hear the lecture in honour of the great London neurologist of the last century. Hughlings Jackson himself would have been most appreciative of the theme so close to his own manner of thinking. In the closing stages of the lecture there were references to neurological insights provided by the basic ideas. There were considerations for example of standing, of movement and posture, of stepping and the scratch reflex, which are rhythmic responses that can be elicited by stimulation of the spinal cord. In closing he gives a premonition of his future dedication to the brain-mind problem, which will be the theme of a later chapter of this book.

> Hughlings Jackson in his writings, turns back and forth between muscular co-ordination and mental experience, as if for him they were but aspects of a single theme. It may be that to decipher how nerve manages muscle is to decipher how nerve manages itself. If so, not without significance should be what we have just glimpsed, that there are in the nervous system heights of excitation and depths of inhibition higher and deeper and with grades of adjustment ampler than muscle with all its subtleties can commensurately express.

Meanwhile in 1930 Sherrington arrived in the laboratory one morning with the news that he had been asked the previous evening to write a book on his Oxford work for publication by the Clarendon Press. This request had been made during the meeting of the Press Board of which he was a member. His reply had been that he would agree if he could persuade his associates in the laboratory to join him in the project. So here he was gathering four of us – Creed, Denny-Brown, Liddell and myself, with the invitation. We were happy and excited in various degrees according to our characters! We soon had outlined the division of labour, which was in accord with our research experiences. Sir Charles was to do the final chapter on reflex coordination of the spinal cord after the groundwork had been laid by chapters on spinal reflexes of various types and on central inhibition. Liddell was to be coordinator and editor. It turned out to be an arduous task because his colleagues had many other commitments. I remember my disappointment at the slow progress. Since I had less distraction and an excess of enthusiasm, I was able to write my three chapters before anybody else had started! I was to have the advantage of their criticisms and I learnt from them. I think it was my third rewrite that eventually was published. We never saw in advance Sir Charles' contribution. As he finished one section after another he would deliver each directly to the Clarendon Press for printing! Because of the delays *The Reflex Activity of the Spinal Cord* was not published until 1932, about two years after its conception. Sir Charles' seventh chapter, "Lower reflex coordination"' was the longest (fifty-five pages) and occupied about one-third of the book. It was to be his last purely scientific writing and the book came at a time when it could be regarded as the crowning achievement of the Oxford School.

When Sherrington was writing his great chapter in the book he must have realized that it was in the nature of a farewell to his lifetime of experimental studies of the nervous system. In it he gathered together the fruits of almost fifty years of research and related this to all that was known about the simplest part of the central nervous system, the spinal cord. All his life he had been concerned in the management of muscle by the nervous system, particularly when studied at the simplest level, namely the spinal reflexes. He introduces the chapter by some important general statements:

> By nervous coordination we may agree to understand that cooperation of nervous processes which secures with a normal muscular system the due performance of a muscular act. By due performance is here meant, since we are dealing with animal reflexes, execution of the act in such a manner as appears to an observer correctly to secure its end. Such normality will include normality of time relations, of spatial relations, and of tension development. Thus a movement must appear correct in speed, extent, direction, duration, and work done. Reflex acts of the simple kind considered in this book do not involve coordination of the highest and most delicate grades. For that reason they are likely to reveal explicitly some basal elements fundamental to all coordination.

He is aware that the usual laboratory technique of evoking reflexes by electrical stimulation of nerve can mislead, but throughout he is careful to recognize and evaluate the distortions introduced by a technique that has many advantages, particularly in respect of "nicety of adjustment in strength and time". The first section is a prologue that elaborates on the reflex artificialities that derive from electrical stimulation of bared afferent nerves. Yet in conclusion he wisely states that data of inestimable value have been furnished by this technique.

The second section deals with "Quantitative adjustment of reflex contraction" and covers much the same ground as in the Hughlings Jackson Lecture, but with more wealth of illustration and with his characteristic vivid presentation. The essence of the story is the gradation of reflex excitation in a motor centre. Two factors are concerned in the strength of a reflex: the fraction of the motoneurone pool that is discharging impulses; and the frequency of this discharge of the individual motoneurones. In an illustrative figure (Fig. 4) it can be seen on the base line that, as in the Hughlings Jackson Lecture, the level of excitation is classified in four categories: zeros, subliminals, subtetanics, maximal tetanics. With the latter the frequency of firing gives the maximal tetanic tension of which the motor unit is capable. The two subtetanic frequencies illustrated were based on studies of muscle responses at different frequencies. The picture above shows a motoneurone pool, as in Figure 3, but with the four classes identified. Graphically represented by the dotted lines are the grades of excitation of the neurones of the pool from zero through levels that fail to evoke discharges, the subliminals, to levels of degrees of subtetanic and eventually to maximals. Note that with the maximals the frequencies of discharge go on rising above that required for a maximum tetanic contraction of the muscle.

On the basis of this diagram Sherrington is able to account for the whole range of reflex responses, for example by graded skin pressure evoking flexor reflexes or by graded muscle stretch evoking postural reflexes. All you have to do is to imagine the sloping dotted line of Figure 4 moved to the

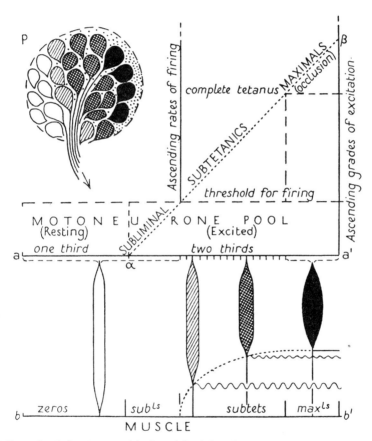

Fig. 4. From the *Reflex Activity of the Spinal Cord.* Creed, Denny-Brown, Eccles, Liddell and Sherrington. Oxford University Press, 1932. Scheme of distribution of excitement in a reflexly active motoneurone pool of a muscle. Grades of excitement plotted against numbers of motoneurones [abscissa a a'] and of motor-units [abscissa b b']. α β denotes excitements in active fraction of pool

right with progressively weaker reflexes and to the left with progressively stronger. In the former case there will be fewer or no maximals, the fraction of the subtetanics will decline and be at slower frequencies and a larger fraction of the pool will be in the subliminals or zero classes. In the latter case there will be the reverse adjustment in the pool fractions. As he states, "... adjustment of amount of contraction ... proceeds by extensity and intensity". As already stated the experimental basis for these two factors had been demonstrated by Adrian and Bronk and by Denny-Brown for the individual units. There would seem to be two defects inherent in the system illustrated in Figure 4, but both are illusory: the subtetanic units have a tremulous response, but the muscle contraction will be smooth because the various subtetanized units will be out of phase with each other; it appears wasteful that maximals can be excited above the level necessary for giving a maximal contraction, but this powerful excitation has functional importance because it ensures an enhanced resistance to inhibition.

The diagram also accounts for the characteristic time courses of reflex responses produced by a steady excitatory input. Some start abruptly at full strength, having what is called a *d'emblée* character. Others start small and progressively increase, having a recruitment character. These characters derive from the time courses of the grades of excitation in the motor centre, but of course there is the further problem of interneuronal inputs to the centre of both excitatory and inhibitory character. So the conclusion is that

> ... the motor centre even at its spinal simplest is more than a mere passive relay forwarding impulses on their way out to their muscle. It is an instrument which always actively summates the excitatory effects of its incoming impulses, and quantitatively adjusts the reflex contraction. Thus is varied the number of motoneurones engaged, and thus a whole scale of grades of excitement are exerted on the individual motoneurone. Under full natural conditions the grading does not end with that. We have then to envisage the further interplay between the graded excitation and graded inhibition coincident concurrently on the centre.

It will be apparent that the conclusions in these last scientific contributions by Sherrington are variations on the same motif or theme. As in music they become more elaborated, but never lose their identity. We can recognize that his imagination had a poetic and thematic expression.

The subsequent sections of his chapter are devoted to a review of a large number of reflex phenomena, that need only be enumerated here. Reciprocal innervation is the expressive name given to the central effects of afferent inputs that often excite the neurones of one motoneurone pool, say the flexors, and reciprocally inhibit the antagonistic motoneurones, the extensors. There is much complication of this simple happening with complex muscle arrangements such as occur with double joint muscles. Other reflex phenomena are the several varieties of rhythmic or alternating reflexes such as stepping, scratching, shaking. As Sherrington recognized, these were beyond present explanation, so he had to be content with a phenomenological treatment. In the concluding sections there are reviews of the states of the spinal cord resulting from ablation at higher levels – decerebrate rigidity and the spinal state. In these very valuable reviews it is as if Sir Charles was having his last word on these phenomena to which he had contributed so much.

Some quotations from the concluding remarks are in order. He asks whether anything like a general principle emerges that is fundamental to coordination and answers in a partial affirmative, as is illustrated in these quotations.

> Under intact natural conditions we have to think of each motoneurone as a convergence-point about which summate not only excitatory processes fed by converging impulses of varied provenance arriving by various routes, but also inhibitory influences of varied provenance and path; and that there at that convergence-place these two opposed influences finally interact. The two convergent systems themselves, one excitatory, one inhibitory, make of the entrance to the final common path, which we may accept the motoneurone as constituting, a collision-field for joint algebraically summed effect. In the higher vertebrate rarely is either member of this paired system, excitatory-inhibitory, wholly quiet when its fellow is active, for their relation to stimuli is reciprocal. The opposition between the effects of the two on the motoneurone is quantitative, and the grade of functional activity or inactivity of the motoneurone reflects this quantitative interaction.
> The foundation of the quantitative grading is based on the individual motor unit. The musculature as a whole being composed additively of motor units, the coordinative taxis takes expression in the musculature as a whole as an additive effect.

The final paragraph continues in this same mode. The thought remains focussed at the level of the spinal cord without even a glance at the higher levels.

> Heights of excitation therefore occur in the nervous centres greater than the skeletal muscle-fibre can commensurately express. If this seems wasteful of central activity we may remember that additional excitation exerted on a motoneurone whose muscle-fibres are already driven maximally for tetanic contraction is not necessarily wasted. That surplus remains still a contribution to coordination because further excitation offers a further resistance to inhibition. Conversely, an added inhibition in the case of an already quiescent neurone although in one sense wasted, is a further protection which coordination may need against excitation. In times of crisis the dilemma lies between strong actions and the very strength of the action taken may serve to safeguard it against interruption.

Yet a year later in the Rede Lecture Sherrington concentrated on the higher levels of the nervous system, venturing into the mind-brain problem that was to be central to his thought for the rest of his life.

F. The Nobel Prize

Despite the great achievements of Sherrington from the 1890s through the 1920s and into the 1930s it was surprising that the Nobel award did not come his way. The story of this long delay is told with surprising frankness by Professor G. Liljestrand in the official publication (1962) of the Nobel Foundation, *Nobel, the Man and His Prizes*. There we are told:

> The exceptional importance of Sherrington's contribution had been generally recognized for a long time. In many of the nominations, submitted by altogether 134 persons, representing thirteen countries, this was stressed with an emphasis that was unusual even in such cases. As early as 1902, E. A. Schäfer declared: 'There is no one who in my judgement has furnished greater and more accurate additions to our knowledge of the nervous system (physiology) than Professor Sherrington', and in 1921 F. G. Donnan wrote to the Committee: 'In the field of physiology and medicine, Professor Sherrington's works remind one of that of Kepler, Copernicus and Newton in the field of mechanics and gravitation'.
>
> That in spite of the high esteem Sherrington enjoyed, he was not awarded the prize until 1932, was due to several circumstances. In the first special investigation on behalf of the Committee, which did not take place until 1910 the examiner (J. E. Johansson) found that some delay was advisable, while in 1912 and 1915 he came to the conclusion that Sherrington's discovery of the reciprocal innervation of antagonistic muscles deserved a prize. To this view the objection was raised in the Committee that this discovery, as Sherrington himself had stressed, had already been made in 1826 by the brothers C. and J. Bell, though it had happened to be forgotten. By the time the first World War broke out, several members of the faculty as already explained, wanted to apply more strictly the stipulation in Nobel's will regarding a definite discovery, and consequently the examiner (Johansson) did not feel he could support Sherrington's candidature. After Johansson had retired in 1927, there was a certain change in opinion, but it took a few years more before the new attitude could assert itself.

It was at this stage that Professor T. Graham Brown was invited to make a nomination for the Nobel award, and naturally he concentrated on his old associate, Sherrington. In November 1931 he wrote to me (J. C. E.) asking for assistance in drafting Sherrington's claims so that there could be inclusion of the discoveries made in the Oxford period. I asked advice from John Fulton, as well as Liddell, and a most helpful letter from Fulton enabled me to send to Graham Brown on 22 December a comprehensive draft of Sherrington's claims with special emphasis on his recent work. This is reflected in the Nobel report which very felicitously summarizes the analytical work of Sherrington on the spinal cord, though it leaves out his definitive studies on the mechanical tension of motor units, which are the unitary components of all muscle contractions.

> In careful studies of the strength, duration and distribution of the muscle reflexes in relation to the same parameters of the stimuli, Sherrington and his co-workers obtained functional characteristics of the relay stations in the spinal cord. The information-processing that takes place in these junctions, represented by the synapse is based on both

addition and subtraction, and Sherrington found expressions for the excitatory and inhibitory processes which participate in these processes. He thus showed how, for the resulting reflex activity, the balance between excitation and inhibition are determining factors. The description of synaptic excitation and inhibition, which Sherrington was able to give, influenced subsequent studies of what happens in the membranes of the nerve cells at the synaptic junctions.

Graham Brown – and no doubt others – had sent in their nominations in January 1932, but in the pressure of work at Oxford this episode was largely forgotten. There had been so many unsuccessful nominations. So our surprise and delight were all the greater when the announcement came over the B.B.C. late in October. Ragnar Granit was living in an apartment opposite our house. He burst in with the news late in the evening. So we immediately telephoned the Sherrington home. Lady Sherrington told us that the Swedish Embassy had telephoned that afternoon, but Sir Charles told nobody and in his accustomed modesty had gone off to a dining club at Merton College, where he kept silent on the award so as not to disturb their pleasant conversational evening. We planned a big surprise. The telephone gathered in all his associates and their wives to his home to await his return. He was overwhelmed by the enthusiasm and rejoicing. Granit as a Swede was the leader of the celebration. I remember the call to drink to Sir Charles and Lady Sherrie (as we affectionately called them) in sherry! Sir Charles delighted Granit by saying, "The Swedes are great poeple". This is my last memory of the wonderful occasions at 9 Chadlington Road. Lady Sherrie already had the affliction she was so sadly to die from the next year. In December she was too ill to travel to Stockholm for the prize award. Sir Charles was therefore accompanied by his daughter-in-law, Margaret Sherrington.

During November Sir Charles had the task of writing his Nobel Lecture "Inhibition as a coordinative factor", and in early December set off for Stockholm. The award was on the appointed day (December 10). Linked with Sherrington in the award for Physiology or Medicine was his dear friend Adrian "for their discoveries regarding the functions of the neuron". The elaborate citation for Sherrington and Adrian was excellently given by Professor Göran Liljestrand, who in 1928 had visited Sherrington at Oxford during the Harvey tercentenary celebrations.

The Nobel Lecture was delivered on December 12, and is a masterly review of the role of inhibition in the central nervous system from the earliest suggestions of Descartes up to our most recent investigations. In characteristic manner there is a superb discussion of the nature of the central excitatory and inhibitory processes, which so well foreshadows the discoveries by intracellular recording two decades later:

It is commonly held that nerve-excitation consits essentially in the local depolarization of a polarized membrane on the surface of the neurone. As to 'central excitation', it is difficult to suppose such depolarization of the cell-surface can be graded any more than can that of the fibre. But its antecedent step (facilitation) might be graded, e.g. subliminal. Local depolarization having occured the difference of potential thus arisen gives a current which disrupts the adjacent polarization membrane, and so the 'excitation' travels. As to inhibition the suggestion is made that it consists in the temporary stabilization of the surface-membrane which excitation would break down. As tested against a standard excitation, the inhibitory stabilization is found to present various degrees of stability. The inhibitory stabilization of the membrane might be pictured as a heightening of the 'resting' polarization, somewhat on the lines of an electrotonus. Unlike the excitation-depolarization it would not travel; and, in fact, the inhibitory state does not travel.

We are indebted to that same lecture for an inspired summing-up of the essence of his life's work on the nervous system:

The role of inhibition in the working of the central nervous system has proved to be more and more extensive and more and more fundamental as experiment has advanced in examining it. Reflex inhibition can no longer be regarded merely as a factor specially developed for dealing with the antagonism of opponent muscles acting at various hinge-joints. Its role as a coordinative factor comprises that, and goes beyond that. In the working of the central nervous machinery inhibition seems as ubiquitous and as frequent as is excitation itself. The whole quantitative grading of the operations of the spinal cord and brain appears to rest upon mutual interaction between the two central processes 'excitation' and 'inhibition', the one no less important than the other. For example, no operation can be more important as a basis of coordination for a motor act than adjustment of the quantity of contraction, e.g. of the number of motor units employed and the intensity of their individual tetanic activity. This now appears as the outcome of nice co-adjustment of excitation and inhibition upon each of all the individual units which co-operate in the act.

G. Farewell to Oxford

After the Nobel Award in 1932, Sir Charles was to suffer two grievous blows from which he never fully recovered. For us all it was a period of overwhelming sadness. Lady Sherrie died in 1933 after many months of illness. Then Sir Charles himself was stricken by very severe rheumatoid arthritis. For more than a year it caused him severe pain in the most afflicted joint, the acromio-clavicular, and the movements of his left arm were permanently impeded. He spent many months being treated at Droitwich Spa. I once visited him there. His indomitable spirit triumphed over his adversity, and to meet him was still a joyful experience. On returning he found the laboratory carrying on after his long absence and decided to retire because he felt he was no longer needed. But we pleaded with him to stay, and he agreed for a while because he felt his presence would help the status of the laboratory and its support by grants. A photograph (Fig. 5) was taken

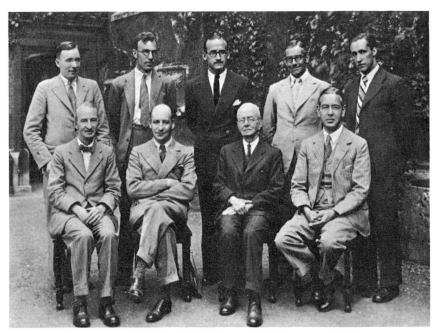

Fig. 5. J. H. Wolfenden, J. C. Eccles, J. B. Odoriz, J. P. V. D. Balsdon, S. Obrador, C. Wilkinson, H. M. Carleton, C. S. Sherrington, E. G. T. Liddell. Photograph taken outside the Hall of Exeter College after a lunch given by two research students in the Physiology Department: J. B. Odoriz and S.Obrador. Exeter College, Oxford, 1934

at this time (1934) and shows his good recovery. Finally in early 1935 he announced his impending retirement. Number 9 Chadlington Road was sold and most of his valuable collections of books were dispersed. At that time he gave to the British Museum over two hundred incunabula that they did not have. He was to retire to Ipswich, his original home town and Miss Ethel Davis, Lady Sherrie's niece, was to be his housekeeper in this new (and old) environment. We did so hope that he would have continued to live in Oxford, but Miss Davis had decided on her home town, Ipswich.

It is important to realize that in the whole Oxford period there was no secretarial assistance in the laboratory. Sir Charles did all of his enormous correspondence by hand, and had to do his filing of all records and letters. I went up to his study on his last day to see if I could help him in the immense task of clearing up the office. There was little I could do to help as he sorted and discarded, but he was full of memories of the past.

I listened enthralled when he talked about his earlier years. In retrospect he felt that he had concentrated too much on anatomical studies, particularly in his long investigations on motor and sensory roots and their detailed peripheral destinations. He was referring to his massive anatomical publications of over 300 pages in 1892 and 1894. But he went on to say it was necessary in order to give an assured anatomical basis for all of his later physiological studies on reflexes. He spoke with regret about the time he had wasted in demolishing Pfluger's laws on spinal reflexes, but again it was necessary to clear all this rubbish away before he could advance in his chosen field of spinal reflexes. He spoke with extraordinary modesty about his whole scientific accomplishment, saying that at best he could claim to be a forerunner. He hoped he had laid a good foundation, and he prophesied that the future investigators would have undreamed of success because of the great advances in technology that had already begun with the amplifier and cathode ray oscilloscope. It was a very moving experience at the close of his great scientific career to witness this humility and this generosity with no taint of jealousy for those of us who were to spend our lives building upon what he had built so well. So the Oxford laboratory of the Sherrington era came to an end in June 1935. Research continued, but we sadly missed the leadership and the friendship of the great spirit that had departed. Contacts were continued with letters and with visits of Sir Charles to Oxford, and of ourselves to Ipswich. But the sense of loss was ever-present.

As mementos of the past I had in my study at the laboratory numerous drawings on the wall. When Sir Charles came to discuss some of the results he would take out his pencil and move over to the white plaster wall to make an explanatory diagram. So in the course of some years the walls of my room were covered with Sherrington's drawings and he had to search to find a spare place for another drawing! I used to frame each one with a line and date it. Sad to relate there was no photograph of this treasury of drawings, and when I returned in 1952 to give the Waynflete Lectures all trace had disappeared under a re-painting.

Regretfully for many years no attempt was made to conserve the equipment from the Sherrington days. The Ashmolean Science museum was not interested. Astrolabes were their chosen field, not the experimental equipment of a great Oxford scientist. Some twenty years later Dr. Sybil Creed collected what she could find and that is still conserved in the Physiological Laboratory. In 1976 Professor Whitteridge rehabilitated some equipment for display at the Centenary meeting of the Physiological Society in Cambridge. The most notable was a falling table used in the stretch reflex investigations by Liddell and Sherrington in the early 1920s. It was truly the end of an era.

(J.C.E.)

Chapter 6

Major Correspondents in His Later Years (Oxford and Thereafter)

No picture of Sherrington would be complete without a sampling of his more concentrated correspondence with a group of long-time friends. In this chapter we shall follow his ideas, hopes and fears as he writes to Harvey Cushing, Osler's two bibliographers William Francis and Archibald Malloch, Sir Geoffrey Jefferson, A. V. Hill, Edgar Adrian, John Fulton, Howard Florey and John Eccles.

Harvey Cushing corresponded with Sherrington from 1901 to 1939. While the letters were often on purely personal matters they give a picture of Sherrington which it is important to view. For example in 1927, before setting out for the centenary celebrations of the University of Toronto Sherrington wrote to Cushing that he hoped not be be "a plague to you" by visiting Boston and giving a Dunham lecture as well. On his return to Oxford he sent his love to Cushing's daughter Barbara "whose exemplary return to school first thing on Monday morning threw my late rising into relief".

As Sherrington was crossing from Britain to Boston, his Oxford pupil and Australian Rhodes Scholar, Hugh Cairns, was crossing the Atlantic in the other direction. Cairns wrote to C.S.S. of his Boston training:

> I had a remarkable year's experience with Dr. Cushing. I realized what it was to be in the very 'front line' of surgery. The memories of it are not unlike the best memories of the front line in France, and I am wholly won over to brain surgery. I feel almost that I want nothing more than to be allowed to do this for the rest of my life in the way that Dr. Cushing taught me to do. I shall never forget that this joyous existence was opened up for me by you to whom I owe my job with Dr. Cushing.

One of us (W.C.G.) was associated with Cairns ten years later when he became Nuffield Professor of Surgery at Oxford, and brought the distinguished Spanish neuropathologist Pío del Río-Hortega to work in his laboratories as a guest of the Nuffield Foundation. Late at night I would hear the stories of Cairns' first weeks with Dr. Cushing in Boston. His ship was late, and he arrived outside Cushing's operating theatre rather apologetically and announced himself to Adolf, the *major domo* of the operating suite. A voice boomed out from the operating room, "Cairns, you're two days late. Get in here". It was six weeks before Cairns managed to get off the service long enough to pick up his trunk at the dockside. He told me that he had once contemplated buying a pistol either to shoot Cushing or to shoot himself, so arduous were his early weeks in Boston.

Throughout the Sherrington-Cushing correspondence runs the wonderful bond established by the Oslers. In 1928 Lady Sherrie wrote: "I fear Lady Osler is anything but well. She seemed so tired, and now has been in bed some time, as no doubt you know, but Dr. Gibson's report is much better this evening, and she seems brighter again". Cushing was right in thinking that Sir William Osler's collection of 7600 books, ranging over the entire history of medicine, would not leave Oxford for McGill University in Montreal as long as his widow lived. From 1919 when Osler died to 1928 when Lady Osler followed him, Dr. William Francis, Dr. Archibald Malloch and Reginald Hill of the Bodleian perfected the catalogue raisonnée which Osler had begun so many years before. Sherrington was a frequent visitor to the team working at 13 Norham Gardens. On 13 January 1929 however, Lady Sherrington wrote to the Cushings, "For some time to come I shall avoid going near Norham Gardens as much as possible, that dear half-way home to me . . . Oxford life can never be quite the same to C. and me".

After the books had left for McGill and the handsomely produced *Bibliotheca Osleriana* was published by the Oxford Press, Sherrington received a copy as a gift from the cataloguers. He wrote to W. W. Francis, by then installed with the books in the Osler Library at McGill:

> Let me make a small enquiry about the Osler Library . . . it does not seem to contain copies of the following:
> i.   Alb. Haller: Sur la formation du coeur dans le poulet, etc. Premier memoire. Lausanne. MDCCLVII.
> ii. Second memoire.
> iii. Marshall Hall: On the Circulation of the Blood. (with plates) London, 1831. 8 vo.
> iv. Observations on Blood-Letting. London, 1836. 8 vo.
> v.   Marshall Hall: Synopsis of the Spinal System. London, 1850. 40.
> If you would wish to have these for the library, I have copies and would be very pleased to send them.

On 15 June 1933 Sherrington wrote to Cushing about Lady Sherrington's death from cancer:

> Her gallantry and her patience never faltered to the last – even for a moment. She looked back with deep satisfaction to the happy glimpse she had had of you when she was convalescing from her first operation. She had been ill for longer than her brave spirit was

willing to acknowledge, even to friends. Her second operation was a short-circuit for a recurrence of the growth in the lower duodenum . . . her emaciation became extreme; her spirit always bright and indomitable! Everyone round us was thoughtful, helpful, and understanding to the uttermost; and her thoughts were of, and for, her friends right through.

Sherrington's letters to Cushing are full of the lore of ancient books, their publishers and illustrators. He speaks of being able to buy rare items at a ". . . market stall with quite usually incunabula exposed on it – often in the rain! I have a Laurentius Valla Elegantiarum, 1476, from it still. Venice"[1]. In another letter Sherrington told Cushing: "Henry Viets told me you are interested in Etienne Dolet. I copied out the items of his which are in the British Museum and think you may like to have the list". Then follows a detailed account of *thirty-three items* from the years 1535–1557. Though Cushing was suffering some circulatory ills he kept energizing people. Sherrington told him: "You just pump fresh air and zest into everyone. You galvanize one as Galvani – or was it Signora – did the frogs' legs". He reminded Cushing of their Liverpool exploits, thirty-seven years before:

It is good news to hear that you have been dealing with the motor cortex – no one can know so much about it as yourself – and found some of the old material useful. I remember very well the drawing you made – wonderfully good, and done before the impressions of the actual experiment had got 'cold'. How you did brighten us all up – and improve us. You will be grieved to hear that dear George Cox died last Monday. He was one in a thousand. Cancer of the bladder with secondary growths . . . He was very brave, and talked of you as one of his heroes.

Your letter speaks of Lyons and the barber surgeons . . . I fear I know little of the story. But you prompt me to enclose some quaintly picturesque transcripts (translated) from 2 old volumes I have . . . One of these transcripts – from dear old Laurent Joubert to his mother – I found quite touching. A great writer L. Joubert – with a Rabelaisian touch – friend of Rabelais as he was.

In the Spring of 1938 Cushing was inciting Sherrington to publish another volume of poetry, to which Sherrington replied:

What I have is very slender! . . . You tell me a lot of intriguing things. Diane de Poitier's book! You know Jean Fernel saved her life: she was thought to be 'gone' but he pulled her through. Catherine de Medici, poor woman, wouldn't allow Diane into the room when Henri lay dying, after his tournament wound from Montgomery. Fernel had died the year before, or he would have been there . . . My edition of Joubert is 1598 . . . a witty old boy.

With war threatening even in November 1938, Sherrington sent greetings to Cushing – a mixture of memories, political news and – as usual – medical history:

No, it is not *hebitude*, not inherent vice, nor temporary aberration which has been the cause of my blameworthy delay in writing, but sheer pressure of footling little jobs claim-

---

1 Now in the Woodward Biomedical Library, The University of British Columbia, inscribed on a sunny day at Ipswich in June 1938 to Wesbrook's memory.

ant to be done . . . the Hunterian Museum and 'all that' have been under threat of air attacks. It does seem scandalous. The Bibliotheque Nationale all sand-bagged, and the Louvre and National Gallery strewn with sand and halfstripped. We hear it is doubtful whether the Sudetens wished to become Germans at all! . . . I picked up the other day an 18th century Barber-Surgeon's licence granted under the Regents of the Fac. of Medicine in Paris. You may like to read how it runs.

On another occasion Sherrington said to Cushing:

Boxing Day yesterday, why does it always remind me of Pickwick and Sam Weller? Snow all round us – what we call 'deep' – i.e. 6 inches on the level. My thoughts have over and over been with you, but 'that or this' has often seized me by the coat-sleeve and stopped my getting the note-paper out and writing. A shameful way of life I admit. In my short experience (December 1938) if one wants to know what it is to be busy 'retire from your business'.

On 29 March 1939, Sherrington wrote: "Dear Harvey, A bird of good omen has whispered to me that if our desirable planet keeps on turning it will bring us all the heartfelt delight of an anniversary of your birthday in the 2nd week next month".

To which Cushing replied:

Dear Sherry, I have passed my 70th mile-stone without accident and though Hitler and Mussolini have set back the clock the 'planet kept turning', and on the 8th inst. came your welcome cable of greetings and also the photostats of Henry 5th privilege for the surgeons of Paris – a fascinating document . . . Thanks for your lovely letter and the pleasant things said therein. Always affectionately, Harvey Cushing

Cushing died on 7 October 1939.

The Sherrington-Osler connection was maintained by Osler's nephew, Dr. William Francis at McGill. Sherrington kept up a steady stream of gifts to the Osler Library and Francis sent Sherrington his thanks and usually a piece of doggerel as well. In one of these exchanges Sherrington wrote: "It delights me to think that you interested your neighbours in Montreal of the French Faculty with the *De Homine* of their 17th century compatriot. A great person he was. There is that magnificent portrait of him in the Louvre by Franz Hals".

Sherrington had good reason to remember Descartes' *De Homine* in the Osler collection. He had loaned it to Sir William in 1914. Two years later Sherrington needed it and went to Norham Gardens to retrieve it, but found that Osler had written in it, "Given to me, August 16, 1914 by C. S. Sherrington". Sherrington immediately wrote in it "E libris Gulielmi Osler 1914" and replaced it on the shelf!

To Francis he confided: "I often *read* – yes *read* – your *Bibliotheca Osleriana* – a charming mine of information. I always come on something fresh." On another occasion he told Francis:

I get so much pleasure from the *Bibliotheca Osleriana* of an evening . . . I fancy it is not unlikely I may have to turn out from my house here (Ipswich) – the soldiers may want it and also may want to be disembarrassed of people my age. The air-fights are frequent about this place and our planes and 'personnel' are always the superior – but the enemy have the numbers.

Two unusual gifts by Sherrington to the Osler Library were the medical tracts by Jean-Paul Marat, who was assasinated in Paris in 1793 in his boot-shaped bath by Charlotte Corday. Sherrington was wrapped up in the story and would lean forward in his little rotating summer-house in the garden at Ipswich and describe the stealing of the collection of gold coins from the Old Ashmolean Museum at Oxford by Marat, the self-professed doctor-lawyer, pamphleteer and, alas, thief.

The peregrinations of Marat in England, one jump ahead of the law are still being studied by scholars, so many aliases did he use. Sherrington's interest was in the defence used by Marat in his trial at Oxford. He held that theft was a capital offence when the aggrieved party was an individual, but that stealing from a public institution was not theft at all! Instead of hanging or 'transportation' to Australia, Marat's penalty was five years' hard labour on the hulks at Woolwich, dredging sand, gravel and mud from the bed of the Thames. He was the paranoid writer of *The Chains of Slavery* which, to his disgust, not many Britishers took seriously. He arrived back in Paris in time to incite people to revolutionary extremes with his newspaper *Ami du Peuple* and his book *Plan de Législation criminelle*. Sherrington would have smiled had he known that Marat is memorialized today in the name of a Russian battleship.

Dr. Archibald Malloch, the other Canadian who worked on the *Bibliotheca Osleriana* team, was a frequent correspondent of Sherrington. Malloch's father had taken in Osler as *locum tenens* in Hamilton, Ontario in 1874 while he waited for a McGill appointment. On New Year's Day 1932 Sherrington wrote a remarkable letter to Malloch, who by then was librarian to the New York Academy of Medicine:

Best thanks for the delightful letter. I wish we were able to expand it by some conversation; alas! that is not *yet* practicable . . . Yes, very interesting what you say about "incident" in scientific discovery. You remember when someone said to Pasteur that Lister's tracing of wound suppuration to "germs" owed itself to L's coming across P's papers. P remarked: L. would not have profitted unless he had prepared himself for such a view – been nearly there already. Poincaré makes the remark that a solution to a problem that had held him for several weeks suddenly occurred to him as he was *getting out of a taxi-cab* in Paris. Walter Fletcher says his best ideas have come to him in the bath! Newton's phrase was that his solutions came to him by "constantly thinking unto it". Galsworthy says he writes by going alone into his study after breakfast and thinking what his characters have been doing since he left them the day before. One point only seems common to all these modes; i.e. absorbing *interest*, so that the mind voluntarily or involuntarily cannot let the theme alone – cannot relinquish it – gets a background which is creative when the suitable event arrives in the foreground. But I must not bore you thus.

Later in the year Sherrington told Malloch: "If here our two Royal Colleges along with the Royal Society of Medicine could put their libraries and library resources [together] London would have a really good – i.e. first-rate – Medical Library. But they are not yet *near* doing so. I admire your success at the [New York] Academy".

An interesting aside was Sherrington's remark: "You raise the question whether 'TB' connotes any enhancement of the mind. I take it that you dismiss that – and so should I – Keats held that no sick man should write poetry; therefore to write poetry he must be at his best, and forebore to do so when he knew he had 'TB' and so the sonnet, 'Bright star would I' etc. was his farewell to verse".

Not far from the Osler's era was the friendship of Sherrington and Sir Geoffrey Jefferson, Britain's leading neurosurgeon in the 1920s. Lady Jefferson, Gertrude Flumerfelt, came from the far side of the world, Victoria, British Columbia, to study medicine at Oxford. Her father, a financier, was the first Treasurer of the University of British Columbia. To Sherrington and to Osler she was always 'Trotula', the name of a woman surgeon from the ancient School of Salerno.

In June 1939 Sherrington told Jefferson: "I enjoyed your fine notice of Harvey Cushing. What you tell me of his treatment of an application to him . . . years ago for a testimonial tickles me and my vanity. I expect I wrote to him when the chair at Oxford was vacant – but in fact the University kindly invited me thither, so no testimonials were sent in".

In 1949 Sherrington told Jefferson:

I knew Ramón y Cajal personally – he was once a house-guest with me in London – a guest bristling with oddities – but a *great* man. His foremost pupil Hortega you may remember died 2 years ago in Buenos Aires, and his collected works of the 'silver method' are about to appear, translated into English by Dr. Wm. Gibson of Sydney (Path. Dept.), a past-master of the technique. Your typescript should reverse its present order of mention. Cajal was senior – as well as more eminent than I. Most of the silver technique was Cajal's own invention – it interpreted the nervous system. But I shall bore you – excuse it and believe me, sincerely yours.

From the nursing home in Eastbourne Sherrington addressed "Jeff":

And now may I ask you the question whether you would yourself see your way to undertake a broadcast on *The diseases described by our writers of fiction*. I am asked by the BBC to suggest names whom they could invite with confidence in 'knowledgeability' and a combination of medical along with literary learning . . . and will you please transmit to Mistress 'Trotula' my thanks for her help.

In the world of research was Sherrington's faithful friend, the gifted scientific catalyst, A. V. Hill, F. R. S., Foulerton Professor of the Royal Society, and one of the truly great minds behind Britain's defence in two wars. In

1926 Sherrington told him concerning his research: "Delighted you have actually trapped and measured the elusive 'nerve action' heat. Byron, you remember, spoke of it as 'a fiery particle' – perhaps you won't agree with his next line which said it could be 'snuffed out by an adverse article' – in a Quarterly Review!"

In 1929 Sherrington wrote to Hill, who with his assistant had personally delivered to Oxford a new type of stimulator – based on the neon tube:

> That you, with all your other interests and occupations of mind and time should remember my 'stimulation' difficulties – well kindness surely is not the adequate word! And then that you should prepare and demonstrate it to me 'in the flesh' and say 'here you are'! It is simply more than aboundingly good of you . . . All yesterday we were working with your 'stimulator' – it answers beautifully . . . We had *power* for a whole room full of cats . . . The potential divider with its delicate wire shall have our respect.

During a very active period in 1931 Sherrington told Hill: "Eccles is busy with an arduous question of his own just for now – and it is hard to switch off the tune. As for him and me in conjunction, when we can, we have to try to finish some not very refreshing trials of interaction between inhibition and excitation – they should not take long now."

One year later Sherrington sent Hill this note: "I enclose a brief paper for the Journal of Physiology. I hope you will find its statement in better form than that one you so blue-pencilled two years ago – or was it a year ago? I have lived and I hope learnt since then!"

With the announcement of the award of the Nobel Prize in Medicine and Physiology to Adrian and Sherrington in 1932, the correspondence which Sherrington was called upon to answer was mountainous. He wrote to A. V. Hill:

> That one's best friends are pleased is surely the gayest of all accompaniments to a slice of good fortune! And there must accrue to yourself that particular "bonhomie" in this instance of a genial conspirator whose plot has thickened to a solid issue. Take once more my heartfelt thanks for your much too generous kindness and pains. It is an added delight to me to be associated with Adrian – I feel it a true distinction to be so treated – also to be linked (at an interval) on to yourself. Really our Editorial Board is becoming choked with Nobellites!

A. V. Hill had received the prize in 1926. As already pointed out (p. 70), it was to be many years before the secretary to the Nobel Committee made known the fact that Sherrington had been nominated by 134 scientists before the award was made. The physiologist on the Nobel Committee had been unalterably opposed, because of Sherrington's outspoken views on 'Prussians' according to his son Carr. Again a note to Hill on his recent paper: "I have been enjoying your 'Chemical Wave Transmission in Nerve', some of it is beyond me in the sense that I follow you humbly, and am delighted in that process, but can go only where your hounds lead, not otherwise knowing the country. I have not enjoyed any reading so much for a long time – challenging ideas that make me 'buck up'!"

By 1934 the eight years of carrying the editorship of the *Journal of Physiology* were beginning to weigh heavily on Sherrington, who wrote: "I am not doing my fair share". However, in response to his colleagues on the Board, especially Sir Henry Dale, he agreed to serve for one final year. He sent a note to Hill from a Bournemouth 'hydro':

> If ever man were blessed with generous friends and colleagues he is now writing to you . . . Thank you very much for the offprint of the 'lecture' – admirable and unanswerable – a most convincing and appealing setting out of the ethics and logic of internationalism in science and scholarship . . . This thin snow with strong sun here suits me – it makes a sadly sophisticated sea-side place quite bracing. Nothing can sophisticate the *sea* itself.

To Henry Dale he explained: "I received marching orders to come on here from Droitwich [spa] and get some sea-air". Contributing greatly to his recovery from a year's rheumatism which immobilized each arm in turn, was a visit from his Boston pupil Alex Forbes: "Forbes blew in very delightfully for a night last week – then left for Italy. You had enthused him immensely – he said the Journal would contain the three most outstanding papers for this decade in its next number. We sat up talking till 'next morning' and he had a great go with Eccles."

From White House, Graham Road, Ipswich, he again wrote to Hill:

> I wonder whether you feel I make a mountain of a mole-hill. I feel so sure that 'Abstracting' is a problem of great importance for science generally and that we live in a transition stage of it at the present time. With 36,000 current periodicals of science, and the publication of over a million original papers annually, and a *rate* of increase which grows greater year by year, scientific work and reading are being more and more snowed under by scientific papers and records. Hence the 'abstracting' journals. But these latter have not yet settled down to understanding their true job.

In arranging for the International Physiological Congress proposed for Oxford in 1941, A. V. Hill wrote to Sherrington on 13, November 1938:

> I don't think you know – your humility prevents you – how great are the affection and regard which your colleagues have for you. But I know you will not charge me with being given to overstatement, so I hope you will listen to what I say – and said yesterday. It is *true* that you could do the greatest possible service to physiology and to British physiology and Oxford at the same time, by allowing us to name you as president of the Congress in 1941 . . . I know what a difference it would make to Oxford . . . and how much difference it would make to the 'Congressists' old and young alike.

One is reminded of the effect of Sherrington on the First International Congress of Neurology at Berne in 1931 when Leon Asher presented him as the "philosopher of the nervous system". The two thousand Congress members rose as a body and cheered him to the echo. Some could not believe he was still alive, so much had he done for so many years.

On 19 November 1938 Sherrington replied:

> I have been chewing the cud of your kind suggestion and now write to say about it, 'yes'. That is, if you and others wish we to serve as President at Oxford for the Congress, I would accept and would do my best to fill the bill. I cannot give you real hard work, but you tell me you know me too well to expect it of me . . . If I do not live up to it, let the reason be the excusable one that I shall not be living at all.

A. V. Hill then wrote happily: "I had almost sent one of the 'Greetings' telegrams to Mellanby in a golden envelope. Nothing could be better"[1].

As the second World War began, Sherrington looked forward to visits from Hill who had 'radar' duties in the Ipswich area from time to time, with other physicists whom Sherrington welcomed as long as the military authorities allowed him to retain his lovely new house 'Broomside', overlooking a tranquil and beautiful valley. The trans-Atlantic ships were still active, one bringing his friend Alan Gregg of the Rockefeller Foundation. The mail from Forbes at Harvard and John Fulton at Yale was a great tonic. When Hill decided to seek one of the university seats in the House of Commons Sherrington wrote at once: "So far as *one* vote carries, you have mine". Hill had transported him to Caius College, Cambridge, from London where he had been temporarily lodged with relatives. He had been found on the roof of the Royal College of Surgeons cheering on the Spitfires in the Battle of Britain and Hill wisely took him to Cambridge for safety. By 20 June 1941 Sherrington was writing: "That Germany now attacks the U.S.S.R. seems proof of the mess in which she finds herself".

On receiving from Hill a congratulatory letter on his ninetieth birthday Sherrington wrote:

> Dear A. V., . . . You undo the high opinions I have been holding of you; you *can't* be the really busied man I have supposed. However, there I know you *are*, and therefore I must set it down to goodness of heart! . . . As to myself, when King Lear cried, 'Ripeness is all' – he was speaking in character . . . There is a ripeness which one sees on the ground *under* the trees. I begin to understand *that* ripeness – it's good for the ground and nothing else!

At the age of almost ninety-one Sherrington wrote to Mrs. A. V., the onetime Lady Mayoress of Cambridge and a member of the distinguished Keynes family:

> I am impelled to write by remembering so vividly a splendid supper which you gave . . . at your house a number of years ago. A feature was 'Chinese eggs' – which I was myself a trifle afraid of, but on the example being set by our host himself, I greatly daring greatly enjoyed . . . a frivolous mortal like this present correspondent of yours, has it still freshly before him . . . I thought it might amuse you to be reminded because the tiresome features seem to fade and the amusing seem to stick longer.

---

1 The Congress had to be postponed because of the war, but took place in Oxford in 1947, when every member received a special re-issue of *The Integrative Action of the Nervous System*. For the entirely new introduction by Sherrington, see Appendix 11.

Edgar Adrian was of a younger generation than Sherrington, and, until his death in 1977 was still active at Trinity College, Cambridge in which he made his home. In 1924 he wrote to Sherrington asking if he might come over to Oxford ". . . to watch you preparing a reflex experiment. I have ventured into mammalian work without having learnt the technique and I am always regretting that I have never been over to Oxford to see the right way of going to work".

After his long-planned visit he wrote back to Sherrington, thanking him for a recent reprint: "I wish I could tell you adequately how splendid it is to see the way in which your work has been going ahead – and how much more accessible the neurone has become in your laboratory".

On the announcement of the Nobel Prize in October 1932, Adrian wrote:

> This letter is intended to reach you just as you are starting for Uppsala so as to preclude any reply. I won't repeat what you must be almost tired of hearing – how much we prize your work and yourself – but I must let you know what acute pleasure it gives me to be associated with you like this. I would not have dreamt of it, and in cold blood I would not have wished it, for your honour should be undivided, but as it is I cannot help rejoicing at my good fortune.

Sherrington was having considerable pain in his joints on his return from the ceremonies in Stockholm and Adrian wrote: ". . . your sciatica must be making you feel the limitations of neurology". To Sherrington, languishing in the mineral baths regime at Droitwich, Adrian sent a note after receiving a Royal Medal in 1934: "Your telegram was the culminating pleasure of the day . . . For a neurologist to have your approval is really worth all the medals that were ever awarded. We miss you on the Medical Research Council"[1].

Much to Sherrington's delight, Adrian was made professor of physiology at Cambridge in 1937. To a letter which C.S.S. sent Adrian replied: "If I had anything like your power of carrying on research, running classes and laboratories and yet finding time to encourage and be kind to all of us, I should have no misgivings about taking the chair here . . . When you publish your Gifford Lectures I am going to ask you for a copy. They will be the first Gifford Lectures that I shall really read all through".

On receiving an honorary degree from Oxford, Adrian told Sherrington: "I am glad that my achievements are likely to be extolled in Latin, for in that language the most commonplace record can be made to sound mysterious and dignified".

---

1 Sherrington had resigned in 1934 after serving since 1925.

The final exchange took place on 29 November 1951, two days after Sherrington's ninety-fourth birthday. He told Adrian:

> Yes, to my own surprise, I am in a sense ripe for re-reading that fine old tale of Victor Hugo's 'Quatre-vingt treize!', where, in V.H. manner he describes the cannon getting loose in the rolling brig and threatening to beat a hole through the ship's hull, and the passenger (the 'hero') climbs down with a noose rope and single-handed lassoes the mad thing . . . It is now some little time since I actually was in Cambridge but one of my most lasting and vivid pictures of it is a double one – the outside and the inside of the Trinity College Library – a Wren masterpiece.

With that he enclosed a poem (see Chap. 7) and the correspondence came to a quiet close.

Two of Sherrington's pupils were young Rhodes Scholars who arrived at Oxford in 1921. They were members of Magdalen College, John Farquhar Fulton and Howard Walter Florey. Their lives were to be closely interwoven with Sherrington's from that year on. Fulton came from Harvard Medical School and Florey from the University of Adelaide in South Australia.

From 1922 to 1952 Fulton exchanged approximately 200 letters with Sherrington and his household. His Rhodes scholarship having finished, he returned to Boston to complete his neurosurgical apprenticeship with Harvey Cushing. On leaving Oxford in 1925, Fulton and his outgoing and charming wife Lucia, a Bostonian, expressed their sadness to the Sherringtons, to which Sherrington replied:

> If your bidding goodbye to Oxford brings you regrets, so does it to your Oxford friends nonetheless. We shall all miss you and Lucia badly and the laboratory without you will. I don't like to think of it . . . Your generous gift of the old original 'ballot sheet'[1] of the Royal Society will be very much appreciated and when the Society's Council meets you will receive a formal acknowledgment.

Fulton had already become a collector of rare and significant medical books, and soon after returning to Boston he sent a first edition of Descartes' *De Homine* to Sir Charles, who wrote:

> This first and difficult to get, Edition is . . . my favorite one. It has the 'flap' plate of the heart which so pleased Osler, and has also the little sketches – by Descartes' own hand . . . The post-humous appearance of the *De Homine* is itself significant of Descartes's personality. I myself fancy he considered himself as truly following the Church of Rome which he consistently professed; I fancy that it was conscientious aversion to publishing what he felt might be distasteful to that Church which led him to withold the MS, and that it was not any pusillanimous fear of punishment which actuated him as motive for witholding the book. The portrait of him by Franz Hals, which you may recall in the Louvre, looks a little cynical but bears no trace of cowardice. A fine painting it is.

A long correspondence ensued concerning Fulton's book on muscle, then in preparation. Sherrington summed up his view on the inclusion of nerve:

---

1 Fulton found this unused 1662 ballot folded between the leaves of a second-hand book on a stall in London, on his way to a Royal Society lecture.

After all, muscle is the main exponent of the whole nervous system. Hence it is but logical not to omit one from the exposition of the other; but on the contrary by setting forth the characters of each to make the characters of the other emerge more clearly and interestingly. Doing this you correct a tendency obstructing present neurology and fill a gap which wants filling.

Fulton soon returned to Oxford to a Magdalen College fellowship in natural science and remained in the University Laboratory of Physiology until the summer of 1929, when he was appointed Sterling Professor of Physiology at Yale University in New Haven, Connecticut, at age thirty. He wrote from the *Mauretania*: "I could not bring myself to come and see you yesterday. I hope you will understand. These two years have slipped away, I scarcely know how, and we leave with broken hearts". However, a Sherrington group was being assembled at Yale including Dusser de Barenne, Kirby, formerly George Cox's assistant animal keeper at Oxford, ("a model of industry"), ten monkeys and prospects of three chimpanzees and five African catatryx monkeys. To add to the mixture Alex Forbes flew his floatplane into New Haven for lunch at the new laboratory. Fulton felt so homesick for Oxford that he told Sherrington: "I broke down the other day and subscribed to the *Times*".

In a protracted discussion on muscle Sherrington gently reminded Fulton of the early work at Liverpool in 1898 on "isolation alteration" with muscle changes "amounting to dystrophy". The question of primates for localization of brain function brought Sherrington to the very practical matter of support for such a colony: "I shall have opportunity to speak to Gregg (of the Rockefeller Foundation) about your observation and will urge the necessity for gorillas". Scarcely a letter went to Fulton without some esoteric information, as on 17 October 1932: "We can remember that it was on the heath near Tunbridge Wells that [John] Evelyn was robbed of his silver shoe buckles and left tied up by the highway pads".

Following his wife's death, Sherrington sent her delicate necklace to Lucia Fulton saying: "Will you . . . forgive my offering you by this letter, instead of personally, the accompanying little memento of dear Ethel – a tiny keepsake which, you may remember, she sometimes wore, and would, I know, like to think carried its token of recollection to yourself"[1].

From the Worcestershire Brine Baths Hotel at Droitwich, Sherrington wrote to Fulton: "I think the modern world is going back – I mean disimproving in some ways while going forward in others. Aesthetically, letters

---

1 For the opening of the Sherrington Room at the University of British Columbia by Sir John Eccles in 1970, the necklace which passed from Lucia Fulton to Catherine Ann Gibson was added to the display of Sherringtonia.

show much blunting of 'values'. I think departure from 'truth' by exaggeration seems a great weakness of literature today; a blunting of appreciation and sensitivity".

By September of 1934 Sherrington was asking Fulton to remind him of the opening date (27 September) of "Penfield's new laboratory, for I should like to send him a little cable-message on the day and occasion". Little did Sherrington know that his name would grace the 'neurological hall of fame' at the entrance to the Montreal Neurological Institute – along with Cushing, Horsley, Hughlings Jackson, Ramón y Cajal and Camillo Golgi.

The opening day was graced by the silver-haired Cushing – speaking most engagingly, but probably anxious to slip down the hill of the McGill University campus to see the beautifully housed Osler Library. The Institute which Penfield was opening in Montreal was what Cushing had, unsuccessfully, tried to build at the end of the first World War in the United States – to treat and to study soldiers returning with severe injuries to the nervous system.

At about this time Sherrington sent to Harvey Cushing, through John Fulton, two issues of the first edition of Florence Nightingale's *Notes on Nursing,* and old books continued to dominate the Sherrington-Fulton correspondence into 1935. Sherrington told Fulton of coming on some works published in 1516 in Venice on the 'morbo gallico' – syphilis. He said: "I was interested to see that Aquilanus there was always writing it as *lues venerias.* This is the *earliest* use of that phrase I have met with. No mention in any of them of the notion that the *morbus* came to Europe with Columbus' sailors".

By 1935 Sherrington's new house at Ipswich was ready and he wrote to the Fultons: "I shall look forward to welcoming you in one which is at the top of this hill, with a view to the south, east and west – and a little pinewood scenting the whole place". Ethel Davis reported many Oxford visitors to the new house in its first year – Eccles, Carleton, Franklin, Gibson and Hoff, ". . . all delighted to see Sir Charles looking so well and cheery; it is wonderful what our East Coast air and climate has done for him."

For several years to come the chief subject of letters was Jean Fernel, Sherrington's hero – the first 'physiologist' some would say, and first 'pathologist'. Before long Fulton had put his book collector's talents to work and had found works by Fernel in the most unlikely places. Of neurological interest was Fernel's mention in 1542 of the small central canal of the spinal cord which Sherrington believed both Vesalius and Estienne missed when they did their work slightly later. Sherrington's knowledge of

the early printers was encyclopaedic. He said, for example, of the Estien-
nes: "They had, you remember, ill fortune; Charles dying in prison; Robert
fleeing from religious persecution to Geneva – as later did Andreas Wechel,
I think to Francfort".

Following a flying visit by Fulton to Ipswich, Sherrington wrote:

> Thank you for mentioning again that the old *Integrative Action* still floats. I know how
> generously you regard it, and am very grateful. But looked at rigidly I cannot but recog-
> nize that it has 'had its day'. Its best future is for what lives of it to be incorporated –
> unobtrusively – into what is written with similar scope now and after, for a time.

The Estienne printing odyssey kept recurring, and on 25 August 1936
Sherrington wrote:

> As to Robt. Estienne, Kenyon, who is versed in the history of the Bible, told me recently
> that Estienne's edition of the Greek text of the New Testament [Paris, 1546] was so
> excellent that it was *the* text for the next three centuries, and was what our so-called
> Authorized Version in English (1611) was translated from – the translation which held on
> both sides of the Atlantic up to the Revised Version of the Anglo-American Commission
> in 1880 – the occasion when the Oxford Press sold and despatched one million copies on
> one day, it is said.
> You ask about Geofroy Tory? He was a professor of philosophy, a poet and a critic, *as well
> as* being an artist, craftsman and reformer. The booksellers' catalogues have a habit of
> speaking of Fernel as 'the teacher of Vesalius'. I feel sure this is a 'guess'.

From Yale Fulton was telling Sherrington: "Under your stimulus I acquired
several [Fernels] this summer on the continent and returned to find a
number of others that I had rather forgotten about". Fulton was also receiving in his laboratory students from laboratories around the world which
Sherrington's early pupils had developed. Thus Leon Extors came to Yale
from Bremer's laboratory, Gibson from Penfield's, and so on. Alfred
Frohlich (after whom the adiposogenital syndrome was named) and a
Liverpool pupil of Sherrington's, passed through New Haven to see Cushing in 1939 en route to Cincinnati where he was able to find refuge in the
Ben May Laboratory of the Jewish Hospital. In fact, the Sterling Labora-
tory of Physiology at Yale became a working partner with the Laboratory of
Physiology at Oxford in many ways.

When a newly discovered work of Fernel appeared in a dealer's catalogue, Sherrington was quick to bring it to Fulton's notice:

> There is . . . a fine copy of the 1st edition of Fernel's *Medicina* at Davis and Orioli's now –
> in beautiful early binding. The vol. is not common. There is one copy in the Surgeon
> General's and in the Bibliothèque Nationale. Not in the British Museum or Vatican. The
> B.M. will be having my copy, which you may remember is in contemporary binding.

Fernel was being incorporated into the Gifford Lectures which Sherrington
was preparing at Ipswich late in 1936, so that Fulton frequently received
notes on what Fernel had to say on an amazing range of subjects: "Fernel is,

by the way, the first to record – perhaps to see – 'ulcerative endocarditis'. He speaks of three cases. This is surely the earliest record of it – 1554 – in the *Pathologia*".

Not only news of Fernel went both ways across the Atlantic. Books were warmly given and received. Thus, on 6 February 1937, Sherrington wrote:

> Please accept from me the accompanying little copy of the *De Abditis Rerum Causis*, because I know from your list which you sent me, you have not yet a copy of this edition. I' must apologize for the worm holes – but the worms are *not* active I know. I have had the copy a long time – picked it up in Paris. I have, however, another copy of this edition. I came across it in London this week – it is bound up with the 1st Frankfort edition of the *De Luis Venereae Perfectissima Cura Liber*, . . . *so that frees my old copy of De Abd. Rer.,* and I should wish the latter to be with you.

The Gifford Lectures are 'played down' so often in Sherrington's correspondence that one suspects he was remarkably shy about mentioning them at all. This was not so in personal conversation (as both of us can testify) but in written communication he was very diffident, as Fulton was to learn in 1937:

> I have been in the north wandering . . . My early summer was rather cut into here by lecturing at Edinburgh. No, my lectures there are not published, but I have next year to give some more, and the idea will be for them to be published all together. I fear they are *not* interesting . . . my Edinburgh jaunt had rather interrupted my correspondence, and now I will get down to it again.

In the Royal College of Physicians Library in Edinburgh he found incunabula "of great interest and rarity". In Glasgow he found what he thought must have been an illuminated copy of his writings given by Fernel to his princely friend and patron, the Dauphin of France.

Following the conclusion of the Gifford Lectures he told Fulton: "I got back after a short course of lectures at Edinburgh, at early part of June – a milieu of philosophy and divinity which I found very pleasant".

Soon, however, the correspondents were back to Fernel, Sherrington telling Fulton:

> Vesalius left Paris for Louvain in 1538. The frequent statement that Fernel was his teacher I can not find substantiation for – but probably Fernel was *one* of his teachers, and Fernel's own interest in and advocacy of dissection of the body with his pre-Vesalian teaching of it, shows that Vesalius' work was just part of – and not the source of – a 'modern movement' at that time . . . What you point out about the 'appendicitis' case appearing first in the 1567 edition of the *Pathologia* is most interesting.

Sherrington was asked to serve on the editorial board of the gestating *Journal of Neurophysiology,* and he promised that Fulton would have his ". . . co-operation as a 'sleeping' partner . . . I wish you and the new *Journal* all success . . . I hear Río-Hortega is in Oxford with an appointment there and means of getting on with his researches".

It was not long before Sherrington's pupil, Professor Hugh Cairns – the 'spark-plug' of the Nuffield scheme to produce a full medical school at Oxford – asked one of us (W.C.G.) to drive Don Pío del Río-Hortega over to see Sherrington at 'Broomside' on the Valley Road into Ipswich. The day was bright and Sir Charles was tanned and active. He had met Cajal only once, but to meet one of the 'younger generation' of Spanish neurohistologists was also an extreme pleasure. While they conversed in French, Sherrington kept interjecting little Spanish phrases, which brought smiles and approbations from Río-Hortega. The two men – separated by twenty years – were of much the same build – slight but sprightly. Coloured moving pictures were taken in the garden, showing them strolling arm in arm. Sherrington's phrases in Spanish carried him back more than fifty years and he laughed at himself as he tried to resurrect a little of his once-familiar vocabulary. Río-Hortega could hardly believe that Rámon y Cajal's friend and host of 1894 was not only alive but full of humour and high spirits. All the way back to Oxford he commented on Sir Charles' hospitable reception and especially upon the quality of the China tea offered him! All the cares of his own country and his own sad losses of two institutes and many students in the Spanish Civil War were forgotten in the glow of such a visit with Sherrington. Next day at Oxford he proudly told the visitors to his laboratory that he had just had tea with Britain's greatest scientist. Sherrington was greatly pleased when Harvey Cushing and Río-Hortega received honorary degrees at Oxford in June 1938.

Sherrington's summer of 1939 was interrupted – as he says – "I have been torn away from Fernel and all that" because "I had some Edinburgh lectures to finish (for the press) – involving natural theology!" In fact, he and Ipswich were agog over the excavation of a grass-covered tumulus, which instead of containing a Viking boat as expected, produced a tomb of Anglo-Saxon royalty . . . "of the early 6th century – with a boat 82 feet long and treasure – gold and silver – fibulae, a gold buckle weighing 4 oz., an embossed shield, coins and also 'loot' from the Mediterranean!"

Nevertheless Sherrington added to Fulton on 26 July 1939, "I fear the Copenhagen congress will be poorly attended. Hitler's madness acts very disadvantageously for it. If he attacks Poland there will be war *at once* and he is such a liar, no one can believe a word he says". With Harvey Cushing's death at age seventy Sherrington felt keenly the loss of a pupil, a bibliophilic friend and a world leader in neurology and endocrinology. Sherrington wrote:

> What a likeness between him and Osler! as well as profound differences, these latter almost complemented in the two natures, giving together an extreme richness. I sent a few

lines to the British Medical Journal on Tuesday . . . We have spent only 3 'nights' in the trench at the top of the garden . . . I have 2 lads from Ilford near London, as billets. They are an amusement and an 'interest'. They spot the different types of airplanes which fly over with a skill which leaves me astonished. We have 20,000 children billetted in the town here – their school teachers have come with them and they have their gas masks slung across their backs as have we all.

Sherrington told Fulton that the medical school of St. Thomas's Hospital had sent its pre-clinical classes to Oxford. The Royal Society moved its offices to Trinity College, Cambridge, where the city was "full of khaki and sandbags". With his knowledge of German Sherrington often listened to the radio broadcasts from Nazi-occupied Europe: "This week it has been boasting, Germany killed 100,000 Poles within one month! True it is that thousands of Poles must be dying of starvation in the snow now".

As 1940 began Sherrington was back with his hero Jean Fernel, reading prodigiously on the geographical background and the times in which he lived. "He seems to have been the one to launch not only the word 'physiology' in its modern use but also 'pathology'." He wrote to Fulton: "You spoke in your letter of the book Denny Brown has so devotedly 'produced' from my scattered things. It really *overwhelmed* me to receive it, and there he thanks *you* for the bibliography which re-overwhelms me when I turn to it. I blush when I see these items which I supposed would have escaped even Fracastoro's bibliographer".

"To Lucia Fulton Sir Charles sent in February 1940 a domestic account of the knitting that Ethel Davis and her Ipswich friends were doing. They had received a letter from a mine-sweeper thanking them for their product. The garden at 'Broomside' was filled with Brussels sprouts and potatoes. If the German invasion did not materialize Sherrington said that his household would eat the crop and plant more! Occasionally he was able to get away to hear a lecture – as when he listened to Adrian speaking at the Royal College of Surgeons on "Pain": "He was admirable, but, as he stressed, pain (physical pain) remains a biological enigma – so *much* of it *useless, a* mere curse!" Sherrington complained ". . . the times are sadly delaying – you will smile – my booklet of verse [which] has run to a second edition!"

Eventually the galley-proofs of the Gifford Lectures were at hand, and John Fulton was asked to store one set of them in safety at New Haven. Sherrington noted that there would be some illustrations – ". . . an innovation for the 'Giffords'". He added, "Alas – as for my lectures[1] on Fernel – there seems now little chance of their appearing, although they are finished".

---

1 Thomas Vicary Lectures, Royal College of Surgeons, London.

On Osler's birthday, 1940, Sherrington told Fulton how he and his household had spent five nights in the past week in his garden trench. With the collapse of France the military forces required 'Broomside', and Sherrington was forced to move to his ageing brother's home in London, and into his crowded shelter by night. Of the fall of France he wrote sadly:

> To the regret and astonishment of us all we have lost our great ally. Many of our French friends are as distressed and surprised about it as are we – e.g. Rudler of Oxford, my old colleague writes me his bitter amazement at the armistice, following the giving way of certain of the French armies . . . I cannot believe it is the real France which has defected.

His friend John Beattie had returned from 'Dunkerque' with a leg wound acquired when his ambulance was attacked from the air. He was returning to work at his laboratory at the Royal College of Surgeons in Lincoln's Inn Fields, and Sherrington said, "I hope to join him there". It was from this daytime observation post that A. V. Hill wisely removed Sherrington, taking him to Cambridge. Through all of this war activity he was delighted that the reading room of the British Museum had remained open to the public! As 1941 began Sherrington wrote from Cambridge to Fulton about the Yale work on 'the bends' in aviators and in resurfacing divers – ". . . dear old [John Scott] Haldane used to wax eloquent to me on that theme". It was during Sherrington's professorship at Oxford that J. S. Haldane and his son, J. B. S. Haldane, carried on their hair-raising researches on anoxia, simulating high altitudes with gas mixtures piped into a cabinet about the size of a telephone booth.

The Physiological Society meetings in Cambridge provided an opportunity for Sherrington to see his pupil Howard Florey, whose film he was able to view on the ". . . control of capillaries – a striking demonstration – not by any special cells, but by the ordinary nucleated endothelium. William Harvey would have been intrigued".

Yale was to know something of the war through the children who came from England for the duration. The Florey children's coming to the Fultons freed the parents in Oxford to work, with a large and devoted team at the Sir William Dunn School of Pathology, on penicillin – of which more presently. John Fulton met large numbers of displaced children – some with their mothers, who came to New Haven, as other British children did to parts of the United States and to Canada.

Once more on Jean Fernel, Sherrington wrote to Fulton that only 30% of the normal paper supply for books could be made available because of the war. This occured at a time when the measurable demand for reading material reached an all-time high. At the same time Sherrington worried about the printing of the Philip Maurice Deneke Lecture which he had given at Lady Margaret Hall, Oxford, on "Goethe on Nature and on Science".

The German bombing of the British Museum caused much anguish on Sherrington's part for he was a Trustee who took his work seriously and lived for that institution. He estimated that 150,000 volumes had been destroyed. He was nearing the end of his writing on Jean Fernel and anticipated that he would feel the loss of his constant friend after so many years of scholarly association. Fernel too would have enjoyed that association. Not only was Fernel about to desert him, but his long-time friend and rival book-collector, Arnold Klebs, died at Nyon in Switzerland. With this, another of the Osler circle was gone.

With the end of the war Sherrington felt that he might utter a small complaint without giving comfort to the enemy – he wrote of the increasing stiffness in his 'neck-joints'. A year later, in a reminiscent mood, he told Fulton of his long association with Kronecker, the outstanding continental physiologist, and of Bowditch's mutual respect for him:

> On some excursion in the hills from Berne (after the Leipzig days) both B & K being of the party, a large pool was met with – from melted snow at the top of a 'col'. K. deliberately halted the party and christened the 'pond' Lago di Bowditch in honour of N.P.B.! Years later when K. was a guest at B's summer camp . . . Bowditch, map in hand, told the company that such and such a hill-crest – pointing to it, was still unnamed, and went on, with all ceremony, to celebrate its christening as 'Peak Kronecker'.

In 1947 Sir Charles celebrated his ninetieth birthday at Eastbourne, having retired to a nursing home where he could get constant care for his rheumatism. He told Fulton: "When in the course of yesterday forenoon I opened the *British Medical Journal* I got a shock of surprise . . . With the best will in the world I cannot persuade my own conscience that to reach the 9th decade is an act that has merit!"

His son, Carr, daughter-in-law Margaret and their daughter Unity, gathered for the celebration with a special cake, since Unity's twentieth birthday fell on the following day. Margaret's assessment, written to Lucia Fulton was: ". . . found the dear man surrounded by letters, parcels, telegrams, etc., looking amazingly fit and young, saying he would get them all answered personally in time".

Howard Florey was another correspondent who kept Sherrington's teachings uppermost in his mind throughout his life. He never forgot that Sherrington had been first a pathologist, and then a physiologist. When Florey received a note from 'Sherrie' in July 1923 he could hardly believe its content: "Let me congratulate you on the excellent work you have done . . . I shall be very pleased for you to come on in October as a Demonstrator for the mammalian class".

Florey always spoke of his 'good luck' in life – as when, fifteen years later, he began his penicillin work with the most active strain of the mould. Certainly the appointment to Sherrington's staff, albeit in the most junior post – demonstrator – was good fortune. From 'ship's surgeon' to 'demonstrator in physiology' may not have seemed a quantum leap into medical research, but it signalled the beginning of an odyssey unusual in physiology and in pathology.

As his demonstrating year came to a close, Florey began to worry about his future and Sherrington proceeded to chat with him about good pathology being really abnormal physiology. One can imagine these rather tentative discussions in the spartan quarters which Sherrington occupied in the University Laboratory of Physiology. Each man was waiting to find out what the other thought. Florey could be vociferous but in the presence of Sir Charles he stood in awe. Finally Sherrington told him that the John Lucas Walker 'studentship' – in fact a fellowship which had nourished some of the greatest pathologists in their younger years – was open at Caius College, Sherrington's Cambridge home. Florey gave in and said that he would like to apply. Sherrington clapped him on the shoulder, telling him his name had already been submitted and remarked that clearly he had always been an abnormal physiologist at heart! Years later Florey was to retell the story with bursts of laughter, wiping the tears from his eyes, mimicking the two players in the drama – little knowing that at Ipswich Sir Charles was also re-enacting the interview – with that quiet smile breaking over his face, and a chuckle as he finished the account – as always, rotating on the arm of his chair and shaking all over.

After his pupil had gone to Cambridge Sherrington wrote to him to know if he could help to bring his experimental results on brain capillaries before the Physiological Society, or his publishable manuscript to the attention of the editors of the highly respected journal *Brain*. It became clear to Florey, as to other students who were associated with Sherrington, that no matter what one studied, or where one set up his research laboratory in later life, that bird-like quiet catalyst was anxious to help, to open doors, to provide references to great scholars and to assist with appeals to funding bodies. His loyalty to his students was legendary – always benign, and tinged with a diffidence which was proverbial.

In February 1925 Sherrington wrote to Florey not only offering to 'introduce' his paper at the Physiological Society, but explaining to the young scientist:

> The Society would form a means of securing a somewhat earlier date for such facts as can be shortly stated and where there is similar enquiry going on by a number of other workers

which might prejudice future views as to the originality of your own personal findings . . . Inflammation: No doubt you are conversant with the Madrid neuroglia results – but look at the pictures again. They must have high significance – for capillary changes and inflammation. The sucker foot that attaches itself to capillary wall – the view taken of them when Cajal first showed them was that they were means of transport of nutrient from blood to perikaryon's perilymph spaces.

Eventually the professor of pathology at Cambridge recommended that Florey spend a year at Philadelphia with A. N. Richards on capillary pathophysiology, and wrote to Sherrington asking him to find for him 'another Florey'. Soon Sherrington was helping Florey to condense the historical introduction to a paper on the 'contractility' of the lymphatic vessels. Not only was he assisting – he was drafting the introduction – and in parentheses adding: ". . . or something of this kind. C.S.S." Sherrington warned him in a later letter: "There have been such a series of congratulatory events in regard to you recently that my pen is running out". Invitations to the anniversary dinner of the Royal Society were sometimes mixed in with remarks on an unusual finding in the venous system of a cat. As to a muscular reaction never before noted by Florey, Sherrington wrote: "The phenomenon you so interestingly describe is . . . the 'idiomuscular contraction' of Maurice Schiff (1851) then of Berne, later of Florence. It has gone out of fashion for modern physiological textbooks . . . The best account is still, to my mind, an old one by Schiff, in his little handbook *Physiologie*, published at Lahr, 1858, . . . 17–25".

Florey must have taken to heart Sherrington's reliance on the microscopic anatomists of Madrid, for we find Sherrington writing for him a note of introduction: "Enclosed a note to Cajal – delighted to furnish it. I think it a capital idea, your visiting his Institute . . . Se habla Español? Bueno-Mañana por la mañana". However, as Florey told us years later, it was the perpetual cry of 'Mañana' that drove him out of the Instituto Cajal! He could get no satisfaction, no animals (rats or mice) to work on, at the times promised. So he gathered up his books and walked out. Halfway across the Retiro Park he was overtaken by a messenger sent to bring him back. He was met at the Institute door by a distraught Director, waving in his hand a little phial of methylene blue, said to be from Paul Ehrlich's laboratory, as a peace-offering. If only Florey would return, all the animals he required would be provided!

On his return home Florey found a letter from Sherrington asking if Exercise XXI, pages 126–128, of the *Mammalian Physiology* laboratory text should be dropped from a new edition being prepared. Florey must have smiled as he read the words: "Do you think it too pathological?" He did not, and made certain revisions to the exercise, "Amoeboid Movement,

Phagocytosis, Intravenous Injection of Bacteria". Florey was thoughtful enough to refer to Sherrington's work in this field which appeared in *Journal of Pathology and Bacteriology*, 1:258–288, 1894. He might have cited also, Ramón y Cajal's early paper on the subject in *El Diario Catolico*, Zaragossa, 1885.

By return mail Sherrington then asked Florey for further advice on the practical exercises in physiology concerning the modification of the heart beat, and thus of the cerebral circulation through carotid sinus stimulation – as shown so classically by his pupil Bremer. Then, on learning of a visit by Florey to the continent, Sherrington gave him three written introductions, and "a spare card which might be handy". He commended to Florey the "ability and energy" of René Leriche, the French neurosurgeon.

Following the death of Professor Georges Dreyer in 1934, the electors to the chair in the Sir William Dunn School of Pathology were named and the usual round of consultations began. Florey was strongly supported by Professor Dean of Cambridge and by Sherrington, who wrote: "If there is anything you think I can do in any way just let me hear – and don't hesitate to suggest". Three weeks later Sherrington reported to Florey that Lincoln College, to which the chair was attached, had named Sir Edward Mellanby of the Medical Research Council to act on its behalf on the Electoral Board. Sherrington gave up his place on the Board to Sir Farquhar Buzzard, the Regius Professor of Medicine at Oxford. It has been said that the chair was about to be awarded to someone other than Florey when Mellanby burst into the meeting of Electors. His train from London had been so late that he almost missed the most important meeting in Florey's career.

Mellanby was a very distinguished scientist and a man with great administrative experience. When he had finished speaking Florey was invited to fill the chair, much to Sherrington's satisfaction.

As Florey settled into the Sir William Dunn School of Pathology more than a gentle breeze began to blow. Some reported it as a hurricane – but Florey had learned a great deal from Sherrington – that sound argument quietly put was better than baseless bluster. Sherrington warned: "It is good to hear from you, and to know you and your wife have found a house convenient for getting to and from the laboratory . . . I hope it is *not so* convenient that you will get daily no sufficient exercise and out-of-door 'refresher' in passing to and fro".

On Christmas Day 1937 Sherrington complained: "I am pretty well myself – rather *more* deaf I fear. Sight if it fails, you get sympathy for, but *hearing*, 'Oh, he gets *so* stupid!'"

What Sir Charles was to hear in 1937–1938 of Florey's lecturing to the first clinical class – eight of us – was to delight him. He would chuckle when Florey's salty phrases were reproduced: "Here you'll get pathology as process – the abnormal physiology of the human body. In London you'll get all the undertakers' pathology you'll ever want". As students we were taught by excellent lecturers in this trial six months in Oxford, spent at the Sir William Dunn School in South Parks Road, at the Radcliffe Infirmary and at the Osler Pavillion for tuberculosis cases up the hill near Headington. Florey and Chain were the first to impress upon us the anti-bacterial effects of lysozyme, isolated by Fleming, and of penicillium moulds – known since Pasteur's time but not yet successfully harnessed.

By January of 1941 Sherrington was expressing the hope: "May you have the children home again [from Yale] when next Christmas is on us, is my earnest wish". This was not to be realized before the end of a long war. Sir Charles was greatly interested in the penicillin story, both as a biologist and former pathologist and bacteriologist. He had heard of the month-long struggle in Oxford to save the life of a policeman dying of massive streptococcal and staphylococcal infection. The first dramatic improvement in his condition could not be maintained because the pitifully small supply of penicillin was too soon exhausted. The cynics, however, had a 'field day', learnedly predicting the end of "this test-tube nonsense".

However, Florey and his team finally accumulated enough penicillin to treat five children, whose individual requirements were smaller. Their upward course excited everyone who witnessed the trials, but Florey chose to describe the results conservatively in August 1941 in the *Lancet*. Sherrington asked if he might put up his distinguished pupil for membership of the Athenaeum, to be seconded by Rudolph Peters, and proceeded to muster the long list of signatures required.

With the help of the Rockefeller Foundation, Florey and his 'right hand', Norman Heatley, went to the United States to seek help in mass-producing the new substance of such promise. Help was quickly forthcoming when Florey encountered his old teacher of Philadelphia days, Dr. A. N. Richards, wartime chairman of the medical research branch of the powerful Office of Scientific Research and Development. On his return to Oxford Florey reported to Sir Charles in his characteristically low-key fashion in a hand-written letter, reproduced here with the kind permission of Lady Florey.

Sherrington wrote briefly to Florey congratulating him on his election to the Council of the Royal Society – the first step on his rise eventually to the Presidency. "I think you will find it an opportunity to get a view of the organization – a very loose organization – of scientific research in this

Telephone: Oxford 2273.
Telegrams: Pathology—Oxford.

SIR WILLIAM DUNN SCHOOL OF PATHOLOGY
UNIVERSITY OF OXFORD

Aug 2nd 1942

Dear Sir Charles,

Thank you very much indeed for sending me a copy of your lecture. It is most kind of you to have remembered me in this way. I was most disappointed that I did not see you when you were in Oxford but was delighted to hear that you were in the best of spirits.

We are all pretty busy here — we've had 48 weeks of teaching this year, finding through the medical students. A certain amount of research is going on but it is a matter of filling in large numbers of forms three days to keep anyone on the job.

The penicillin work is moving along & we now have a fairly substantial plant for making it here. It is most tantalising really, as there is, for me, no doubt that we really have a most potent weapon against all common sepsis.

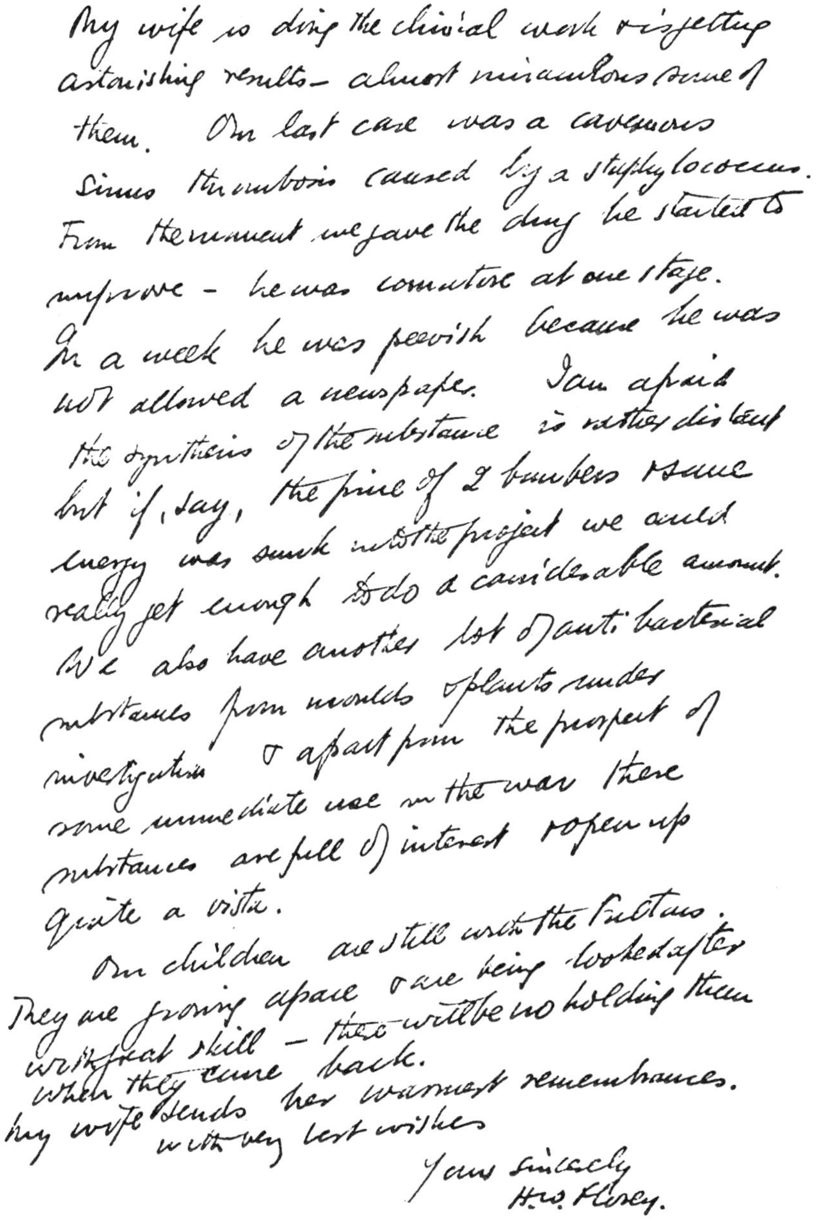

My wife is doing the clinical work & injecting astonishing results — almost miraculous some of them. Our last case was a cavernous sinus thrombosis caused by a staphylococcus. From the moment we gave the drug he started to improve — he was comatose at one stage. In a week he was peevish because he was not allowed a newspaper. I am afraid the synthesis of the substance is rather distant but if, say, the price of 2 bombers & same energy was sunk into the project we could really get enough to do a considerable amount. We also have another lot of anti-bacterial substances from moulds & plants under investigation & apart from the prospect of some immediate use in the war these substances are full of interest & open up quite a vista.

Our children are still with the Fultons. They are growing apace & are being looked after with great skill — there will be no holding them when they come back. My wife sends her warmest remembrances.

with very best wishes

Yours sincerely
H.W. Florey.

Fig. 6. Howard Florey's letter to C.S.S. on Penicillin, 1941

country which is a great help for judging it. All success to you! The responsibility is not a light one in these stirring times".

When Florey gave the Lister Lecture on penicillin, Sherrington assured him: "Lister would have been delighted. It is long since a surgical discovery of such an order has been made. The last 'Lister Oration' I heard was given by Harvey Cushing . . . Much has happened since that short time ago – a great quickening in interest, and you have helped to bring that about". When Florey wanted to visit Sir Charles at Eastbourne there was a war-time accommodation problem: "I have been able through the kind intervention of the Revd. Mother here to get you a room at the Victoria Cross Hotel . . . nearly all the hotels are closed – many of them are too damaged to be open".

An Honorary Fellowship at Lincoln College, Oxford, for Florey produced another note from the Esperance Nursing Home at Eastbourne: "My dear Howard, If you go on like this I shall have to treat myself to a special secretary to write congratulatory letters to you". As he entered upon his ninetieth year Sherrington wrote again to the Floreys:

> Howard can truly look back and think that Oxford has a role in world medicine today which she would never have had but for his own work and outlook there. And Ethel's share in that has been a noble one. What an incentive for young Charles – and lest it seem at first a bit overpowering, he has the poets to remind him that to 'envisage circumstances all calm, that is the height and top of sovereignty'.

For the ninetieth birthday of Sir Charles the Floreys sent a special message as did a host of friends. C.S.S. replied: "The kind message from you and your wife is a great contribution to my small domestic fete . . . Your own laboratory, I hear, is full of young researches, I wonder what Rhodes' among them. I used to like meeting Allen of Rhodes House; he seemed of much ability and character". Soon he was to be writing again:

> Yes, I *like* the mild weather, though I am told it is unseasonable. A friend the other day wished me a 'good old-fashioned white' Christmas. No, I said, please retain it for yourself. I am glad you are composing an authoritative book on antibiotics – there is great need for it. I can suppose there is a temptation to go on and on adding to it as new literature appears. But it might be better to put your foot down at a certain date, and there cut it short – leaving all since that date to a new edition . . . Insist on making your own opinion felt about it . . .

The old fire was there as surely as it was when Sherrington was discussing editors and publishers with Florey twenty-five years previously!

A year later Sherrington was congratulating Florey on having hired a retired brigadier to handle routine administration at Oxford. Many are the stories of the post-war rivalry by department heads at Oxford, each seeking to engage a retired officer outranking that of his neighbour. Sherrington was back on the theme of the three-volume handbook on antibiotics, repeating the warning: "I hope you have chosen a business-like publisher . . . I am sorry to hear of your difficulty about 'demonstrators' – if the price of bacon has gone up so of course should that of science teaching".

One degree ceremony which Sherrington regretted missing was that at the University of Lyons in France in 1946. As Edgar Adrian wrote to him:

> I promised to tell you how sorry they were not to have you at Lyons on Tuesday. You will, no doubt, receive the highly decorative hat to add to your collection. I am sorry to say that Florey got an even more decorative one than ours, for his is an M.D. and that has a lot more gold braid than a D.Sc. . . Florey lectured in the evening – a first rate lecture which kept one's attention all the time. You were quite right in saying what a pleasant companion he would be on the journey. We spent an idle day in Paris together last Sunday and went to a concert after looking at the book stalls along the river.

Adrian continued after a digression on country houses seen en route with Florey:

> I finished Jean Fernel in the train coming back from Lyons . . . You have certainly made Fernel live in the round and altogether. I can't help feeling what a disappointment it must have been for him to lose faith in astrology after all his mathematics and astrolabes. He must have been a comfort in a sickroom. Your book makes me want to learn much more about those times. I have always found it so hard to imagine dinnertable conversation in Latin – mainly, I suppose, because it seems now to be so much more suitable for Public Orators.

Sherrington would be reminded by Adrian's closing remark of the amusement which Ramón y Cajal felt at the ponderous Latin orations which he heard when he received his honorary degree at Cambridge. He would also be reminded, by the reference to Florey receiving a Lyons M.D. degree, of the Nobel prize-winner's consternation when he found that a Lyons medical student, Duchesne, had published in his graduation thesis in 1893 an amazing description of the value of penicillium moulds in treating infections. Florey's eye for rare medical books was second only to that of his class-mate Fulton, and one can see Sherrington pressing Florey on his return from Lyons for a report on the Paris book stalls which C.S.S. had prowled so long ago.

Needless to day, Sherrington's death in 1952 in his ninety-fifth year brought sadness to Florey as to all pupils of Sir Charles. To the last Florey was a faithful correspondent and visitor to Eastbourne. These visits sent one away refreshed and amazed, such was the range of Sir Charles's interests. One of us (W.C.G.) visited Sherrington in September 1951, on the return journey from Copenhagen to Vancouver following upon the International Congress of Poliomyelitis. I described the hope that some held that a study of the various strains of the virus would sooner or later lead to a vaccine. Sir Charles cocked his head as he sat by the blazing fire: "How many doctors did you say were there?" I replied, "Six hundred, Sir Charles". He smiled and asked, "Did any good ever come of *six hundred* doctors getting together?" Then he questioned me about 'Frank Wesbrook's University' – was Dr. R. E. McKechnie the surgeon, still Chancellor? "No," I said, "He was for twenty-six years, but no longer". The fact was that McKechnie had been dead for years, but Sir Charles called off the names of his friends in British Columbia as if his visit in 1897 with Lord Lister were yesterday. He wanted to know about Río-Hortega's pupils and the Instituto Cajal – a remarkable conversation for a man of such years. His deafness was marked and his limbs rheumatic, but his eyes still sparkled.

Coming up to Oxford four years after Fulton and Florey, John Carew Eccles, a Rhodes Scholar from Melbourne, Australia, began a firm friendship with Sir Charles and a ten-year apprenticeship which ended only when C.S.S. left the Waynflete Chair. From 1937 when J. C. E. went to Sydney, Australia, as Director of the Kanematsu Institute, there was close contact by correspondence and in February 1952 there were two personal visits to Eastbourne.

Sherrington's letters to the future Nobel laureate were a great mixture of personal news and discussion of new scientific discoveries. He was always supportive and helpful to a scientist trying to establish medical research in untilled ground – not to say stony ground sometimes. While Eccles was still at Oxford he could expect that for every manuscript submitted to Sir Charles there would be one, and possibly several letters in reply – from Droitwich if ill, or from Ipswich in retirement. The detail in these notes was very full. He would begin his criticism by such a phrase as: "Am I not right in thinking that . . .". In 1934, from Ipswich C.S.S. wrote:

> For your theme it would be helpful if there were some word which expressed the process (a) of exciting as distinct from (b) the state of excitement which (a) produces. There does not seem any unequivocal word to hand. I expect I am not clear. What I mean is: suppose a stone flung at a board producing a sound from latter. Then the horizontal momentum of the stone, decreasing as it goes, serves as (a) *exciting process*, which starts in the board on arrival there (b) the *excitement* whence the specific effect under observation, i.e., the sound. It is difficult to find words distinguishing (a) from (b) to the reader . . . I hope you have had a fine holiday.

In November 1936, C.S.S. wrote to J.C.E. at Oxford concerning a manuscript: "It makes a most interesting story". He added: "I suppose you are justified in accepting" certain anatomical assumptions – gently raising a key question. He continued: "Not the least interesting part of your article is the critical summary of the position of neuromuscular transmission especially in striped muscle – it gave me real pleasure to read it . . . the whole article is admirable, clearly written."

Then with the voice of experience C.S.S. added: "If a spinal root ganglion would serve, remember the 2nd cervical in the cat lies outside the vertebral canal altogether and could be reached easily."

In a later letter the same year C.S.S. reminded Eccles of what Ramón y Cajal said of the spinal cord. "Cajal used to speak of it as the 'mare magnum'". Then after several questions as to the spinal cord, to which Eccles had returned, Sherrington asked: "By the way, do you regard the Berger Rhythm[1] as intrinsic in origin, i.e., automatic?"

When in March 1937 Eccles decided to take up the new post in Sydney Australia, which had been under discussion for some time, C.S.S. wrote: "I am pleased in some ways and especially because *you* are pleased, but I cannot help feeling sorry for Oxford . . . I expect you are right in wishing it – but we shall *miss* you – and many will do so besides 'us' . . . However, you will form your 'school' and group and the Southern Cross will shine on you, and we shall have the greater exchange of young people and new ideas travelling back and forth".

No sooner had Eccles been installed on the top floor of the Kanematsu Institute overlooking Sydney Harbour than Sherrington wrote him a long and wonderful letter, saying in part: "With the clean air and sun the operating will go well, and strong light a great help". C.S.S. probably had in mind the contrasting Oxford weather and his own diminutive 'animal operating room' set into the roof of the Physiology building. Sherrington's quarters had a wooden ring of electric light bulbs over the operating table which seared the ears of pupils as tall as Penfield, Eccles or Cairns.

Sherrington reported to Eccles that Río-Hortega, Wilder Penfield's Madrid teacher – discoverer of the 'microglia' in the brain – had now set up a laboratory at the Radcliffe Infirmary ". . . working at the microscopy of brain tumors – the material coming from Hugh Cairns". Further in this long letter C.S.S. said:

> Dear old Rutherford's death was very sad – I mean such a loss! I went to the service in the Abbey. Baldwin and Eden were among those there.
> Old books are still an attraction for me – I mean 15th and 16th centuries. As for reading I have been re-reading Descartes. He is wonderfully clear – a pleasure even when one does *not* agree with him. Kant is 'woolly' compared with him. Also my Greek has come back to me a little and I am slowly enjoying – yes, *enjoying*, Aristotle's 'De Anima'. Well, you have had enough of me.

On New Year's Eve of 1938 C.S.S. told Eccles, among other items, that: "I have started reading Lawrence of Arabia's letters – an amazing person. . . .

---

1 Hans Berger had just reported on what today we would call the electroencephalogramm. Caton in Liverpool, Forbes in Boston and Beck in Poland were forerunners.

Fulton has managed to get some 'Tarsius' over to New Haven [from Bohol]. It has just turned up among the very few Eocene mammals, so that our family stock is 'ancient'".

Two further letters to Eccles, by then in New Zealand, may be quoted briefly – one of 18 November 1945: "Does your colleague Popper take any interest in that borderland between psychosis and physiology which I used to be attracted to? Hardly, I expect. Binocular fusion (both of spatial and colour) is surely a fine field, and I think quite out of fashion now".

On 10 December 1946, nearing the age of ninety C.S.S. discussed the latest discoveries by his friends:

I have been reading Hevesy's results with isotope labelling of complex molecules. It gives me a new picture of the constant shuffling of the atoms in molecules which I had supposed 'stable' for the time being – so that a sugar will take up, and then shed and then take up again a labelled atom while waiting in the liver; a particular type of molecule can evidently be renewed in various ways. Hexose monophosphate present in red blood corpuscles is largely renewed in a few minutes. The labile P of adenosine triphosphate is renewed very quickly and the second P atom rather more slowly. Hevesy was a pupil of Rutherford and began the work under him.

The foregoing selection of letters written by Sherrington, it is hoped, will give some idea of his wide variety of interests, his interest in his pupils around the world, and his transparent sincerity. His corrspondence with Wilder Penfield is being edited by Penfield's biographer, Professor William Feindel at McGill University. It, also, shows the strong and inspirational ties between teacher and pupil for close to half a century.

(W.C.G.)

Chapter 7

Sherrington
The Philosopher of the Nervous System

A. The Rede Lecture

The Rede Lecture "The brain and its mechanism" was delivered to the University of Cambridge on December 5, 1933. In contradistinctin to the earlier lectures of Chapter 5.E it is oriented to the brain not to the spinal cord.

> Inside the animal's form sits the brain, its work broadly to increase the animal's grip on the world about it, and hardly less the grip of the external world upon the animal. Grown up with the animal it fits the motor mechanism of the animal much as a key fits its lock. A question the curious ages never fail to ask is, who turns the key?

This question is soon answered: "The outside world . . . in commerce with the animal."

The neural machinery of the brain is believed to operate in much the same basic manner as the spinal cord.

> These two opposed processes, excitation and inhibition, cooperate at nodal point after nodal point in the nerve-circuits. Their joint operation at any moment settles what will be the conduction pattern, and so the motor outcome, of the signalling going forward in the brain.
> A little more or a little less of inhibition or conversely of excitation on a nerve-net and the pattern of the reflex shifts like the pattern of a tapped kaleidoscope.
> Nerve management of muscle resolves itself largely into management of nerve by nerve, expecially by brain, more and more so as evolution proceeds. With no greater equipment of muscle the super-imposed amount of nerve becomes greater and greater; each new nerve-growth seems to entail further nerve-growth. Fresh organization roofs over prior organization. Brain is an example. 'So on our heels a fresh perfection treads'. But were it a Government Office we might be suspicious. This brain of ours is a perfect excrescence although our endowment in muscle remains but moderate.

After considering the complexities of brain performance in control of behaviour, there is a tentative introduction to the brain-mind problem.

> We have seen the brain as an input-output signalling system. The signals entering it are not mental, nor are the executant signals which issue. But signalling which travels certain ways in the brain for instance through the great new nerve-net seems to get, so to say, mental

existence, though losing it again before even the penultimate exit-path. No microscopical, no physical or chemical means detect there anything radically other than in nerve-nets elsewhere. All is as elsewhere, except greater complexity. The aggregate of cells is enormous. The biologist microscoping this nerve-material, 'the stuff that dreams are made of', is struck by the seemingly, reckless profusion of wealth of nerve cells.

Sherrington still had misgivings: "But indeed, what right have we to conjoin mental experience with the physiological? No scientific right; only the right of what Keats, with that superlative Shakespearian gift of his, dubbed 'busy common sense'".

Nevertheless the dilemma grows:

The two, for all I can do, seem to remain disparate and disconnected. I recognize that, from observation which becomes more and more precise, the time and place of the two sets of events seem to be coincident. All goes to show that they do in so far correspond. Mental experience on the one hand, and brain happenings on the other, though I cannot correlate together, I nevertheless find to coincide in time and space.

But when it comes to the enigma of how this can happen, Sherrington states that the biologist ". . . although he have no answer . . . speaking in all humility . . . has to make it plain how far or near he is from answer". This is a most salutary comment. It has been a common failing of scientists to pretend to a greater knowledge than they have, and thus to mislead mankind.

Then follows an account of nerve actions so far as they can be understood even at the highest levels of the brain. However, the quest for some unique structures or actions fails. "There is, so far as I know, in the chemical, physical properties, or microscopical structures no hint of any *fundamental* difference between non-mental and mental regions of the brain."

It should be noted that here there is introduction of the concepts of non-mental and mental regions of the brain, the latter being the *liaison brain* in a later terminology. However, later he states: "But, strictly, we have to regard the relation of mind to brain as still not merely unsolved but still devoid of a basis for its very beginning. I am not a defeatist, for I would urge active pursuit of the enquiry".

There is amusingly enough a statement redolent of Gilbert Ryle's ridicule of the mind-brain problem by referring to it as the ghost in the machine, when Sherrington wittily states: "A ghost may be a very weak visual stimulus and yet release a large mental reaction".

The final conclusions are worth quoting because of the arrogant attack they evoked by his old friend Pavlov. Sherrington said:

If nerve-activity have relation to mind, we can hardly escape the inference that nerve-inhibition must be a large factor in the working of the mind. The problem I have too grossly touched to-day has one virtue at least, it will long offer to those who pursue it the comfort that to journey is better than to arrive; but that comfort assumes arrival. Some of us – perhaps because we are too old – or is it, too young – think there may be arrival at last. And when, and if, that arrival comes, there may be still regret that the pursuit is over. If only for this, that man, the best among us, having found how the brain does its thinking, will certainly try to improve its ways of doing so, restraining some parts, amplifying others, introducing short-cuts, and, certainly increasing speed and aiming at economy and devising as seems to him best. We need not be prophets to foresee that then will come the long-told speedy extinction of man. The planet will then be re-liberated, free for the next era of animal domination. May I be forgiven for mentioning the hope that the new dominant may not be anything of the social insect type!

Presumably it was this last wish that in 1934 aroused Pavlov to the attack in a seminar session taken down in a stenographic record in 1934 and reported in an interesting paper by Volicer (1973).

I shall now turn to a criticism of Mr. Sherrington. He has been a neurologist all his life, engaged in the study of the nervous system, though, more of its lower part, the spinal cord, than the higher part.
Comparing the laws of the brain and its mechanisms, he draws a very strange conclusion. It appears that up to now he is not at all sure whether the brain bears any relation to our mind. A neurologist who has spent his whole life studying the subject is still not sure whether the brain has anything to do with the mind. If nerve activity have relation to mind . . . I did not trust my knowledge of English and so I requested others to translate it for me. How can it be that at the present time a physiologist should doubt the relation between nervous activity and the mind? This is the result of a purely dualistic concept. This is the Cartesian viewpoint, according to which the brain is a piano, a passive instrument, while the soul is a musician extracting from this piano any melodies it likes. Obviously this is his viewpoint. Probably Sherrington is a dualist who resolutely divides his being in two halves: the sinful body and the eternal, immortal soul. I am all the more surprised that for some reason or other he regards knowledge of this soul as something pernicious and clearly expresses this point of view; according to him, if the best of us acquire some knowledge of the nervous system this would be a most dangerous thing threatening the extinction of man on earth. He makes the following statement, which appears to me rather strange: if man learns to know himself and on the basis of this knowledge to govern himself in a economical way (such economy is not bad since it means that he will preserve himself for a longer time), then our "planet" will be reliberated, free for the next era of animal domination. What do you think of that? What does it mean? Why, it's simply preposterous!
If nerve activity have relation to mind, then he is inclined to think that this concerns only inhibition. Thus, positive work is of no significance whatever, while inhibition, discontinuance of work seems to go very well with the soul. He literally says: 'If nerve activity have relation to mind, we can hardly escape the inference that the nerve inhibition must be a larger factor in working of the mind'. Why is, then, the essential positive activity rejected as having no relation to intelligence, while inhibition is regarded as having such a relation? Gentlemen, can anyone of you, who has read Sherrington's booklet, say anything in defence of the author? I believe that this is not the matter of some kind of misunderstanding, thoughtlessness or misjudgement. I simply suppose that he is ill, although he is only seventy years old, that these are distinct symptoms of old age, of senility.

As a comment on the senility, Sherrington had just turned seventy-six when he gave the Rede Lecture and he was to continue in active intellectual work for nearly twenty years, writing two of his greatest books, whereas Pavlov was eighty-five and died two years later. In the ensuing discussion in

Pavlov's seminar Kupalov puts up a defence of Sherrington, but is beaten down by Pavlov.

It should firstly be noted that Pavlov was in error with respect to his misunderstanding of the role of inhibition in the brain. Pavlov had never been able to assimilate the fundamental discoveries of Sherrington in the operation of neural machinery. He had misused the words 'reflex' and 'inhibition', as Sherrington had often remarked. Conditioned reflexes are not reflexes, but very complex behavioural responses. The word 'inhibition' in Pavlov's theories has no relation to the precise synaptic mechanisms, which Sherrington had studied and defined theoretically. Sherrington's final position with respect to the fundamental role of inhibition is expressed in the last quotation given above from his Nobel Prize address (Chapt. 5.F). After over forty years of intensive study, we can still fully subscribe to that position.

Today we can appreciate better the prescient fears of Sherrington about the abuse of knowledge. Already we can see it in the threat of human genetic engineering and again there are the programmes by Skinner and others for conditioning and controlling, so as to give security and happiness in the manner of Huxley's *Brave New World.* But Sherrington was thinking also of the rigorous enslavement of the Soviets under Stalin and of the threatening Nazi control in Germany, where the attempt was being made to fashion whole peoples on the model of the social insects.

I do not know if Sherrington ever saw the text of this Pavlovian diatribe. He had better memories of earlier days. In his visit to St. Petersburg in 1912 he visited Pavlov and told of his simple patriarchal life. He, supported by his wife, made a strictly Orthodox family, having meals at a long table with Pavlov presiding. Along one wall he kept some of his dogs with their salivary fistulae so that they could be carefully tended like children. In 1929 Pavlov and his son visited Sherrington at Oxford. There I also met them. I recognized and appreciated the cordial atmosphere of the reunion of these two great scientists, leaders at that time. Pavlov was still very critical of the Soviet totalitarianism. In 1923 he had publicly denounced Soviet communism by stating: "For the kind of social experiment that you are making I would not sacrifice a frog's hind legs". However, in the last two years of his life he succumbed to the blandishments of the Soviet government; hence we may account for his criticism of Sherrington. Pavlov was to have his great occasion when he was President of the International Union of the Physiological Sciences that was meeting in Moscow and Leningrad in the summer of 1935 a few months before his death. Then followed the disastrous period for Soviet scientists during which Pavlov's science posthumously became the revealed truth, never to be questioned, and to be defended as a dogma against all threatening deviations. This strictly imposed orthodoxy crippled Soviet neuroscience for decades – right up to present time. Ironically it was a fate that Pavlov would not have wished or enjoyed.

B. The Gifford Lectures: Man on His Nature

Throughout his long life as an experimental scientist, Sherrington's imagination was creatively engaged in the building of theories and concepts that have come to be recognized as the secure foundation for future developments in the brain sciences. This work is generally regarded as his great achievement. But his creative imagination was also actively engaged in attempts to explore and redefine in the light of the new scientific knowledge the great enigma of the brain-mind problem – the world-knot of Schopenhauer. As early as the 1890s he was carrying out experiments on binocular fusion that were designed to reveal the relationship between the visual input and the subjective experience. This work was fully described and discussed in the last chapter of *The Integrative Action of the Nervous System* (1906). There he concludes that:

> Our experiments show, therefore, that during binocular regard of an objective image each uniocular mechanism develops independently a sensual image of considerable completeness. The singleness of the binocular perception results from union of these elaborated uniocular sensations. The singleness is therefore the product of a synthesis that works with already elaborated sensations contemporaneously proceeding.
> Pure conjuction in time without necessarily cerebral conjunction in space lies at the root of the solution of the problem of the unity of mind.

The course of the last decades of his life was foreshadowed in the final sentence of *The Integrative Action of the Nervous System:* "It is then around the cerebrum, its physiological and psychological attributes, that the main interest of biology must ultimately turn" (cf. Appendix 8).

Only at the end of his full experimental life did he turn to this long-submerged philosophical interest, tentatively in the Rede Lecture, which we have already considered, and then in that great imaginative and creative work, *Man on His Nature*. These Gifford Lectures were delivered at Edinburgh University in May 1937 and June 1938. Lord Gifford had founded the lectures for the purpose of having Natural Theology "considered just as Astronomy or Chemistry". In his initial considerations of what was required Sherrington states:

> The Natural Theologist, if we may so address him, in his effort from consideration of Nature without appeal to revelation to come to a conclusion about the existence and ways

of God has thus to include himself as part of the natural evidence. He then sees himself as a piece of Nature looking around at Nature's rest.

Nature, in virtue of himself, has now entered on a stage when one at least of its growing points has started thinking in 'values'. This comes before him as part of the evidence to be considered.

The province of Natural Theology is surely to weigh from all the evidence derivable from Nature whether Nature taken all in all signifies and implies the existence of what with reverence is called God; and, if so, again with all reverence, what sort of God.

The general theme of *Man on His Nature* is the dualism of man's nature, body and mind. This philosophical position is completely antipathetic to the established philosophy of this materialistic age; hence preceding biographers have, we think, underestimated this great book, and have been very critical of its philosophy. In the manner of Ryle, who at that time was very much in fashion, Lord Cohen (1958) argued that Sherrington's linguistic usage of such words as 'mind' and 'matter' is fraught with dangers and prejudices. It is the familiar and now discredited 'category mistake' that was used with such assurance by Ryle. Granit (1966) is also unhappy with Sherrington's dualistic philosophy, and is at pains to emphasize the evolutionary pantheism that is tentatively expressed by Sherrington at several places in the book. Granit's final conclusion is that Sherrington is not "the philosopher of the nervous system" as stated by Asher in 1931, but that he had ". . . the mind of an artist, complex, intuitive, rich, visual in the extreme". By contrast the mathematical physicist Schrödinger (1958) regarded *Man on His Nature* as one of the great books. The criticisms have been based on a rather superficial and cursory survey of this great book. We think it deserves a much more considered evaluation.

In embarking upon this task we have to enter into the spirit in which these lectures were given. It was an enquiry into Natural Religion by a scientist who had spent a lifetime in the rigorous discipline of trying to establish the basic principles of operation of the central nervous system, and by a scholar well versed in the classics and with a deep sympathy and understanding of European man in his cultural pursuits. In the four hundred years from the Renaissance, natural science had had enormous successes in its programme of understanding nature, and man as a part of nature. In this great enterprise man's special status had become diminished. For example it was Sherrington more than anybody else who had shown that man resembled other animals in having a central nervous system with the same basic principles of operation. The methods of physics and chemistry had served well in the attempts to account for the propagation of nerve impulses and the transmission across synapses. So much so that it was optimistically predicted that even the most subtle reactions of the brain ultimately would be reducible to physical and chemical explanations. Thus at the time of the lectures there was the prevailing scientific belief that man in all his most unique mental characters – thoughts, imaginings, memories, decisions, creativities in the arts and in the sciences – would ultimately be explicable in a materialist and deterministic mode. There would then be no residue pointing to a mental or non-material component in man's makeup. This promissory triumph of monist materialism was the confidently expected goal of the scientific study of man. The brain-mind problem would then become a non-problem after over 2000 years of fruitless philosophical enquiry. And the principal interest of Natural Theology – the uniqueness of man – would evaporate at the same time.

This was the dominant climate of opinion that provided the challenge to Sherrington when he accepted the invitation to deliver the Gifford Lectures. He could have chosen a closely reasoned disputation on the prevailing philosophical mode. *The Concept of Mind* by Gilbert Ryle was to win a considerable but ephemeral acclaim in that manner. It was the academic security of philosophical professionalism that Cohen and Granit regretted missing. We can be grateful that Sherrington avoided that academic pitfall. There have been enough erudite and dull performances of that kind which have contributed no illumination of understanding. Instead he chose to give his creative imagination full play with its resources of poetic expression and with the richness of visual imagery. These were the means used to display and marshall his enormous resources of scientific knowledge that are always in evidence and that are used most tellingly in reasoned arguments.

These lectures can best be appreciated if they are understood as Sherrington communing with himself, or in the intimacy of a select group of scholars. He raises questions that often are the means to further questioning. So in lecture after lecture we may hear reversions to earlier themes that are now re-explored with newly fashioned questions. It is the very antithesis of the rigorous didactic method and it has the great advantage that there is no confrontation of his audience with dogmas that can repel and so close down the communication. There is an openness and flexibility and one feels one is participating in the enquiry and so is carried along with it. The aim is thus not to instruct or to dominate, but rather to commune, utilizing for this purpose the attractions of the language and the enticements offered by the resources of one of the most cultured minds of the modern world.

The critics have been unhappy with the device adopted right from the outset of having the sixteenth century French physician, Jean Fernel, introduced for the purpose of reference to an earlier almost prescientific age where there was no conflict between natural knowledge and religion. We would suggest that Sherrington did this to heighten the drama devolving from man's changing beliefs about himself and Nature with the consequence of a growing feeling of cosmic loneliness. But there was also another reason. As I can remember from conversations at Ipswich where he was preparing the lectures, he had misgivings about how he could present the stark message of modern science to an audience composed largely of clergymen. The frequent references to the beliefs of Fernel would relieve the spiritual bleakness of so much of his story by introducing little vignettes from the Age of Faith as represented by Fernel.

Lectures 1 to 6 were given in Edinburgh in May 1937 and were in their content almost entirely fundamental biological science. Their role is to lead up to the biological nature of man. As such they form the background for the much more controversial questions of the second set of lectures and so will be dealt with in summary form.

i. Nature and Tradition

Fernel is introduced early in relation to the characters of his dialogue: Brutus is ". . . a cultured man in the street of sixteenth century Paris"; Philiatros is a senior doctoral student; Eudoxus is Fernel. Fernel came at the end of a period where Natural Religion and the Christian Religion were combined by harmony into one religion.

> He is one who cannot be content to hold his beliefs about Nature and his spiritual creed apart the one from the other, in separate chambers of his heart. He must have them meet and rejoice together. It is a feeling which commends him to us; it would seem, too, a feeling which the cultured of his time shared with him, to judge by the large and lasting circle of the readers of his book.
> But we notice also how, with the drift of science, knowledge has moved since then.

It is interesting that during the lectures Sherrington repeatedly refers to himself as "the man in the street", that is, as a Brutus of the twentieth century, and as such he carries on his questioning and his dialogue.

ii. The Natural and Superstition

Despite the sophisticated academic dialogue of Fernel it has to be recognized that the sixteenth century was rife with superstitions – astrology and the occult. Fernel contributed much to the relief of medical practice from superstitions, but necessarily he continued with the old beliefs in the four elements and in his explanations of disease on this basis. There was as yet no chemistry or physics as we know them. He came to be increasingly critical of astrology, but the elimination from Nature of the occult came long after Fernel. As Sherrington says at the end of this lecture:

> The world's horizon is new to the degree of offering a wholly new perspective. The eyes which look at it are new. The old Walpurgis night is over; its company is disbanded; its votaries are fled, its dance will never be resumed; its festival has lapsed, because deserted. The half-gods are not only vanished, they are by nigh forgotten; matter for labels and a museum-shelf.
>
> Yet not for us to forget is our escape from a long nightmare – the exchange of the monstrous world for one relatively sane. To see, and where we can to disentangle, the facts of Nature free from those perplexing mysteries which were in truth not there. There remains and to spare of deeper mystery. The mystery of Nature needs no superstition. We can interrogate the natural world with a confidence drawn from riddance of misunderstanding no less than from extension of understanding. We can see with whom it is we talk. What wears a divine livery can without fear or favour display it to man's gaze. The position for reading from Nature's lips what she may have to say to Godhead never yet in the past was what it is for us today.

He had in mind his audience!

iii. Life in Little

The theme of the third lecture is 'life' as exhibited by single cells. Later questions arise about 'life' and 'mind', so life is studied in detail in order to give a clear picture of a living energy system. We give one sample of the imaginative writing:

> Essential for any conception of the cell is that it is no static system. It is a material system and that today is to say an energy system. Our conceptions of it fail if not dynamic. It is a scene of energy-cycles, suites of oxidation and reduction, concatenated ferment-actions. It is like a magic hive the walls of whose chambered spongework are shifting veils of ordered molecules, and rend and renew as operations rise and cease. A world of surfaces and streams. We seem to watch battalions of specific catalysts, like Maxwell's 'demons', lined up, each waiting, stop-watch in hand, for its moment to play the part assigned to it, a step in one or other great thousand-linked chain process. Yet each and every step is understandable chemistry. The cell has proved to be a perfect swarm of catalysts, or of trains of catalysts, each a link in a serial suite of chemical action.

This is immensurably far from Fernel, where the body was vivified by the "immaterial life-principle tenanting the body", which left at death. In the forty years since this was spoken by Sherrington the dynamic picture has become immensely more complicated with interacting feedback systems of control. Yet this visionary account is still valuable and exciting.

iv. The Wisdom of the Body

This lecture begins with a moving and felicitous appeal to his audience.

> We dismiss wonder commonly with childhood. Much later, when life's pace has slackened, wonder may return. The mind then may find so much inviting wonder the whole world becomes wonderful. Then one thing is scarcely more wonderful than is another. But, greatest wonder, our wonder soon lapses. A rainbow every morning who would pause to look at? The wonderful which comes often or is plentifully about us is soon taken for granted. That is practical enough. It allows us to get on with life. But it may stultify if it cannot on occasion be thrown off. To recapture now and then childhood's wonder, is to secure a driving force for occasional grown-up thoughts. Among the workings of this planet, there is a *tour de force*, if such term befits the workings of a planet. Wonder is the mood in which I would ask to approach it for the moment.

The occasion is the formation and growth of a living being (ontogeny) from the process of fertilization onwards. Some examples serve to illustrate the brilliance of the exposition.

> With the lens of the eye, a batch of granular skin-cells are told off to travel from the skin to which they strictly belong, to settle down in the mouth of the optic cup, to arrange themselves in a compact and geometrical ball, to turn into transparent fibres, to assume the right refractive index, and to make themselves into a subsphere with two correct curvatures truly centred on a certain axis. Thus it is they make a lens of the right size, set in the right place, that is at the right distance behind the transparent window of the eye in front and the sensitive seeing screen of the retina behind. In short they behave as if fairly possessed.
>
> But the chief wonder of all we have not touched on yet. Wonder of wonders, though familiar even to boredom. So much with us that we forget it all our time. The eye sends, as we saw, into the cell-and-fibre forest of the brain throughout the waking day continual rhythmic streams of tiny, individually evanescent, electrical potentials. This throbbing streaming crowd of electrified shifting points in the spongework of the brain bears no obvious semblance in space-pattern, and even in temporal relation resembles but a little remotely the tiny two-dimensional upside-down picture of the outside world which the eye-ball paints on the beginnings of its nerve-fibres to the brain. But that little picture sets up an electrical storm. And that electrical storm so set up is one which affects a whole population of brain-cells. Electrical charges having in themselves not the faintest elements of the visual – having for instance, nothing of 'distance', 'right-side-upness', nor 'vertical', nor 'horizontal', nor 'colour', nor 'brightness', nor 'shadow', nor 'roundness', nor 'square-ness', nor 'contour', nor 'transparency', nor 'opacity', nor 'near', nor 'far', nor visual anything – yet conjure up all these. A shower of little electrical leaks conjures up for me, when I look, the landscape; the castle on the height; or, when I look at him approaching, my friend's face, and how distant he is from me, they tell me. Taking their word for it, I go forward and my other senses confirm that he is there.
>
> A wonder of wonders which is a commonplace we take for granted. It is a case of 'the world is too much with us'; too banal to wonder at.

Here is a vivid statement of the mystery of the brain-mind problem that will exercise us when we consider later lectures.

> Does the wonder then lapse of which we spoke at the outset? The cell's doings are affairs merely in routine conformity with ascertained ways of 'energy'. To apply the term *tour de*

force, as at the opening I ventured to apply it, to any of these phenomena is out of place. Nor can we regard the 'human' as more wonderful than any of the rest. But a wonder is there still. True, we can understand Keats' sighing against science, 'there was an awful rainbow once in heaven!' Yet he was 'to find', as has been written of him, 'material in the scientific view of the world for the highest achievements of poetry'. Could we foretell the rose-bud from its chemistry, would that make its beauty less? Does such knowledge impair the beauty of the world? Surely the reverse, for we then know that such as the rose-bud are neither accident nor miracle. The wonder is there still. It rests on different ground. Nature is not made less wonderful because her rule of working begins to be intelligible. If it be a question of wonder, rather the more wonderful.

Sherrington finishes this inspired lecture by a gesture to the audience and the promise of exciting challenges, but there is a final word of warning.

When we are told that the modern chemist and physicist cannot get on without the hypothesis that matter explains everything, a position is reached akin to that of initation into a faith. A rigid attitude of mind is taken as an orientation necessary for progress in knowledge. Is there anything different between that and the efficacy of the spiritual exercises of St. Ignatius as introductory to mystic convictions expected to follow? What either expedient may possibly gain in intensity of insight is surely at disproportionately greater cost to breadth of judgment.

v. Earth's Reshuffling

The lecture on ontogeny is followed by an evolutionary lecture. The theme was broad, touching also on cosmic evolution, and leading on to the origin of life and its evolution. Again the attitude of wonder permeates the whole lecture:

Does it seem strange that an unreasoning planet, without set purpose and not knowing how to set about it has done this thing to an extent surpassingly more than man has? It is to be remembered that Earth's periods of time have been of a different order from man's, and her scale of operations of a different order, and that man's cunning in this respect dates but from yesterday. Yet, we agree, it does seem strange.
It is enough here that evolution by rearranging old parts is constructing new harmonies, chemical and biological. It is composing new melodies from some of the same old notes.

New questions arise with the increasing complexity of living forms that:

. . . was the work of evolution. Often the more complex evolved from the less complex. What does the progressive change to greater complexity, which often accompanies evolution, do for life?
Does such integrated complexity, as we might call it, bring into being anything absolutely new?
We should hardly expect so. Yet it does seem to be so. The complexity introduces recognizable mind. It does so gradually, and nurses it into flower.

After this statement of crisis in evolution there follows a long conventional account of evolution and of evolutionary genetics that has in part been superseded by the cataclysmic happenings of molecular biology in the subsequent decades. Then there is a return to the question of the origin of mind, which is of particular interest in relation to the later philosophical lectures. The statements are quite emphatic:

> Evolution of the mind is as incontestable as evolution of the body.
> Ours is an earthly mind which fits our earthly body. It produces percepts of earthly things from an earthly view-point. It helps the besouled body to deal with terrestrial things, thereby to live.
> Let us not disown mother Earth; rather let us rejoice to call her 'mother'. Earth's nature is our nature. We owe to earth the entire gamut of our mind's wonders, whether of joy or pain. Life's story has been an unfolding of germinal powers of the planet bringing emergence of mind. Let us give thanks where thanks are due.

But Sherrington goes on to have a slight misgiving with respect to this conventional dogmatism, so he introduces an alternative theme.

> ... there have been other views. Our mind wondering about itself has at times indulged the thought that it is not earthly. It has judged itself to be of 'heavenly' origin. It has so judged sometimes apart from any special revelation of faith. Therefore it is that such a view comes before us here.
> What has led it to regard itself as not of earth? What signs of unearthliness attach to it? Its own experience is the entire gamut of all knowledge; if evidence of this alleged unearthliness is anywhere it must exist there.

In this questioning, reference is made to Fernel, who held that our mind derives its nature from the stars. For others it was preternatural. Thus no satisfying answers seem to be forthcoming. A pre-established harmony with miraculous intervention is rejected provisionally in favour of a monistic interpretation. But there is later some rethinking:

> Kant seems to assume the human mind to be a finished thing, a completed item of existence. But the human mind is part of a tide of change which, in its instance, has been latterly and, we may think, still is, running like a mill-race.
> We do not know that it ever will be finished. We see it as a provisional *ad hoc* arrangement of the present. Often will it be reminded of this when prosecuting its latest task of establishing the 'values' (*cf.* Chapter XII, *Man On His Nature.*)

This suggestion of values leads on to the later philosophical chapters, to which the next is transitional. The whole of this last quotation shows how Sherrington recognized cultural evolution – "running like a mill-race" – that has an unimaginable future if we can preserve the essential conditions – freedom for full play of the creative imagination.

vi. A Whole Presupposed of Its Parts

The theme of this sixth lecture is the motor act, with contrast between reflex and voluntary action. We are introduced to the term 'recognizable mind' from behaviour of man and higher animals. Naturally Descartes is a principal character in the story of automata and the analogy with human action.

... Descartes, developing the doctrine of mindless motor acts in man and animals, put it forward with a force and clearness which caught the abiding attention of the world. He said in effect 'the bird or dog of which we imagine as it flies or runs, that its act is conducted by thinking, willing and so on, is not so actuated. Its movements are in truth just the running of a wound-up clock. So likewise with many of our own motions, yours and mine'.

Sherrington tries to see how far this Cartesian concept can be interpreted on the basis of modifications of modern neuroscience.

Let us here take a liberty with our subject. Let us suppose processes in the brain which correlate with mental processes, these latter, not the purely sensory but processes more complex, concerned with relations between the items of our experience. Let us think of these as possibly arising locally in the brain. In order to distinguish them from those (the extrinsic) which arise outside the brain in the receptor or sense-organs let us label them 'intrinsic' and think of them as, especially in ourselves, belonging to the roof-brain. Assume for the moment, against the position of modern science, that the correlation of brain and mind amounts to what we may call a *contact utile* between them . . . The two are not, however, in watertight compartments. Thus, the 'intrinsic' can be evoked via the sensory, for instance, in the elaboration of these latter perceptually. The 'intrinsic' are, however, quasi-independent of the sensory. The sensory are similarly quasi-independent of the cerebral 'intrinsic'. Each can occur without the other.

Let us suppose that both the 'extrinsic' and the 'intrinsic' are in touch with the organs of movement and can operate them. When the 'extrinsic' do so independently of the 'intrinsic', that is reflex action. When the 'intrinsic' do so independently of the 'extrinsic' a form of 'willed' action results. Our normal motor behaviour would then consist in a harmonious combination of the 'extrinsic' and the 'intrinsic'.

Many problems arise from this model of human and animal action, as will become evident in much of our later consideration.

Sherrington has many interesting comments on Descartes:

Descartes' 'automatism' was a great event in physiology. And it had notable repercussions beyond. We need not, even were I competent to do so, enter upon them here. For one thing it re-equipped 'materialism'. At the same time it freed the finite rational soul from obligations to matter as rarely had it been freed before. It took from it the burden of operating matter. The course of scientific discovery has since then conspired with this view of Descartes to cut the individual into two disparate halves, mind and body. That severance is pronounced a paradox by Nature and by Evolution. Nature and Evolution deal with the individual, body and mind together as unity.

He wrote his *De Homine*, sometimes called a physiology, to describe how man moves as an automaton. It was a work of genius. Thus, purely *a priori* it assumed that the motor act required an inhibitory process along with an excitatory. This idea was original with Descartes. Experimental physiology 250 years later confirmed it.

If Descartes

... meant, and in various passages he does seem to mean, that, just as man is an automaton with superadded mind, his opinion lies today where he left it. In some ways the medieval adhered to Descartes. The medieval view generally denied to brute kind any loftier status than that of terrestrial furniture provided for man's use during his probation here. The Cartesian lack of sympathy and understanding in this matter of creature-kind went further, an unaccountable trespass both against our fellow-creatures and against common sense.

Sherrington was deeply imbued with a sense of the brotherhood of animals and strongly rejected the Cartesian puppet analogue for man or animals. He recognized its dangers when applied as a political dogma.

> Today his conception of the doings of man still finds its echo in official Russia. The citizen there, taken *en gros,* seems to be viewed as a system of reflexes. The State can 'condition' and use these systems of reflexes. 'Reflexology', as it is there called, becomes a science of man on which the State leans. In 'reflexology' Descartes would find Ivan Pavlov of Petrograd his greatest successor; and the successor was an experimentalist as Descartes was not.

The present-day programme of Skinner in *Beyond Freedom and Dignity* would have been anathema to Sherrington.

An important aside is worth quoting in the light of Sherrington's great contributions to the reflex.

> As to the term itself, Descartes in describing his automata did not say 'reflex', or rather he scarcely did so. It is to be found once, and then not in substantival form. It was Willis, Professor of Medicine at Oxford, who writing, rather later, on the nervous system, gave numerous instances of automatic acts, where stimulus was promptly followed by movement without conscious participation of the 'will'. He spoke of this action as being 'reflex'. Historical importance attaches to the conception of reflex action. At a time when nervous function lay involved in mystery, and therefore at the mercy of the occult, the 'reflex' introduced a category of nervous action so simple and straightforward as to be free from the mysterious. It made an excellent start for scientific analysis of nerve.

Sherrington actually had been the scientist to do this *par excellence* in the 1890s: "The real importance of Descartes' step was that it handed the work of the nervous system over to the nervous system itself".

However, Sherrington never did fall victim, as did lesser scientists, to the temptation to give a complete account of human behaviour on the basis of reflexology, as is done by behaviourists even today.

"To subsume the whole of human behaviour under what has been called 'reflexology' might further be taken to mean that that roof-organ of the brain reacts simply on the reflex plan. But that there is much which contradicts. Our inference has to be that we are partly reflex and partly not."

But then we have a statement of parallelism as a solution of the mind-brain problem:

> As to the mind and the brain one supposition is that mental experience running with the physical act, though wholly disparate from all material events and therefore from the physical act, the two series of events, mental and energetic, yet somehow keep step together, their doing so being evidence that they are related, but with no suggestion as to 'how'. As Bergson insists, to speak of parallelism between the two is hardly allowable because they are incomparable. There remains yet further the non-possumus inference that mind is an epiphenomenon, and that the mental and physical do not interact.

Yet mind is effective, as Fernel opined, and not a mere ineffective shadow as in parallelism (which is a kind of dualism). It is because of mind's effectiveness that it has prospered in evolution.

The influence of mind on the doings of life makes mind an effective contribution to life. We can seize then how it is that mind counts and has counted. That it has been evolved seems to assure us that it has counted. How it has counted would seem to be that the finite mind has influenced its individual's 'doing'! Lloyd Morgan, the biologist, urged that 'the primary aim, object and purpose of consciousness is control'. Dame Nature seems to have taken the like view.

This raises the enigma of interaction between mind and the matter-energy world of brain that will be so much considered in the later lectures. The evolutionary argument for the effectiveness of mind has been completely overlooked by the many schools of modern philosophy that deny the influence of the mind on the brain.

vii. The Brain and Its Work

A year later Sherrington continued his lecture series. He introduced his seventh lecture with two quotations:

The chief function of the central nervous system is to send messages to the muscles which will make the body move effectively as a whole. (E. D. Adrian)

L'homme n'est qu'un roseau le plus faible de la nature; mais c'est un roseau pensant. (Pascal)

He built upon the elaborate introductory course of the preceding year, and so was able to concentrate his attention on the specifically human problem of human brain in liaison with the mind. However, he does not distinguish sharply between human and non-human brain in their mind-like association. He has to avoid the dilemma of trying to define how far down the animal scale there is a mind. In order to accomplish this he introduces the term 'recognizable mind'.

Among the phenomena of life, mind is one which, as we were noting, seems of more restricted distribution than at one time was currently supposed. But in so saying we use 'mind' in the meaning 'recognizable mind'. Mind as in everyday parlance we understand it. Mind presupposing of it what each of us experiences as 'mind', feeling, knowing, wishing and so on.

He admits that on these criteria grades of mind shade off to the undecipherable, but at least much of life is excluded. A related question is: ". . . what part of all the action, of which the individual is the scene, does mind go with?"

The answer is the nervous system, primarily in certain motor acts. This is a surprising answer because one would have anticipated a sensory and not a motor identification. But he goes on to specify the motor acts as being those central to the individual and of paramount importance at that time: "It is this one main doing which has an accompaniment of mind".

After this decisive statement there is much discursive talk and some homely examples as he calls them; but eventually there is an amazingly clear and decisive example told in his characteristic vivid manner, particularly so as he describes a situation he so often had experienced. We have often been in the position of the friend.

> An act, from the point of view of *mind*, is a doing with a definite aim. It is integrated from parts and some stand nearer to the aim than others. If I have under the microscope an object which I want a friend to see, my hands move the preparation to bring the tiny object into the centre of the microscopic field of view. I am seated; my head is stooped, one of my eyes is looking through the microscope-tube, my other is, by practice, sufficiently detached from the other's act to be not convergent with it, and I am unaware for the time being that it sees anything. The fingers of both my hands are tentatively pushing the glass-slide slightly this way and that, with the 'purpose' to move the object to the desired spot. I would regard the search with my fingers as the focal part of the integrated act. The sitting, the stooping, the looking, although parts of the act do not dominate it as does the search by the fingers. The rest is background. It is to the focal act with the fingers that mind particularly attaches. Not to the fingers as such, still less to the executant mechanism moving them, which is away up the arm. What the mind is concerned with is not the act but the aim. It is more aware of the finger-part than of the rest because the fingers' part stands nearest to the aim. The rest is mental fringe, even submental. Finite mind is like a moving focal point which wanders restrictedly within each of us, with an aim. Never at any time pervading much of us. At all times most of us is impenetrable to it. Clearly we must not suppose 'life' and 'mind' are one and the same. The finite life is a phenomenon accessible to sense; the finite mind is not.

On this basis he excludes recognizable mind from being an attribute of the countless activities of living organisms. As to its evolutionary origin he states:

> Mind, recognizable mind, seems to have arisen in connection with the motor act. Where motor integration progressed and where motor behaviour progressively evolved, mind progressively evolved. That kind of motor integration which arrives at concentrating the complex mechanism on doing one thing at a time offers a situation for mind; and the doing of that one thing finds mind alongside it. But not the whole of the doing. The integrated act has its focus, and there mentality has its focus.

Despite the sophisticated example of the controlled movements of the microscope slide Sherrington is at pains to recognize mind in higher animals. He illustrates the grave injustice of separating man from other animals by the criterion of recognizable mind. He cites with disapproval the beliefs of Fernel:

> For Fernel man has a whole category of the soul which nothing else earthly has. By that right he is in truth *not* of the earth. It seems to escape Fernel that man's life of all lives is the most completely and fully bound to earth because life's experience, wholly earthly as it is, is in man's case the most complete and full. Being the completest of its kind, and its kind being that of the planet's side, it is more thoroughly earthly than is any other. And it is subordinate to 'zest-to-live' as an aim. It is the most complete and full nexus between life and earth that we know. Man is the most, not the least, earthly of all creatures. His knowledge, feeling, strivings all conspire with his body to make him so to a degree unknown to other life.

It will be remembered that this overwhelming earthly tie was also emphasized earlier. The illustrations given make it clear that these earthly ties cover the whole range of mental experiences in relation to our total surroundings. We might say that earthly stands for everything except the province of astronomy, but that restriction is now absurd in the light of the revelations of modern astronomy and space travel. What is implied must be the whole matter-energy system of the cosmos, with special concentration for most of us on our immediate material environment, both living and non-living.

The bond of sympathy with all life raises severe problems for Sherrington as he explores the competitiveness that seems necessary for survival.

> We and they are all comrades in one same great adventure – life . . .
> All of us were launched and are steered by one same urge-to-live.
> With each life in its own thinking, so far as it have thought, its living is what the world is for; its own life is its first charge in the world; where it *has* mind, that mind endorses the view. Thus each life is a harmony of acts attuned to zest-to-live. Should that make life a sacred thing as between lives having the 'values'?
>
> It might seem so. But the world of life shows another picture. Is life sacred? Life conflicts with life, even to the death. Life, feeds on life. Man's own life feeds upon other lives. Life finds its direst enemy, the planet over, is other life. In the world-order, at least as instanced by our planet, life is not sacred.
>
> Is life a 'value'? Surely a means to 'value'. Is life then sacred? This life conflicting with life even to the death? And there are grades of life. The question would seem not whether life is sacred, but how far sacred. That question looms as one likely to grow a sterner and sterner problem. A question which we may think the future of this planet turns upon. A part of it is this, whether the planet in its approaching phase is or is not to be *the human planet*. That one life, human life, seems on its way to something, natural truly, but nevertheless super-human. What means shall bring it about? Mind serving 'zest-to-live'? How? By ruthless conquest or beneficent mission. As to which, it lies with the 'values' to decide.

Sherrington reveals his deep emotional attachment to living creatures, but it can be suspected in this feeling of communal fellowship that he is concentrating on those creatures that could have recognizable mind. This is confirmed by a later passage:

> Did conceptual thinking come to the human mind *de novo* and fully fledged, a new gift? Or did it come climbing the sub-human ladder? The man-like ape clearly has symbolic thinking. It has 'thatness' as well as 'thereness'. What is the conceptual in rudiment? Has the dog no such rudiment? With such queries we may do well to carry ourselves back in thought to man in his primeval setting; man shaping a stone into a tool. That of the pre-human and sub-human chapter preceding the notion 'tool'? The chimpanzee is a tool-user and tool-deviser. He will, untaught, take a crooked stick to bring a banana within reach. Where one stick is not long enough he will, untaught, join together two end on for the purpose. May we not think his experience has brought to him some adumbration of 'tool' as a concept? Would not the sub-human and pre-human record if we had it lead us along degrees of mind which link us without break to frankly infra-human ways of thought, to brute mind whence human mind has come?

> For Fernel man's mind was another order of mind created by heaven and placed above the rest. For us man's mind is a recent product of our planet's side, produced from mind already there long previously, yielding man's mind by gradual change of previous mind.

This last sentence is his final opinion on the natural history of mind, and one that we can respect and remember during the later philosophical explorations of these lectures.

Now the attention moves to the brain considered simply in its neurophysiological activity of impulse discharges and synaptic transmissions. In trying to convey some concept of this to the audience Sherrington elaborated a remarkable model that he described so wonderfully. So we quote a section of his long description in order to exhibit an excellent example of his imagination in action. We can be sure he had Keat's poem on "Fancy" in mind. He invites

> ... fancy to help itself by recourse to a model. So with our conception of the brain; if we may let our fancy run and follow an engineering bent, it may contrive us something, however crude, not too remote for pictorial service.
>
> A scheme of lines and nodal points, gathered together at one end into a great ravelled knot, the brain, and at the other trailing off to a sort of stalk, the spinal cord. Imagine activity in this shown by little points of light. Of these some stationary flash rhythmically, faster or slower. Others are travelling points, streaming in serial trains at various speeds. The rhythmic stationary lights lie at the nodes. The nodes are both goals whither converge, and junctions whence diverge, the lines of travelling lights. The lines and nodes where the lights are, do not remain, taken together, the same even a single moment. There are at any time nodes and lines where lights are not.
>
> Suppose we choose the hour of deep sleep. Then only in some sparse and out of the way places are nodes flashing and trains of light-points running.
>
> Should we continue to watch the scheme we should observe after a time an impressive change which suddenly accrues. In the great head-end which has been mostly darkness spring up myriads of twinkling stationary lights and myriads of trains of moving lights of many different directions. It is as though activity from one of those local places which continued restless in the darkened main-mass suddenly spread far and wide and invaded all. The great topmost sheet of the mass, that where hardly a light had twinkled or moved, becomes now a sparkling field of rhythmic flashing points with trains of travelling sparks hurrying hither and thither. The brain is waking and with it the mind is returning. It is as if the Milky Way entered upon some cosmic dance. Swiftly the head-mass becomes an enchanted loom where millions of flashing shuttles weave a dissolving pattern, always a meaningful pattern though never an abiding one; a shifting harmony of subpatterns. Now as the waking body rouses, subpatterns of this great harmony of activity stretch down into the unlit tracks of the stalk-piece of the scheme. Strings of flashing and travelling sparks engage the lengths of it. This means that the body is up and rises to meet its waking day.

Following this ecstatic display of the wonders of cerebral activity, the discourse turns back to its relationship with the mind.

> If the roof-brain (the cerebral cortex) acts spontaneously, as electrical technique seems to detect, then there occurs action in it *not* initiated through any gateway of sense. The physiologist uses 'spontaneous' here just as he uses it of the heart, which beats 'of itself', i. e. is self-activated. He does not intend any reference to free-will. If 'free-will' means a series of events in which at some point the succeeding is not conditioned by reaction with

the preceding, such an anomaly in the brain's series of events is scientifically unthinkable. When I 'choose' a book from the bookcase I react fundamentally as does my microscopic acquaintance, amoeba, confronted by two or more particles, when it takes one of them. A difference between us is that my fancy conjures up several courses to take. Subsequently I experience my act as doing one of them. That act is, for its time being, my main act. As we saw I am confined to doing at any moment just one main act. From my fancy's plurality of possibles there emerges my *de facto* singleness of act. It leaves me the impression of a decision. Amoeba doubtless is without the fancy; hence without the impression of a decision.

The poetic licence about fancy makes a delightful accompaniment to this philosophical disputation, and serves as a 'cover-up' for evading the free-will issue. The theme of brain and mind is then developed in relation to the ancient hypothalamic regions of the brain that subserve emotional responses or affect in both motor behaviour and mental experience.

To say that this is an ancient piece of the brain is to say that it is part of our brain which still continues that of man's animal ancestral and related stock of long ago. It has meant in them, and still does so, fear, rage and passion; it does so also with man. Doubtless at innumerable turns it has in so doing served them and him well. But over it the roof-brain is a new brain so developed in man as to be the 'human feature'. It stands for knowledge and reason. As we have seen it can govern this old brain of 'affect'. And in man it has developed to be a hundred times the greater of the two. These two in their way epitomize man's complex. Their ratio of evolution in him points significantly. It exhibits the trend of his development. Regarded broadly, the goal toward which animal integration tends, if goal there be, would seem 'mind and more mind', and the immediate meaning of the finite mind in the body would seem to be to influence acts. Its influence upon acts is what, we would think, has given it survival value.

Then the impasse meets us. The blank of the 'how' of mind's leverage on matter. The inconsequence staggers us. Is it a misunderstanding?

The question is not answered, and later there will be much further questioning. But earlier he had raised it in a surprisingly modern fashion when considering whether the activity of the individual were completely accountable to the neuronal complexity of the brain.

Strangely enough, to the reacting individual himself his behaviour normally occasions no surprise. Stranger still, of all people the reacting individual himself is the last to think himself reflex. Such a reflex system, operated by sequences of thousand-patterned stimuli corresponding with total situations of the moment, might well work a Robot for many purposes indistinguishably from a man.

Again this modern Cartesianism is left aside for a later attack.

viii. The Organ of Liaison

In the eighth lecture Sherrington takes his hearers gently through the age-old problem of the "seat of the mind within the body". This has been a topic of misunderstanding and confusion ever since Greek times. Hippocrates gave the correct answer, but not Aristotle, and even Kant was unsure, saying, "No experience tells me that I am shut up in some place in my brain". Despite Aristotle's mistake in localizing the mind in the heart, Sherrington reminds us that we are indebted to Aristotle for general concepts such as 'common sense' and the materialistic view ". . . that the body and its thinking are just one substance". On the theme that knowledge of the brain need not be a prerequisite for advancing original ideas on the mind Sherrington refers to Freud.

> It is far from Aristotle to Freud. They are poles asunder. Yet the work of the two has resemblance in one respect. With both of them their study of the mind is wholly detached from anatomical features of the brain. Even as a background to the metaphors and parables, and classical myths, by means of which psycho-analysis proceeds to tell its story, the anatomy of the brain has no more part there than in the narration of, say, Bunyan's *Pilgrim's Progress*. Widely different from the symbolism and semi-drama of psycho-analytic writing, the compact descriptions of the De Anima are yet similarly remote from reference to gross anatomy; to minute anatomy they had of course no access.

Yet Freud's first publication was an anatomical study of the dorsal roots of the spinal cord! As a student of the brain Sherrington is disconsolate:

> Reference to the brain at present affords little help to the study of the mind. Ignorance of the 'how' of the tie between the brain and the mind there makes itself felt. That is no fault of those who study the mind or those who study the brain. It constitutes a disability common to both of them. A liaison between them is what each has been asking for. That there is a liaison neither of them doubts. The 'how' of it we must think remains for science as for philosophy a riddle pressing to be read. As things stand we cannot be sure that some of the very terms of approach to mental health and unhealth are not still on a plane with the 'humours' of medieval medicine.

> The mind was for Galen, as later for Fernel, a something incorporeal . . .
> The actions of life as far as mind pertains to it, operated the body by the spirits of the anima working the nervous system. The chambers of the brain were for Galen the place of generation and of common assembly of the animal spirits of the soul. Thence and thither they went and came to and from all parts along the nerves. The chambers were therefore the central seat of the operations of the mind and of its spirits.

There follows an excellent account of the origin of the Galenical theory of the vital spirits or spirits of the anima that originally had a basis in Galen's observations on the rhythmic pulsations of human brains exposed in warfare or gladiatorial games:

> Galen's eminence and the subsequent conspiracy of the ages to maintain and exalt it, carried this teaching not only unchallenged but hardened into dogma century after century, down to and beyond Descartes and Harvey. For Descartes however the spirits of the anima were definitely not incorporeal – they were a kind of 'flame', travelling with incredible velocity.

The end of this strangely misleading concept of vital spirits was remarkably slow in coming. Late in the seventeenth century Thomas Willis of Oxford

> . . . shifted the seat of the anima from the chambers of the brain to the actual substance of the brain itself. For him, the crust of the brain, grey in contrast to the underlying white

matter, was the great seat of the animal spirits. The large masses of grey matter bedded in the brain were, in like manner though to subsidiary extent, seats of these spirits of the soul. From the crust of the brain downward the masses of grey matter were threaded together by white matter. Willis's insight perceived that the white matter was fibrous much as nerve-trunks are fibrous.

Sherrington shares with his audience his great admiration for Willis, who on the basis of precise observation gave the first account of the conduction pathways from the brain.[1] "As to the 'localization' of mind, his view was that the higher up toward and into the grey crust of the brain a reflex action occurred the more did conscious mind attach to it."

Sherrington concludes: "Willis put the brain and nervous system on their modern footing, so far as that could be then done".

Sherrington becomes carried away by his imagination in his concluding historical review that is told in a dramatic form with rich poetic allusions. It should be recognized as a masterpiece in the history of ideas.

As for Galen's spirits of the anima, for Fernel, as workings of the anima, they belonged at once both to soul and to body. They were the mind and also what it bodily did. Descartes had brought them down to earth. For him although very subtle they were material, akin to flame. Their death-knell rang when Lucia Galvani told her husband Luigi that the frog's legs prepared for the meal seemed alive on the copper wire. Slowly and surely the ensuing century's analysis resolved this aspect ot the spirits of the anima into transient electrical potentials travelling the fibres of the nervous system. They were no longer 'spirit', but were become a physical event describable under energy.

Their innings had been long. It had lasted from Galen to Galvani. They had dominated medicine and biology through Alexandrian, Christian, Arabian and Jewish learning. Theirs had been a privileged position. The universe, the macrocosm, had its messengers, its 'angels', between the corporeal and the occult. So the microcosm, man, had similar messengers and these were they. They were analogous to the astrologers' 'astral fluid'. The more mysterious they were, the more votaries they had. In his sixteenth century, Fernel could write of them that they are therefore an ethereal substance, tie between the vital heat and the faculties (of the soul), the prime instrument of all function. They had seen much betide. They had seen the Empire become Christian. They had seen the Empire 'fall'. They had seen Christendom reconquer its conquerors; in all those phases they had endured as an abiding belief. They had seen the Mediterranean become, for a time, an Arabian lake, and along with Islam's domination, theirs had spread. They had seen kingdoms shape and nationhood arise, and their place had remained theirs in both. Vernacular tongues had replaced the classical even in Church and Medicine, and they had entered into them. They had been at the law-giving of Justinian and had outlived its decrees. When the known world expanded almost yearly they had expanded with it. They had in the scholastic age been a means of magic, of the basilisk's fascination and of the 'evil eye'. Scholasticism passed but they kept unchanged. They had outstayed wars and pestilence, political convulsion and religious schism. Then, late in the seventeenth and in the eighteenth and nineteenth centuries, their own dissolution had set in. It dated from Nature's coming under enquiry in a new way. It was neither political tyranny nor revolutionary violence which killed them. They expired quietly under the increasing pressure of an effort not

---

1 In conversation at Ipswich Sir Charles used to enthuse about Christopher Wren, Richard Lower and Thomas Millington, who assisted Willis with his dissections at Oxford, all seeking a relationship between brain structures and psychological processes.

consciously directed against themselves, but merely intent on first-hand enquiry into Nature with each step assured by observational experiment.

And so we descend to earth after this great display – actually back to the brain-mind problem.

Galen's spirits had worked the mind as well as the body. They had been a compromise, based on a confusion. They had confounded two incommensurable things. They had given divided allegiance and they fell between two thrones.

Their story is part of a more general one. Life, supra-material though it had seemed, as knowledge got nearer to it, had resolved itself into a complex of material factors; all of it, except one factor. There science stopped and stared as at an unexpected residue which remained after its solvents had dissolved the rest. Knowledge looking at its world had painfully and not without some disillusions arrived at two concepts; the one, that of energy, which was adequate to deal with all which was known to knowledge, except mind. But between energy and mind science found no 'how' of give and take. There was co-existence; that was all. To man's understanding the world remained obstinately double. Busy common sense went forward treating the two-fold together as one.

After much detailed consideration of the brain function such as sleep and waking, tonus, vigilance, as they are understood in modern brain-science, Sherrington returns to the theme of the mind-brain problem at the end of the lecture. His expressions now have a strong dualist flavour.

The two concepts mind and energy, which our experience finds, using the one where the other fails, cover all our experience, are both of course in themselves creations of thought. But what they respectively stand for still remains divided as having nothing in common except time and this curious one and only point of spatial relation, namely 'collocation in the brain'.

...The brain and the psyche lie together, so to say, on a knife's edge. Whatever the solution of the problem we can here feel this. That in the energy-pattern which is the brain, two sets of events happen such as, to human knowledge, happen nowhere else the perceptible universe over. In that universe, sampling it, standing where we do on our planet's side, ourselves compact of energy, nowhere does our glimpse detect in all the immensity of energy any relation of energy other than to energy save in this one instance, the brain. There energy and mind seem in liaison as to place.

Then follows an amusing aside with deep meaning for us in society:

Mind, always, as we know it, finite and individual, is individually insulated and devoid of direct liaison with other minds . . . By means of the brain, liaison as it is between mind and energy, the finite mind obtains indirect liaison with other finite minds around it. Energy is the medium of this the indirect, but sole, liaison between mind and mind . . . Speech, to instance a detail, illustrates this indirect liaison by means of energy between finite mind and finite mind. I have seen the question asked 'why should mind have a body'? The answer may well run 'to mediate between it and other mind' . . . It might be objected that such a view is undiluted 'anthropism'. To that we might reply, anthropism seems the present aim of the planet, though presumably not its enduring aim.

Sherrington continues on this theme to the end of the lecture with a personification, even deification, of the planet and in a manner that is reminiscent of Teilhard de Chardin, though of course not derived from Teilhard, who was later.

It may be that the aim toward which what we observe as progress moves includes the human as step to a further stage, of which we may forecast it will be supra-human. If mind, as we experience it and argue it in others, seem to itself that which the programme of the planet has aimed at, and if communication between mind and mind foster more mind, then to hesitate to read this message because it seem 'anthropic' is to be blind to our cause and to that of our planet, of which latter cause, it would seem for the moment, ours is a part.

ix. Brain Collaborates With Psyche

In the ninth lecture Sherrington begins to grapple firmly with the problem of mind, but always with his characteristic questioning and imaginative asides. The theme of the evolutionary origin of mind leads to an expression of panpsychism. Sherrington is a very strict evolutionist and as such states, ". . . evolution does not create".

> Traced . . . upwards, it would seem that, at least as regards cognition, mind as we know it has for this present its acme in the mind of man. Has the evolution of the brain produced mind out of no mind? But we have seen evolution does not create. All it does is, out of something which was, to construct something further. The fundamental is still unchangeably there. Mind we think of as *sui generis*. Admittedly it seems not physical energy. The energy-concept of Science collects all so-called 'forms' of energy into a flock and looks in vain for mind among them. But mind has evolved. What has evolution had to evolve mind from? What has mind evolved from? Has the evolution of the brain compassed the evolution of the mind or how has the evolution of the mind accompanied that of the brain? It is as though the elementary mental had never been wanting; as though evolution in dealing with the brain had taken that elementary mental and developed it until it blossomed into evidence.

We give this passage in full because it is an indubitable expression of panpsychism. Yet at other times Sherrington is not so sure. On this basis Granit (1966) concludes: "His is a Natural Religion and if a name for describing his standpoint be wanted, it is 'Evolutionary Pantheism'". We will examine this appellation after we finish the detailed consideration of the book. The origin of mind in the evolutionary process raises the related question of its origin in the embryological process. For Fernel there is no problem as he writes: "Created at the beginning by the sovereign Author of all things this part of the soul passes from or comes into the body in a moment. The infant is prepared and formed for it. It is believed that its entry happens in the fourth month, by which time the heart and brain are already there and complete".

"The recital trips along simple as a fairy tale" is Sherrington's kindly aside, and he then goes on to give the most that can be said by modern biology.

> The initial stage of each individual of us . . . is a single cell . . . We have agreed that mind is not recognizable in any single cell we ever meet with. And who shall discover it in the little

mulberry-mass which for each of us is our all a little later than the one-cell stage; or even in Fernel's 40 day embryo? Yet who shall deny it in the child which in a few months' time that embryo becomes? Here again mind seems to emerge from no mind. So, conversely, at death it seems to re-emerge into no mind. Energy is indestructible and that it is so Natural Science finds, in so far, demonstrable. But mind seems to come from nothing and to return to nothing. The devolution into nothing seems as difficult to accept as the evolution out of nothing. If the mental were some form of the energy it so adheres to, the story would be no more than one of energy-transformation. But Science fails us if we ask it for a form of energy which is mental.

The dilemma is complete. The enquiry then moves to the single nerve cell.

That the brain derives its mind additively from a cumulative mental property of the individual cells composing it, has therefore no support from any facts of its cell-structure. For a classroom to exhibit an isolated brain-cell and label it large 'The organ of thought', may be dramatic pedagogy; it is certainly pedagogical overstatement. The cell-organization of the brain may be the key to the secret of its correlation with mind; but not, it would seem, by individual mental endowment of its constituent cells.

So the enquiry returns to the motor act which earlier was seen to have a close tie with mind, but this is not true of simple reflexes.

I cannot by any effort of my will evoke my knee-jerk. Likewise I do not directly experience it ... It is not so with my hand sketching; I do control its act and do directly experience it acting. My experience then is that it is 'I' doing the drawing. If I am told, as indeed science tells me, that I, as mind, have had nothing to do with this act of drawing except as an onlooker, I find that puzzling.
The dilemma goes further. The motor behaviour of the individual is our only contact with his individuality. Indirect indication of him though it be, we in that way interpret him and allow him 'values', moral, aesthetic, etc. We infer he will do a generous act because we have inferred of him a generous mind. We attribute his acts to his mental character which we have inferred from his acts. We even fancy that our mental opinion of him can influence our own motor behaviour toward him. I have come to regard my words as an outcome of such thoughts as I have. When I ask science to tell me how all this is so, science vouchsafes me no reply. If I ask again she tells me it is none of her business; that though spoken words are energy, thoughts are not.

The enquiry is at an impasse as recounted in this simple-minded way, with reliance on the deliverances of materialistic science.
So Sherrington develops a more sophisticated approach to human actions.

The climax of mental integration would seem to be 'attention' ... The 'willed' act is but a culmination of attention. Where is an instance of completer solidarity in a complex organism than a man intent and concentrated upon some act of strenuous 'will'? But the willed act in man presents itself notably in two forms. It may lay under contribution the whole muscular system of the body and every channel of sense. Or it may well-nigh forgo muscular action and well-nigh exclude every channel of sense. This latter kind of integrated act is practically man's alone, as in pondering a problem. The anthropoid primates have not it. But can we imagine man, even primitive man, without it? Rodin's statue portrays prehistoric man erect with hand to forehead essaying abstract thought. His too is that other statue, seated, the 'penseur' absorbed in abstraction.
Nature has dealt with integrated act and integrated mind together; has fostered them together, as a united growth. One tie between them is concurrence in time and collocation in the brain; another is that both compass the same end.

At this stage of the lecture Sherrington reverts to his work of the late 1890s on the combination in visual experience of the inputs from the two eyes.

> It is much as though the right- and left-eye images were seen each by one of two observers and the minds of the two observers were combined to a single mind. It is as though the right-eye and left-eye perceptions are elaborated singly, and then psychically combine to one. The synthesis is a mental one in which the finite mind uses 'time' as synthesiser. We know too that the mind is actively operative in the synthesis. We can take an instance where the two components R and L differ perceptibly; their synthesis on contemporaneous presentation still occurs. With difference in tint between the right- and left-eye percepts the synthesised percept which results binocularly is of intermediate tint. The red and green postage-stamp thus combined is perceived as sheeny bronze. Contemporaneity here finds the percepts no merely passive material but active on each other.

This argues that the perceptual experiences have an independence from the brain events from which they are derived.

> ... the mind integrates the two to a unity not different from either component when the two components are not noticeably dissimilar. And when the two components are noticeably dissimilar they are fused to a compromise between the two. The two components can be so dissimilar as not to fuse. They then alternate in consciousness. In all this there is no evidence that the mind-brain correlation requires in any of these combinings the brain to provide spatial conjunction of the two component processes. All that is wanted is their concurrence in time.

It is suggested that there is a level of independence of mental experiences from the brain events. There is further evidence on this theme from other experiments on perception.

> The mental 'now' is a unity, because whatever its items they conjoin to one significant pattern.
> That unifying of experience of the moment is an aspect of the unity of the 'I'. There are the psychological figures, called equivocal because at one moment they look one thing, at another another. While looked at their 'meaning' unaccountably changes; what is being looked at as a set of steps suddenly without warning becomes an overhanging cornice . . . But it is always the one or the other wholly. Is it to over-simplify to liken to that the mind's interpretation of its 'now' – always a situation with a single meaning? It is an integrated experience which is one situation at a time. Just as the integrated individual, even for those who regard the individual as a machine, is a machine which can do many things, yet a machine which at any time does but one main thing.

The full theoretical implication of the interpretation of such psychological figures has not yet been realized. They certainly indicate an amazing mental construction beyond the triggering brain events. The unity of the perceptual experience leads to the suggestion of convergence with

> ... culmination in final supreme convergence on one ultimate pontifical nerve-cell, a cell the climax of the whole system of integration. Such would be a spatial climax to a system of centralization. It would secure integration by receiving all and dispensing all as unitary arbiter of a totalitarian State. But convergence toward the brain offers in fact nothing of that kind. The brain region which we may call 'mental' is not a concentration into one cell but an enormous expansion into millions of cells. They are it is true richly interconnected.

Where it is a question of 'mind' the nervous system does not integrate itself by centralization upon one pontifical cell. Rather it elaborates a millionfold democracy whose each unit is a cell.

We can agree with this conclusion, but the great enigma remains. How can this democracy be unified in the perceptual experience? After much discussion of this problem there is no satisfying solution. It is all the more disturbing in the light of the detailed considerations of modern neurophysiology. In this dilemma Sherrington quotes from a dogmatic statement of last century when no such problem was admitted:

"The thoughts to which I am now giving utterance and your thoughts regarding them are the expression of molecular changes in that matter of life which is the source of our other vital phenomena" (Huxley.) The terminology is a little 'dated', but is the main position thus set forth altered today? The concomitance in time and place between the 'molecular changes' and 'the thoughts' is still all we have correlating the two. Regarded as a paradox it has become more intriguing; regarded as a gap in knowledge more urgent.
It has its practical consequences. One is that in the training and in the exercise of medicine a remoteness abides between the field of neurology and that of mental health, psychiatry. It is sometimes blamed to prejudice on the part of the one side or the other . . . It has a reasonable basis. It is rooted in the energy-mind problem. Physiology has not enough to offer about the brain in relation to the mind to lend the psychiatrist much help. It has occupied itself largely with what are called the lower levels of nervous action. Results of general value have emerged. The nature of the nerve-impulse, the properties of cell-contacts as one-way gates compelling one-way traffic on nerve-paths, the occurrence not only of action but of active suppression of action, the knowledge that intensity of action means not larger impulses but more frequent impulses, that impulse-effects can sum, or cancel, that there are places where impulses spontaneously arise. Much of this knowledge certainly applies to the brain, and to that part of it which interests us here, the roof of the forebrain. Every nerve-cell of the millions in it is clearly at a glance a nerve-cell. But nerve-cells as a class are elsewhere not specially concerned with mind. It is partly conjecture whether the properties of all these nerve-cells, their fibres, their cell-contacts (synapses), their cell-bodies, have rigidly those characters observed in the more accessible nerve-cells of the spinal cord and elsewhere. That the properties will not differ fundamentally from those elsewhere seems safe to suppose.

Yet the mystery remains – and even is intensified. A consequence is the remoteness between the fields of neurology and psychiatry. With what structural arrangement can recognizable mind be associated is an ever-present and fundamental problem. Sherrington then offers a diversion in suggesting that responses to pain and injury are particularly limited to the unification of the mental experiences. We do not find the appeal to the unifying action of 'affect' convincing.

Sherrington probably also has misgivings, so he continues:

The neural basis of affect we can suppose need not entail much neural superstructure. It might use chemical reinforcement. This lets us stress the roof-organ of the forebrain as especially cognitive, with below it the old kernel-organ of the forebrain especially related to 'affect'; and we remember that every cognition has, potentially at least, an emotive value; emotive, and, along with that, conative effort as a further factor. How do they hang together? What is the significance of their so doing? Not in man alone but infra-humanly in due degrees, no doubt less cognitive. What is the tie which conjoins these several aspects of mind so inseparably? What is it else than 'urge-to-live'? Human cognition may like the winged horse take at times its flights toward the stars and forget earth. None the less it is harnessed to life's car, whose charioteer is 'urge-to-live' sublimed to 'zest-to-live'. It and its fellow-steeds, endeavour, will, emotion, passion or whatever else we call them, pull under the same lash.

Again Sherrington expresses concern at the little help brain physiology can give to the psychiatrist. He asks, "What has cerebral physiology to offer on the whole subject of 'anxiety'?" . . . "The mental is not examinable as a form of energy. That in brief is the gap which parts psychiatry and physiology: No mere running round the cycle of the 'forms of energy' takes us across that chasm".

Sherrington recognizes the impasse, adopting the role of Brutus in Fernel's dialogue!

> In such an impasse it seems permissible for the man in the street, such as myself, to outline to himself briefly, although he can do so but naively, the position.
> What is the reply when to . . . the follower of Natural Science, there comes today someone who asks, 'Mind presents itself as thoughts, feelings, and so on. They are the outcome of the brain. The brain is matter, energy. Matter and energy can only be matter and energy. Therefore thoughts, feelings and so on are matter and energy. Therefore mind is matter and energy?' I trust I do no violence to the argument; I have no wish to do so. The reply by the follower of Natural Science of today, if I as a man in the street may guess it, will be . . . of a different order. As I surmise it, it would say: 'Thoughts, feelings, and so on are not amenable to the energy (matter) concept. They lie outside it. Therefore they lie outside Natural Science. If as you say thoughts are an outcome of the brain we as students using the energy-concept know nothing of it.

So as a student of neurobiology Sherrington finds that he is not helped by orthodox chemistry and physics in his attempts to account for mental phenomena.

> But though living is analysable and describable by natural science, that associate of living, thought, escapes and remains refractory to natural science. In fact natural science repudiates it as something outside its ken. A radical distinction has therefore arisen between life and mind. The former is an affair of chemistry and physics; the latter escapes chemistry and physics. And yet the occurrence of mind – recognizable finite mind . . . appears as a phase of living. If, as is practical, we continue to subsume mind under life, we have to distinguish it as an activity of life selectively and uniquely apart from the rest. The psychophysical difficulty places us in the position of empirics as to much. By ways which may be judged roundabout, we find ourselves at length pragmatically alongside of general commonsense opinion. That may be taken either as sanity or superficiality or perhaps both.

In the conclusion Sherrington returns to the easy position of Fernel with nostalgia:

> For Fernel there was duality but that duality created a situation of no difficulty. Its members, matter and spirit, combined in perfectly satisfying co-operation. Matter was the servant. Spirit, mind, was the master. Perhaps that was from the Phaedo, where we remember the soul rules, the body obeys. Today the duality is there; and combination is

there, but the footing on which the combination rests, so obvious to Fernel, is for our enquiry still to seek. Perhaps the 'servant and master' phrase had in view an assertion of free-will. But where in nature shall we find 'servant and master'? Where our knowledge halts our description will resort to metaphor. Long will man's fancy deal with the tie between body and mind by metaphor and often half forget the while that metaphor it is. Regarding this problem will a day come when metaphors can be dispensed with?

This last very subtle linguistic comment reveals Sherrington's poetic thinking. It appears at so many places in this book, giving it a unique charm. But we can realize that we have been treated to a diversion. It is a temporary expedient. In the next two chapters there is much deep thinking and argumentation on the brain-mind problem.

x. Earth's Alchemy

The tenth lecture begins with a reconsideration of the relationship of the theme of the lectures so far given to Natural Theology:

Our topic of last time asked of and how it is that our thinking is correlated with our brain. If Natural Theology argue from the facts of Nature to a Divine Scheme to which they may point, then that question seems germane to our theme. It lies at the threshold of human approach to the whole Natural Scheme.

Unaided human sight will at best compass but a corner of the scheme. There will be much to which man has not access. The distances are immense and he is near-sighted. He peers into a small patch and what he sees there he submits to his reason which after all is very newly hatched. What wonder if his conclusions be meagre and insecure. What wonder they are narrowly anthropomorphic. Such they must be. That indeed is to him perhaps their chiefest value at this present. Without that they would not yield him, we may think, the zest, courage, ambition, altruism, which they do, or to come to our point, the idea of the Divine.

The great unifying principle of science is referred to by Sherrington as the energy-concept by which he means explanations based on physics and chemistry. Thus the phenomena of biology are reducible to physics and chemistry. Much of this lecture is devoted to building up the evidence and in illustrating the universality of this concept in providing explanations of the whole natural world.

Within the descriptive competence of this unification comes our whole perceptible world, what it is and what it does. The sailing cloud, the bird below it, the setting sun, the coast and sea, the ship and harbour, the lighted window, the flock and the grass down, the voice of the shepherd, it unites these all into one consistent existence whose identical underlying nature becomes through it in so far intelligible to us. Their seemingly endless variety gains thus for man the interest of a concerted system, and, making the interest more poignant, himself is one with them.

The speculations of Democritus and Lucretius cannot be put beside this scheme. They were relatively to it essays in fancy, motivated in their time perhaps chiefly as challenges to the Olympus of the day. The scheme arrived at now by Science is the fruit of patient toil, sifting out facts and in search of more facts, and exercising, it has been said, 'remorseless logic'. It has no tilt against religion as such. It knows its own field to be vast, but also knows it limited.

Thus, a difficulty which ... still haunted our representative of the sixteenth century, Fernel, was the association of 'form' and 'material'. It had exercised Aristotle. Today the single concept, the energy-concept, includes and relates both. Again, in the Middle Ages, and after them with Fernel, as with Aristotle before, there was the difficulty of the animate and the inanimate and the finding of the boundary between them. Today's scheme makes plain why that difficulty was, and dissolves it. There is no boundary.

All of the expositions of the explanatory power of the energy-concept, particularly in its modern form of subatomic particles, have at the same time to recognize that there are limitations.

The energy-concept, we saw, embraces and unifies much ... The scheme seems coterminous with the perceptible. Therein lies its immensity and also its limitation. Immense as it is, and self-satisfying as it is, and self-contained as it is, it yet seems but an introduction to something else.

For instance a star which we perceive. The energy-scheme deals with it, describes the passing of radiation thence into the eye, the little light-image of it formed at the bottom of the eye, the ensuing photo-chemical action in the retina, the trains of action-potentials travelling along the nerve to the brain, the further electrical disturbance in the brain ...

But, as to our *seeing* the star it says nothing. That to our perception it is bright, has direction, has distance, that the image at the bottom of the eye-ball turns into a star overhead, a star moreover that does not move though we and our eyes as we move carry the image with us, and finally that it is the thing a star, endorsed by our cognition, about all this the energy-scheme has nothing to report. The energy-scheme deals with the star as one of the objects observable by us; as to the perceiving of it by the mind the scheme puts its finger to its lip and is silent. It may be said to bring us to the threshold of the act of perceiving, and there to bid us 'goodbye'. Its scheme seems to carry up to and through the very place and time which correlate with the mental experience, but to do so without one hint further.

Thus Sherrington despairs of the ability of the energy-concept to explain thoughts, memories, feelings, reasonings.

So with the whole of mental experience, the energy-scheme leaves it aside and does not touch it. Our mental experience is not open to observation through any sense-organ ... The mental act of 'knowing' we are aware of, but we cannot sensually observe it. It is experienced, not observed ... The attempt to turn observation upon it seems to fail somewhat as an attempt to do two things at one time can impair the doing of each . . . It is an attempt at disintegration of the self. It were probably better to have recourse to memory, and to calling up the memorial traces of the mental act which it is desired to make the object of observation.

This suggestion of Sherrington of recourse to memory would have answered the problem raised by Hume that he could never catch himself in any mental performances. Then follows an example of mental experience that savours of Sherrington's status as Brutus, the man-in-the-street.

Thus we are looking at an aeroplane when we hear a cry from the street. Into the consequent new situation the cry perceived, that is the cry as a mental event, enters as a factor ... It contains (it may be) emotional affect. Leaving that aside let us call it for the moment a 'percept'. As percept it is a complex of certain mental components, a something heard, with 'place' 'in the street', with time 'now', and as to kind or 'species' 'a human voice', it may be 'a child's voice'. Whence is all this? The physical sound in the ear was just a physical vibration. How did it generate this mental complex which seems suddenly to invade mind full-fledged? It cannot have been born full-fledged. It must have gone through a becoming. That is, its activity has undergone some change, in which it would seem various factors were confluent. It has mental structure. How was it produced? Out of what was it constructed? Our experience does not say. It is as we experience it an already constructed complex. We have no awareness of it before then. Its beginnings are unreachable by our mind, though our mind is the only means which could reach them. There would seem therefore to be a grade or grades of mind which we do not experience, as well as the mind which is our mental experience.

By this vivid description and argument we are made aware of the extraordinary problems and mystery underlying a simple experience such as every day we encounter on numerous occasions. Sherrington goes on to develop the inference that there are grades of the mental, a pre-experiential stage, that we are not aware of. He illustrated this idea by stating:

It is as though our mind were a pool of which the movements on the surface only are what we experience. In the situation we spoke of, the cry was a disturbance gaining entrance somewhere at the bottom of the mental pool. Travelling upwards through the pool it shapes itself and accretes to itself and grows, until reaching the surface it contributes in the form of a percept to the general disturbance obtaining there, and is experienced as part of the mental situation or action which for the time being is experienced. The mind we experience, that is, which *is* our mental experience seems to emerge from elements of mind which we do not experience. Here we have not to do with the unconscious of Freud which is only temporarily unconscious, and has been conscious once and may be again. That belongs to a mind of a different grade, and a sphere of reaction other than we are thinking of now. In our rough simile of the pool, the unconscious of Freud would be itself of the surface of the pool, but a piece of surface which lay as it were by a charm restrained for the time from entering activity, and therefore from participating in the general consciousness, a restraint which we might correlate with the inhibition which visits the nervous system far and wide.

This pictorial analogy can help to bridge the gap between neurophysiology and psychiatry – the gap that Sherrington had earlier deplored. Nevertheless he recognized how little we have advanced since classical times in the analysis of mind.

Since classical times physical science has taken the perceptible world and so described its doings as to make of their entirety a new world of thought. But progress of knowledge has not done anything like that where its object is mind.
The complaint is sometimes heard that 'we have learned to control nature before we have learned to control ourselves'. But to bring such a complaint against civilization is to forget that the two theses are not comparable. Their problems do not fall even within the same category. If we are pushed to assess the two comparatively we find the latter not only vastly different but vastly the more difficult of accomplishment.
No attributes of 'energy' seem findable in the processes of mind. That absence hampers explanation of the tie between cerebral and mental. Where the brain correlates with mind, no microscopical, no physical, no chemical means detect any radical difference between it and other nerve which does not correlate with mind.

> The two for all I can do remain refractorily apart. They seem to me disparate; not mutually convertible; untranslatable the one into the other.

Here we have a strong and unambiguous statement of dualism. After this climax of the lecture he goes on to develop the theme and to give specific examples:

> How can a reaction in the brain condition a reaction in the mind? Yet what have we sense-organs for, if not for that? This difficulty with sense is the same difficulty, from the converse side, as besets the problem of the mind as influencing our motor acts.
>
> I would submit that we have to accept the correlation, and to view it as interaction; body → mind . . . then we get surround ⇌ body ⇌ mind. The sun's energy is part of the closed energy-cycle. What leverage can it have on mind? Yet through my retina and brain it seems able to act on my mind. The theoretically impossible happens. In fine, I assert that it does act on my mind. Conversely my thinking 'self' thinks that it can bend my arm. Physics tells me that my arm cannot be bent without disturbing the sun. Physics tells me that unless my mind is energy it cannot disturb the sun. My mind then does not bend my arm. Or, the theoretically impossible happens. Let me prefer to think the theoretically impossible does happen. Despite the theoretical I take it my mind *does* bend my arm, and that it disturbs the sun.

Sherrington seems to regard this as the definitive statement on voluntary action.

The theme of the lecture then moves to such questions as to where the mind is within the brain. Evidently it is not at a Euclidean-point as Kant opined, but can be dispersed over liaison areas of the brain. The final message of the lecture concerns the history of the planet earth. He traces the experimental evidence on psychical experiences and the neuronal disturbances of the brain and eventually comes to recognize the creative contributions of modern neurosciences.

> Nature has evolved us as compounds of energy and mind. The scene of this operation has been the planet where we are. I would submit with deference that for one of like gift to the historian, here is a theme whose telling would be welcome to humanity. A theme which I would still think of as historical although much of it run back beyond tradition. Even if as fact it be too cloudy for history, it is yet worth telling as an available truth: the planet's story with what it has made and done . . .
>
> It is a story not remote for us because it is our own. The planet in travail with its children. With the Universe as heroic background for what to us is an intimate and an heroic epic. A birth in cataclysm. Aeons of seething and momentous shaping. A triple scum of rock and tide and vapour – the planet's side – swept on through day and night. Then from that side arising shape after shape, past fancy. And latterly among them some imbued with sense and thought. And still more latterly, some with thought eager for 'values'. The planet, furnace of molten rocks and metals, now yielding thoughts and 'values'! Magic furnace. Beside its alchemy and transmutations the most impassioned dreams of Hermes Trismegistus and all his fellowship dwindle to paltry nothing. Man in his mood may count himself in his day a brief spectator of his own shaping as it still progresses . . .
>
> Remembering life as a grade of organization he sees progressive organization in the planet include life and promise more life. At one time it had not that organization which means life. He envisages energy as the vehicle for mind, progressing under Progressive organization of those types of system which unfold life. The whole presents itself as one great

graduated scale of surging organization. He reflects that at one time the planet can have had none of his particular variety of system. Now it has. That is, it has evolved recognizable mind. This has issued from its side, at the interface where atmosphere and other physical phases meet, under alternate day and night. The planet has thus latterly become a place of thinking. More, it now harbours mind which values 'values'. It is a planet now with hopes and fears and tentative 'right' and 'wrong'. A planet which is human. What will be to follow? Our pragmatic spectator watching his mother-earth believes that there will come forth from her side more mind, and still more mind. The further evolution of energy-systems will he thinks accomplish that. Perhaps for that they strive. In believing this, he is not doubtful of touch between energy and mind.

Unfortunately this intoxicating prospect of indefinitely extended progress to the suprahuman has become an example of science fiction. Biological evolution has now ceased to be effective. The welfare state has eliminated the operation of natural selection, which even operates in reverse. Terrestrial evolution will never cause the development of creatures with brains superior to the present human brains. We have to remember that biological evolution could be effective only with the most brutal behaviour of beings subjected to harsh conditions that threaten survival. Yet the human future is not without hope, because cultural evolution gives opportunity for the progressive development of mankind.

xi. Two Ways of One Mind

In this climactic lecture Sherrington once again raises the question of the relation between the two concepts 'energy' and 'mind'. It is a remarkable exposition, for he brings his superb imaginative power to bear on this most difficult of all questions.

It has theoretical importance; that is perhaps generally admitted. But its claim to practical importance is apt to raise a smile. Yet the question surely touches the reading of man's situation in his world.
We need not think of it as an issue between idealism and materialism. Nor does it touch so-called 'reality'; our world is in any case an act of mind. It asks rather whether the world, as our mind apprehends it, is for one part of it known to us in one way, for its other part known to us in another, the two ways not of essential parity.

At the beginning of his attempt to answer this great question he returns to the motor act.

In the evolution of mind a starting point for 'recognizable' mind lay in its connection with motor acts. Motor behaviour would seem the cradle of recognizable mind. I incline to endorse the challenging remark (of McDougall) that, 'the most fundamental function of mind is to guide bodily movement so as to change our relation to objects about us.' Moreover the motor act, is that which seems to clinch the distinction between self and not-self. The doer's doings affirm the self.

This introduction to the 'self' prompts him to say:

The concept 'self' taken with all its connotations has become vastly far-reaching and intricate. Yet it would seem to have at its core an element relatively simple, germane to our question here. The awareness or consciousness of each of us, prominent in certain of our motor acts, relates the self to the act. The awareness is of course an example of what in the abstract is spoken of as mind. It seems a law of mind to connect its phenomena by relations. The awareness attaching to these motor acts relates the conscious 'self' to the acts as doing them.

Sherrington then goes on to make a most important statement. The awareness is traceable to two sources: One is sensual with a detailed perception of the act derived from a battery of sense organs and having spatial reference, e. g. of a limb moving; the other is the direct awareness of the 'I-doing' or of the self-doing, and it is not derived from sense. This duality gives the theme for much of this lecture. It forms the experiential basis of the dualism that was central to Sherrington's philosophy.

The sensual component has the unique attribute of projection into a sensual space: "To see a thing is to see it somewhere, and so with all the other senses." This sensual space is always three-dimensional or Euclidean space with the self set central to it.

Projection applies to the radial distance from that percipient self. Awareness, which is the self, identifies together as one 'self' the successive various phases of itself, the I-perceiving, the I-doing a motor act, the I-feeling, etc. Whichever self it is, it is central in sensual space. In no direction of sensual space is the 'I' projected. Yet its centrality is somewhat vague. Perhaps we can put it best by saying that it is always more central than is what it perceives.

The theme leads back to the 'conscious motor act'. It is a field of science in which Sherrington is a master and never has he spoken to such effect as here. He is not content with some text-book platitudes, or with some carefully worded explanations that cover over the great unknowns in these so commonplace events.

The bodily movement is . . . distinguished from the 'I'. The mind, finding relations between phenomena, seeks also to couple some phenomena as cause and effect. This bent or tendency has served it well. Whatever it may mean, it has helped to sift events conjoined by sequence in time. The mind relates the 'I-doing' in the conscious motor act causally with the act. The unprojected 'I' is the 'cause' and the projected motor act is the 'effect'.

It is ". . . one of those unanalysable workings of the mind which are practically tantamount to inference but are drawn unconsciously and often so quickly that the conclusion is reached before there would seem time for full comprehension of the data" . . .
"There seems a whole field, or many fields, of such unconscious mind. Unconscious mind in a meaning, as we said, quite other than the Freudian."

Relentlessly Sherrington develops his train of thought to a clear and challenging expression.

This 'I' which when I move my hand I experience as 'I-doing', how do I perceive it? I do not perceive it. If perception means awareness through sense I do not perceive the 'I'. My awareness and myself are one. I experience it. The 'I-doing' is my awareness of myself in the motor act.

In it my 'self' is not an object which I can examine through sense. As compared with the latter I am at the disadvantage that I cannot submit this to others besides myself to examine and report on. It is private to myself, but each of us can examine his own case. For examining it, all we can do is to attend to what we are aware of in it.

Sherrington shows that he is aware of the criticism and the rejection of introspective evidence that was so fashionable at that time. He even goes so far as to say:

Even if the mind had a sense-organ which were turned inward, so to say upon the mind itself, what would it fulfil? Broadly taken, and briefly, and crudely put, if the purpose of sense be to translate events physical and chemical into mental, what use would it serve in application to the mind which is already mental?

He then reverts to and amplifies an earlier suggestion of the use of memory.

But the mind does experience itself. Memory attaches to that experience. The self can remember and re-live at second-hand and reflect upon its experience of itself. It can think over what its experience in 'doing' was. That perhaps is more effective than the divided effort of trying to examine the awareness actually while the awareness is in process.

At this stage he refers to clinical conditions that provide clear evidence for the duality of the awareness of a conscious act. By disease or injury the sensual awareness of the limb may be stripped away though its motor power is retained in a disordered form. His evidence is convincing.

But the motor act is still evoked and consciously although there is no sensual perception of the limb. The 'I' still experiences itself in acting.

It is true the motor act executed by the insentient limb is clumsy. That it is executed at all and consciously 'at will' is here the point. The launching of it as a conscious act although the sensory basis for it, and the sensual perception of it, are wanting, indicates that this 'I-acting' is not derived from sense-perception but is directly given.

Having disposed of these problems about the effectiveness of I-doing Sherrington reaches the climax of this lecture and even of the whole lecture series. It is an impassioned and even exultant paean for the self.

This 'I', this 'self', which can so vividly propose to 'do', what attributes as regards 'doing' does it appear to itself to have? It counts itself as a 'cause'. Do we not each think of our 'I' as a 'cause' within our body? 'Within' inasmuch as it is at the core of the spatial world, which our perception seems to look out at from our body. The body seems a zone immediately about that central core. This 'I' belongs more immediately to our awareness than does even the spatial world about us, for it is directly experienced. It *is* the 'self'. Yet never has it been seen, or felt, or although it has language has it been heard. It believes it is in daily commerce with many of like kind with itself but never have they any more than itself been seen or felt or heard by it or by any of themselves. Invisible, intangible, imperceptible, it is inaccessible to sense, although to itself directly known. Even if it be in the body it is clearly no part of the body. It contrasts with the body.

The 'I' intuits a special relation between this body and itself. It signifies this by applying to the body the terms 'me' and 'mine'. The 'I' in short is aware of itself as an *embodied* 'I'.

This raises the question of where in the body is the 'I'? Sherrington gives his characteristically subtle replies after illustrating replies to sensually perceived objects, which are always 'there'.

> But 'self' is never 'there'. It is 'here'. If pressed where 'here' is, what will it say? 'In the body?' Were we to demur; were we to expostulate with it and say 'you are not spatial; how can you have place?' I think it might retort slyly, 'have not philosophers complained for me that I am prisoned in the body!'
>
> Descartes, wrote in the *De Homine* after describing the animal as a machine, 'of a truth, I should say, were God to add to this machine (man) a reasoning soul, the place he would give it would be the brain!' We may infer from this that the spatial scene he gave to his famous 'Cogito ergo sum' was cerebral.
>
> Kant . . . says of the soul that it has its seat in the brain; it sits there he says like a spider at the centre of its web. From that seat it puts into movement the ropes and levers of the whole machine. It produces at pleasure 'voluntary movements'. The body is an artificial machine in which the coming together of the nerves is condition for the faculties of thinking and willing – which seems an echo from Aristotle or the Theaetetus.

Then follows one of Sherrington's delightful anecdotes that so often sparkled in his conversation. There is a gentle irony in his aside on the 'true cells'.

> There comes to my recollection an answer given by an authority of international recognition on the brain. He had shown us with his microscope the cells in a tumour of the brain. To the question whether any thinking would be done by them, he replied: 'This tumour is only of the supporting cells, not of the true cerebral cells'. The true cells evidently would think – not perhaps in a tumour because imperfectly organized there. Today's opinion therefore is in this less removed from Aristotle than from Kant. Our interest here, however, is the confirmation from the two philosophers of the want of spatial connotation attaching to the 'I', except as to a certain 'whereness', which sets it within the somewhat indirectly sense-given space-system of the brain.
>
> We, I fancy, shall all agree that the awareness which is the 'I', or 'self' has its different dominant phases. Sometimes it is dominantly the 'I-doing', sometimes dominantly the 'I-feeling', sometimes dominantly the 'I-perceiving' and so on. In all these situations, perhaps especially the last, the 'I' finds itself surrounded by sensual space, but that space never actually attaches to it or gives it extension. Sensual space never gets grip of the 'I'.

The theme of sensual awareness leads on to distinctive features of the external world and the body.

> The external world unlike the body harbours no 'pains'; unlike the body it is not one thing only, but multitudes of things. It is a time-space-frame populated with 'things'.
>
> Visual contour dominates visual space. Perceptually a contour is a line. When we hear that Nature has no such thing as a line, vision answers that all contours are lines. That every contact of fields of light or colour is sharpened and stressed into a line – a psychological line. 'Contrast' develops a 'line' at every contact between abruptly distinguishable areas. If the mind did not deal in 'lines' an outline drawing could hardly be the magical thing it can be.

Sherrington the sensitive appreciator of art is here displayed in this short reference to visual experience. There is well expressed the sensory counterpart of more recent physiological experiments of Hubel and Wiesel and others to the effect that the cells of the primary visual cortex are detectors of lines or edges and exhibit specificity for orientation.

With binocular vision space is oriented in relation to the 'I-seeing' which is looking out through a single eye, a cyclopean eye, that it takes to be ". . . low down in the mid-vertical of the forehead". Its point of outlook it senses as not being in the brain at all, but in the nasal bone! Sherrington goes on tentatively to suggest an experiment.

> It might be interesting to know how far this *locus* given for the mental 'eye' agrees or not with, for instance, that given proprioceptively for a perceiving 'self' reaching out with the arm in various directions. There would be only working agreement between the two. Moreover the whereness of the viewpoint of visual perception changes, as the rifleman knows, when for taking aim he excludes the 'other' eye.

One can hardly imagine how fascinated Sherrington could have been by the exquisite experiments on binocular vision and depth perception carried out by Bela Julesz in recent times.

There is now further development of the theme of the location of the self. It appears to be determined in some subconscious manner as though the whole spatial surround were subtended inwards to a vanishing point. His theme then moves from the spatial to the temporal.

> The 'self' is aware of self not only as 'here' but as 'now'. The 'I' endures in time. Just as space is a continuum for it, so also is time, but time is a continuum which moves . . . In our time-continuum we distinguish brief stationary cross-sections of the flow and speak of each such as 'now'. That such a 'now' is an artefact does not prevent it from serving to integrate the 'I'. The mental items embraced by any 'now' compose one integral whole, which is the 'self' of the moment. Mental contemporaneity, apart from any necessary cerebral conjunction in space, combines them.
> Conation, an attribute of the 'I', deals with a 'now' which has yet to be; and memory, another attribute of the 'I', recalls a 'now' that was. There are therefore future 'nows' and past 'nows'. The 'I' when followed along time has different phases, but it does not question its being one and the same 'I'. It is the same 'I' but in different 'nows' and 'heres'. It remains self-identical in spite of changes.
> In regard to the two indefinables, 'space' and 'time', the 'I' in each of them is central.
> Compared with things the 'I' is largely a negation of all which goes to make things up, yet it is not the less a mental existence even as they. It is based on observations as truly as are they.

The dualism that Sherrington has been at such pains to develop with his rich and vivid argumentation is finally displayed in a form that is reminiscent of Russell's epistemological dichotomy: knowledge by acquaintance; and knowledge by description.

> The one concept is just as much based on factual observation as is the other. Strictly, the observation and fact underlying the non-sensual concept and its 'I', are we may think, more at first hand and more unimpugnable than are those underlying the spatial concept and its 'things'. These latter are after all an inference. If either as fact is more unquestionable than the other it should be the unextended 'I' being the more immediately established. It has it is true one disability as regards evidence, it is impenetrably private.

This is knowledge by acquaintance: "A spatial fact on the other hand can be attested by perhaps millions at first hand". This is knowledge by description: "The two therefore possess as testimony values of a different order". But Sherrington is still concerned to raise the question of the authenticity of knowledge by acquaintance in respect of verifiability: "It is not strictly verifiable by a second person. Hence doubtless there attaches to its class of fact a certain mystery from which the perceptual, observable by many observers in common at first hand, is ordinarily free".

After this epistemological encounter there is a long reference to contrasting views of Fernel, who postulated a spirit-like something in the body, the soul, that also could live outside the body, obtaining then to immortality. Sherrington's empathy with Fernel in his religious beliefs comes through clearly:

> An immense superstructure reared itself upon 'immortality' as an attribute of the finite psyche. There arose the whole of a possible economy for the presumed after-life succeeding death.
> These adjuncts to the soul-concept, persisting for millennia in story and in faith, played their role in history. They influenced civilization. They have, as subject for reflection, not rarely been set forth in language of supreme felicity. Among creations of imagination some of these outpourings stand unsurpassed. For Fernel this inclusion of immortality among the attributes of the psyche was both a tenet of his religious belief and a fact of his science. With him and such as he such faith was no vice of egotism or crude bias of repugnance to cessation. It was with him a conviction which gave just one reason the more for taking life and himself seriously and devotedly.

But also there was created from the concept a whole animistic world that Sherrington describes at length on the basis of Fernel's dialogue and that appears in Fernel's book *Physiologia.* The warning is that: "part of the natural history of the 'I' is therefore its inclination to anthropomorphize the physical world".

Fernel and Kepler both used such preternatural concepts in their explanations of the perceptual world.

In the light of all this philosophical disputation Sherrington reconsiders the theme of Natural Theology, but he has many criticisms and reservations when the 'Cause' achieved a God-like status.

> The naive 'I' observing that things, for instance, 'its' body, appear to begin and end, sought also as to the external world how that world began and was to end. It took recourse to the all-powerful and all-knowing 'Cause' it had assumed, and found there its answer. It attributed the original creation of itself and of all the world to this same all-powerful and all-knowing Cause. It recognized itself as having some likeness to the Cause. Of that its interpretation was that the Cause had created it, the 'I', after its own image.
> It accounted for the universe by means of a Cause imagined after its own type. We need not, for our purpose, follow further this apotheosis. In this ultimate expansion of its scope, the non-sensual concept comes to present an interest for the contemplative 'I' which exceeds that of the whole spatial world itself. We cannot wonder there have been the

recluse, the saint, and the wrapt philosopher who have within these aspects of that concept immersed their lives.

However, the development of Natural Science resulted in more and more successes in explaining natural phenomena. Thus the explanations that had long been offered by the non-sensual concept for happenings in the world of nature came under suspicion.

> As analysis of the natural world by the spatial concept, which we may call the energy-concept, went forward, the explanations of that world by the other, the 'spiritual' concept, were challenged by those which the spatial concept itself could submit. And in this field reason, when it has before it alternative explanations of phenomena, one by application of the non-sensual concept, the other by application of the spatial concept, prefers the latter.

This was particularly true of the phenomena of life which were eventually shown to have an explanation based on physics and chemistry.

> The application of the non-sensual concept has therefore been curtailed in scope. The key positions which it had occupied as ruler of the body it has relinquished. Life, as a principle by which the body lives, has been taken from it. Life as such is found to belong to the other, the energy-concept. With the falling of the stone and the falling of the star, bodily life is counted in the tale of things which energy describes. Finally the whole spatial world, examined by the spatial concept, assumed the appearance of a scene in which 'energy' described it all, all which was and all which had been.

It appeared to be a complete victory for the spatial or energy concept, that is for materialism.

> This in its turn has had further repercussions on the position of the non-sensual concept. The ambit of its excursions has been curtailed. The field to which it aspired was vast. Recent times have taken from it some of its ambitions. It claimed to operate Nature; it claimed to include 'life', an immortal soul, existences which directed whole reaches of the physical world, and a Cause which maintained, controlled, and had indeed created the universe. Some of these claims were set forth by their supporters with a passion and devotion never in literature excelled. Yet time teaches that a number of the claims themselves have in cold truth to be regarded as extravagant.

The phrase of personification "time teaches" can be accepted as a poetic expression by Sherrington, he introduces many such personifications, the most frequent and important being 'Nature'.

Sherrington now returns to the defense and even exaltation of the non-sensual concept after the systematic discrediting it had suffered at the hands of materialism in the last centuries:

> I have been trying to outline as an item of Nature-study the growth and extension, and then the restriction and purification of the applications of this non-sensual concept. When it has been stripped of untenable pretensions, what remains to it? There remains then a residue inalienably its own. A residue more precious than any of its mistaken ambitions. A residue valuable beyond expression, for language, its own half-perfected instrument of expression, is not adequate to express it to the full. A residue which is the source of all of its splendid 'realities' as well as of all its dreams. A residue which contains *all* the 'values' – for space is irrelevant to 'values'. In a word the conscious 'I', called in the abstract 'mind'.

And what a residue! Among its contents are those two same concepts we have been following, creations of thought, embracing between them more than the Universe, for if we call the Universe energy, they embrace mind as well. It may be said this residue, beyond all problematical 'reality', *is* the 'value' of our world.

Sherrington now takes stock of where his relentless enquiry has led him in his quest for a relationship between Modern Science and Natural Theology. It is not encouraging to his audience, but it has some faint glimpses of hope in the strange mystery of dualism.

We have to note then that the result to which we are led in so far, is not a direct endorsement of natural theology so called. The mind by its own unaided vision looking at our world does not find that world resolve into a First Cause and the things which That has created and maintains. It finds, so far as I can exercise 'its' vision, that our world resolves itself into energy and mind.

In continuing the enquiry there is concentration on the nature of mind that so emphatically refuses to be in the energy world. It seems impossible that energy can redefine itself so that the non-sensual mind could be a new form of energy.

So our two concepts, space-time energy sensible, and insensible unextended mind, stand as in some way coupled together, but theory has nothing to submit as to how they can be so. Practical life assumes that they are so and on that assumption meets situation after situation; yet has no answer for the basal dilemma of how the two cohere.

The wave-particle dilemma of physics is not an acceptable analogue, but it gives a guide to behaviour when faced with an intractable dilemma. We can accept energy and mind as a working biological unity, ". . . although we cannot describe the how of that unity".

Practical life regards, for instance, our thoughts as answerable for what we say. It proceeds as though qualities of mind, e. g. memory, courage, rightness of inference, and so on, affect the acts we do . . . Society in general regards mind as productive of acts. While our conception of the mind as unextended seems to preclude mind from interacting with any energy-system, the body inclusive, every-day life assumes there is interaction and that our mind shapes our conduct. Here ethics surely takes the same view as does daily life.

Sherrington then in desperation indulges in a brief flirtation with the psycho-physical identity hypothesis in the hope of finding a unifying principle.

If the 'I-doing', which stands at some disadvantage, as we say, for observing itself, had, instead of assuming that it was the 'cause' of its motor act, regarded itself simply as colligate with the act, a part with it of one event, the seeming inconsistency between the two concepts in this situation would disappear. There would then be no need to ask for interaction.

But there is a penalty as is now illustrated.

Its motor act can be called rightly a 'conscious motor act'. That is exactly what it is. Its awareness is part of it. It can also rightly be called a willed act, unless by that it is intended to say 'will' causes the motor act.

The penalty is that the experienced will is then an illusion the motor act being entirely determined by the energy system of the brain.

> ... 'Energy' and 'mind' although incommensurable become two complemental concurrent parts of one serial event. That is not to say at all that mind is an aspect of energy or energy an aspect of mind. Our concept of energy affirms it as something complete in itself. A self-contained cycle which has no crevice for interpenetration by anything else, let alone mind. Similarly our concept mind excludes energy, for the nature of its own content is non-sensual.

The developing argument leads to a further suggestion of panpsychism.

> We have difficulty in assigning the lower limit of the mental. It may therefore be that its distribution extends to all organisms, and even further.
> It becomes indubitable therefore that our being is a unity whose behaviour we can follow only by including the two concepts and treating them as having 'contact utile' each with the other.

This serves to restrain trespass by one concept into preserves of the other.

> When ... the mind concept is so applied as to insert into the human individual an immortal soul, again a trespass is committed. The very concomitance of the two concepts, which seems a basal condition of our knowledge of them, is thrown aside as if forgotten. Such amplification of the one concept may be legitimate for a revealed religion. Its evidence then rests on ground we do not enter upon here. But as an assertion on the plane of Natural Knowledge it is an irrational blow at the solidarity of the individual; it seems aimed against that very harmony which unites the concepts as sister-concepts. It severs them and drives off one of them lonelily enough, on a flight into the rainbow's end.

Here is Sherrington the poet!

> So too the other concept, the spatial, or rather its devotees, have passed it into fields outside its proper scope. The drive there too may well have been an unbidden urge toward Monism. It represents a natural tendency which in no age has been wanting ... Its immediate *raison d'etre* has often been to dislodge intrusions of the other concept, the non-spatial, from positions, which the spatial concept representing 'matter' was by its advocates felt more adequate to explain. In this in recent centuries it has been triumphantly successful. It has made the energy concept a weapon for man's conquest of the Earth ... But it has had no success with the non-sensual, the 'I-thinking', its ways, and its creations, in abstract the 'mind'. Progress of knowledge, and especially of Natural Science, has only made more clear that the spatial concept's far-reaching notion 'energy' is, as it stands, powerless to deal with or to describe mind.
> Indeed the term 'mental energy' was not rarely used in that belief. This expectation has not been fulfilled.

Sherrington's conclusions after this long enquiry that has been pressed to the limits of knowledge show that he is unreservedly dualistic:

> Mind, for anything perception can compass, goes therefore in our spatial world more ghostly than a ghost. Invisible, intangible, it is a thing not even of outline; it is not a 'thing'. It remains without sensual confirmation, and remains without it for ever. Stripped to nakedness there remains to it but itself. What then does that amount to? All that counts in life. Desire, zest, truth, love, knowledge, 'values', and seeking metaphor to eke out expression, hell's depth and heaven's utmost height. Naked mind ... Mind, yoked with life, how varied in its reaction! It will sit down and watch life acquiescent, or on the other hand take life and squeeze it like an orange.

And that other concept, energy; what of its yield? We saw that Time has winnowed its harvest too. How much remains? The perceptible world. All that the space-time continuum contains; gathered harmoniously into one category, a category which nothing which does not act on sense can enter and which all that does so act does enter.

So we come to the great finale of this momentous lecture.

Between these two, naked mind and the perceived world, is there then nothing in common? ... They have this in common – we have already recognized it – they are both concepts; they both of them are parts of knowledge of one mind. They are thus therefore distinguished, but are not sundered. Nature in evolving us makes them two parts of the knowledge of one mind and that one mind our own. We are the tie between them. Perhaps we exist for that.

xii. Conflict With Nature

Apparently this last lecture was not delivered; being postponed or cancelled because of the impending Coronation. We can think of it as largely being composed later so that it gives a view in retrospect of the whole series. Thus it opens with a reference to Lord Gifford. Sherrington, the collector and lover of old books refers to the *Shorter Catechism* that Lord Gifford once owned and that had his marking slip at a page with the opening paragraph: "Religion is of all things the most excellent and precious". Sherrington is ever mindful of the task entrusted to him in these lectures of treating Natural Theology as a science: "But the desire that facts of Astronomy or Chemistry and the like be taken in examination of, to quote his own words, 'the relation which man and the universe bear to Him' 'the First and Only Cause', is one less simple to fulfil."
He goes on to elaborate:

But direct bearing on the relation of man and the Universe to the First Cause may find little relevance there. More is demanded. There must be considered not only 'masses' and electric charges but such notions as ethical values, ideals and motives. In short the theme embraces as well as the perceived the percipient. That seems of its essence.

Sherrington is concerned that Natural Science now tries to exclude any human element from its view of Nature: "Man as scientific observer becomes an instrument for pointer-readings in the hand of a disembodied intellect."

He feels that the more pure the science the more it needs liaison with the rest of knowledge. With its vaunted purity it cannot approach Lord Gifford's theme. Before attaching itself to Natural Theology it needs this liaison and Sherrington goes on to say that Lord Gifford's own foundation seems to provide this. But Natural Theology has a protean character:

It has articulated itself with the revealed religions, often, I would think, harmoniously, occasionally as though all but it were inessential. At times, I would think, it has proved a ferment of doubt. Regarding it from the standpoint of a famous definition of it as 'that spark of knowledge of God which may be had by the light of Nature and the consideration of created things', the field it enters is a part of the field covered by the great revealed faiths. But in that common harbourage it is not secured by fixed anchors as are they; its anchor is the Natural Science of the time, an anchor constantly dragging.

The view that Sherrington draws of Nature in the light of modern biology is sombre in the extreme.

Today's newer knowledge looking at Nature finds there as wrote Aristotle, 'evil is more plentiful than good; what is hateful is more plentiful than what is fair! . . .
Nature is a scene of interaction, and between living things interaction can be co-operation or conflict. Nature exhibits such co-operation but she is burdened with conflict like a nightmare. Unhalting and blood-stained conflict systematically permeates the field of Nature. Beauties it presents, joys it contains, but a blight of suffering infests it. For that reason whole fields of it are sombre tracts to contemplate.

However, in contrast with the fatalism and despair of classical antiquity, "the reasoned materialism of today is . . . an inspiration for dealing with Nature". Here speaks Sherrington the doctor who had spent many of his earlier years in pathology and bacteriology, even working in the field during cholera epidemics. He gives three instances of hateful diseases that challenge the scientist and that now, since Sherrington's time, have been brought under control. In two there is a complicated life cycle with two hosts. They can be regarded as examples of the 'beauty' of biological design. One is Redia, a worm infecting sheep, with a water snail as vector. The other is malaria with the anopheles mosquito as vector.

Sherrington is carried away in his detailed biological description. It is an attack on the simplistic idea of Cleanthes in Hume's *Dialogue* that pain in Nature is offset by a "coexistent equivalence of pleasure". Sherrington expresses his outrage at this sophism:

Can we by any flight of fancy conceive that this speck of organized slime embodies a grain of pleasure? The mere suggestion, even if unwittingly, rings like a callous levity when heard against the groan of a tortured population.

He continues:

Naive thought might suppose the scheme of Nature would at least value transcendence in life, e. g. a man more than a protozoan speck, or than a parasitic bacillus. But no.
There is for one, that lowly and destructive life, the tubercle bacillus, which martyrs men and animals the habitable globe over. A hundred years ago John Keats, the poet, equally young and great, succumbed to it at the age of twenty-five.

He concludes: "It is for man as critic and censor to interfere". We can take some comfort that this interference has virtually eliminated tuberculosis.

It is today recognized that the charge that Nature is 'immoral' has to be changed to 'non-moral'. The wonder is that non-moral Nature has brought

forth beings that exhibit conscious purpose and that have created concepts
of morality and disciplines of altruism. Yet the way of evolution was beset
with cruelty as we now would judge it. We are still in continuity with the
world whence we have come

> ... but not so long since, as our planet's ages go, we were immersed and submerged in it, a
> part of it not unlike all the rest. Such satisfactions and miseries as we can descry in it were
> then ours too. They were then our lot in life. It is a picture to depict which from the inside
> defies our power. To relive it in imagination is beyond our imagining. So far as it was
> experienced – and we can scarcely gauge what capacity for experience we had then – it was
> experience the like of which we have not now, even in faintest remembrance.
> Studying that other life we do so now with the knowledge that its lights and shadows are
> the kind and order of those through which our infra-human history brought ourselves,
> clambering to man's estate. Remembered they are not. Man's memory never took part in
> them. But gazing at the scene his knowledge can as it were reseize some features of it. It
> was a life of the passing hour containing little yesterday and little tomorrow. Its past and
> future mentally were thin streaks. Its 'now' like a moving spotlight played over an almost
> or entirely non-conceptual world discovering relatively little and ranging relatively little.
> Its world was wanting in variety, for it was mainly meaningless except at points where it
> touched food or sex or danger. Its peak perceptions were food, sex and danger merged
> with motive passions operated instinctively.
> Its world was under a rule of 'might-is-right' imposed by violence and pillared upon
> suffering. But yet the spell of 'urge-to-live' was over it all. Repicturing that life, so far as
> we can, we marvel and rejoice at our escape. The factual history of our past indeed is
> almost antithetically remote equally from the pagan myth of man's descent from the Gods,
> and from the wishful poet's 'intimations' that 'trailing clouds of glory do we come.'

These passages show Sherrington with his realism and biological understanding attempting to experience and describe the brutal way in which our
forebears clambered to man's estate. This attempt at realism is salutary to
an age which often blithely wishes to indulge in the fantasy that this wonderful process of biological evolution has a sacred aura and can be relied on
to continue the upward evolution of man. Put bluntly, biological evolution
involves unimaginable suffering and brutality so that the fittest survive and
the others are sacrified.

> The competition between lives which have mind is in origin one with that between the so-
> called mindless lives of which we were speaking. It overlaps and dovetails in with that and
> continues it on the new plane. It also, because a struggle to live, is essentially a struggle to
> the death.
> Nature in the primeval African forest as observed by a versed and sympathetic naturalist
> of today is found to present an appearance 'sinister, hostile and horrible' (Julian Huxley).
> Nature contains much which is hateful and much of pain. Much 'that spoils the singing of
> the nightingale'.

Here is the thought of Sherrington the poet. But out of all the relentless
struggle for survival came eventually the growing intelligence of man's predecessors, the hominids. There were

> ... groups of related individuals with interests in common organized on a peace-footing,
> the individual as unit contributing social safety and support to the community of units.

Under this organization the mind gradually evinces new qualities of the 'self'. Zest-to-live
takes on new aspects. Thus, in our own human kind altruism, extending to the family and
beyond, to the tribe and beyond, knitting social ties of planet-wide comradeship and
goodwill. Love-of-life extends, so to say, to beyond 'self'. It is sublimated to new aspirations, which in their fullness grow strong and dear as love-of-life itself – pity and charity
and love of others and self-sacrifice, even to sacrifice of love-of-life itself.

We like to think that these virtues of primitive man contributed to his great
biological success, but it has been a long struggle and at times in the
hominid ancestry the issue of survival or extermination must often have
been in doubt. There are examples of extermination in the fossil record, for
instance Australopithecines, that branched off the main hominid line and
ceased to exist about one million years ago. It is presumed that this extermination was due to 'higher' hominids – *Homo habilis* for example.

Sherrington the realist also recognizes the biological success of predatory animals that live on other animals – even animals of higher types. Man
has set out systematically to exterminate or control the predaceous in
Nature. Hence comes the question:

Is life a sacred thing? Is it the right of rational life which has the 'values' to destroy life? Is
that not a trespass against the Spirit of Life? The Spirit of Life! That is what we set out to
find. We could not discover it. We have not found it. Wherever we looked for it it
vanished. We know no Spirit of Life.
Life taken in general can be no sacred thing. It has enslaved and brutalized the globe.
True, life is the supreme blessing of the planet; none the less it is also the planet's crowning
curse.
We think back with repugnance to that ancient biological pre-human scene whence, so we
have learned, we came; there *no* life was a sacred thing. There millions of years of pain
went by without one moment of pity, not to speak of mercy. Its life innately gifted with
'zest-to-live' was yet so conditioned that it must kill or die.
For man, largely emancipated from those conditions, the situation has changed. The rule
and scene are there, and are the same, apart from himself. The change is in himself. Where
have his 'values' come from? The infra-human life he escaped from knew them not. The
great predaceous forms, shark, hawk, panther, wolf, are not blind; they mean the things
they do; they have been given mind. But not with values. 'Wrong' is impossible to them.
More hopeless still, equally impossible is 'right'. Those other creatures than himself, even
the likest to himself, would seem without the values, or it may be at most some 'value' *ad
hoc* for a given situation. Nothing of values as concepts such as are his, constantly
vouchsafing him counsel in situations however variously circumstanced. Whence has he
got them? Inventions of his own? Conventions? How far can he trust them? Can *a priori*
principles suffice to base them? Are they heritable? They are under test. They are in the
making, even more than is the rest that he is.

Here is the mystery of the human situation. Sherrington speaks of this
theme with deep feeling. He reverts again to the obligations of a Gifford
Lecturer, that is, to consider moral aspirations in the manner of science.

... There arises for him a dilemma and a contradiction. The contradiction is that he is
slowly drawing from life the inference that altruism, charity, is a duty incumbent upon
thinking life. That an aim of conscious conduct must be the unselfish life. But that is to

disapprove the very means which brought him hither, and maintains him. Of all his new-found values perhaps altruism will be the most hard to grow. The 'self' has been so long devoted to itself as end. A good man's egotism, it is said, is altruism. Perhaps that indicates a stepping-stone on the way.

For natural knowledge, if we hold natural science to be that knowledge, the natural world as phenomenon becomes a vast thing wholly uninfluenced by 'values'. The appeal to Design has lapsed as an argument and that leaves Nature acquitted not only of good but of evil. More literally than ever 'there is nothing good or bad but thinking makes it so'; and Nature has in that sense no 'thinking' outside man's. He and his ethics stand alone. There is nothing good nor bad except himself.

So man has a strange sense of loneliness not in cosmic space, but here on this planet.

The human mind is strangely placed there . . . All other mind its inferior, and almost incompanionably so. His thinking is thus thrown utterly upon itself. Grappling with its newly found 'values', yet with no experience except its own, no judgement but its own, no counsel but its own. Marked out it would seem, to be leader of life upon the planet, more, willy-nilly set so, he yet has none to seek guidance from. None of whom to ask a question. What wonder his religions seek to supply a Higher Being to meet his need in this?

It is at this stage that Sherrington becomes oppressed by gloom, by ". . . the dreariness that Goethe found insufferable in the materialism of his time 'its Cimmerian grey' ". Almost in desperation with the cruel examples he gives, as in Thomas Hardy's poem *The Blinded Bird,* we feel that Sherrington turns to the theme of altruism, as if it were the last hope for mankind.

Man's altruism has to grow. It is not enough for him to stand and deplore. That is less to mend things than to run from them. A positive charity is wanted; negation is not enough. In effect it needs a self-growth which shall open out a finer self. It requires to absorb into 'feeling' something of the world beyond the self and put it alongside the interests of the very self. That asks biologically an unusual and even a perilous step.

But such altruism would provide awareness of others' suffering with psychical intensity more than that of mere observant intelligence. It amounts to sharing suffering as though another's suffering were the self's. To sense a star is not for our awareness to be the star, but when we sense pain it is that our awareness is that pain. A great gift – some might say divine – comes to the 'self' when perceiving certain suffering external to itself it so reacts to it that that suffering becomes its own, and is shared even as a 'feeling'. That gift is a gift, it would seem, uniquely human.

Altruism as passion; that would seem as yet Nature's noblest product; the greatest contribution made by man to Life.

It may likely mean a human future led by women more eminently than by men.

Sherrington there moves on to survey man in Nature, now that man has in his idealism turned his back on Nature.

Our world is in process of becoming and that becoming is not of peaceful course. It meets on all sides obstacles and perplexities. It engages battle with them. One of those battles is between Man and Nature. Man is in conflict with Nature. We have not here to touch upon man's two other and still greater conflicts; man against man, and man against himself. Our theme is Nature and man as part of Nature. As part of Nature man is deeply involved in conflict with the rest. I would think it a theme even as those others not unworthy the epic and the lyric.

Sherrington now examines very critically various plans for man-made Utopias, or as Hogben writes, plans to make the whole planet subservient to man's need . . . conserving only those [species] which directly or indirectly, contribute the means of food, of shelter, ornament and pleasing prospect". Sherrington condemns this as passionately as a modern environmentalist. He asks: "Are we not, even if masters of our planet, yet its guests; and has it not other guests as well?" It is now suggested that if man

> . . . would render help to his world he has at least one means. That is by his own contribution to human fellowship. The circumambient untraversable which isolates his planet does of its very self serve to compel man's fellowship with man. Man's specific loneliness in the economy of the earth, he alone having the 'values' again compels it. Only amid human fellowship can 'values' be listened to and shared. In him evolution has shaped a social animal par excellence. A man wholly solitary would, said Aristotle, be either a god or a brute. Social life is his opportunity as field for his 'values'. To know that he is a life being evolved which carries with it the 'values' can imbue his social system with a purpose. Human fellowship thus emerges as something of unique worth. Fellow human mind is the sole mind to understand and share to the full with his, and be shared. The loveliest friend of man is man. That theme however demands a worthier pen than mine.

He opines that human fellowship started early.

> Half a million years back he had been flaking flints in the open weather, shaping a weapon, perhaps to destroy an enemy at the cave-mouth, or to be in his turn destroyed; already then it would seem he had felt the beauty of a shapely hand-axe and also had laboured his hand-axe or his scraper not for his own use solely, but for his fellowship, a little group where death kept membership short-lived, and life went direly bare.

The transformation from that time had been stupendous. So Sherrington is moved to take a more embracing view of evolution, which he does in his inimitable style.

> In him, it would seem, evolution had prospered. Other successes it had had. Time had added his to those others. Successive forms of life had arisen, dominating the planet, through certain epochs. They had had each their turn. The record of the planet's rocks told of the ammonites of the warm ancient oceans. They had flourished and swarmed. They had gone their way. They were but fossils now. The great Saurians in their turn had prevailed, battening in the rich river plains, towering prodigies of strength and stature not since repeated. They too had had their day. Their reign had been long, and then they had vanished. Today it is man's turn. A single form and yet the dominant life, so obviously that a glance suffices to show it. What did it mean? Is man one more experiment which Nature makes, later to scrap it? It may be so. Time has brought man his turn to come and then to go? Or did it mean more? Could it be that man would stay? Nothing did stay. The others each had had a spell, in turn to be replaced. There seemed already streaks of sunset across the human landscape. But there is in his instance a new factor, or one at least strangely prominent in it; mind. His oncoming had been an outstripping of other minds. His dominance pillars on mind. Will that ensure its future?

That poetic discourse leads him to survey the histories of past civilizations. He worries about *Homo praedatorius* – predaceous man. As well he might with the present story of the planet.

Predatory war enters then as a feature into community-organization. Since predaceous man is human, in his instance the human mind itself implements predacity. Field after field of human civilized activity becomes a scene of conflict little less internecine than is war. Economic warfare, commercial warfare, class-warfare, are symptomatic of *homo praedatorius*. Serfdom and slavery attach to his régime, in fact when not in name. His régime deals by opprobrium and ostracism with victimized classes in the State. He exploits cruelty on sub-human lives as well as on human life. Predaceous man's rule cuts indeed at the very root of social mankind's organization of life.

We can experience the threat as we see it in the struggle for world domination today. Sherrington's message is for us all. He has also another message which should be projected to those states that attempt a rigid police control in order to preserve the status quo. Thus they fossilize society in the cause of 'security'. There is in

> ... the polity of Nature ... a still older law, namely, change, progressive change, a law older even than life itself. This tells us that the abiding of a *status quo* is not, and never has been, 'lawful' in Nature.
> It would seem that *homo praedatorius* is in a backwater unreached by the tide which set in some millennia since. The great revealed religions bringing their altruism are evidence of that new tide. It may be that the reason why the tide of altruism set in, was as a step toward a re-ordering of life upon the planet. The ascendency of *homo praedatorius* would spell ruin to man's prosperous leadership here. And man must lead or go. To lead is all he is fit for. But leadership does not lie in treating as prey those whom it leads. Man is above all a leader charged with survival of the 'values' which are in his keeping. Man's leadership cannot be tyranny since that would be to forget the 'values'. With the 'values' his leadership must be some form of fellowship. The cement of fellowship is altruism, for that is truth to fellowship. Fellowship cultivates equality of 'selfs', equal respect for values and equal rights in values. It asks man to be watchful against himself that he harm not his neighbour. Altruism as basis of co-operative effort, to guide some of the ways of life to nobler common issues. There is so much for men to do in common.

These inspired messages of Sherrington are needed by the world today as never before – but who of the world leaders takes heed of the deeper biological and philosophical character of human society? We tend to judge all issues on the basis of pragmatic materialism. That short-sighted ignorance may spell the end of our civilization.

So Sherrington comes to imagine a poignant message from Nature to man, where more than ever before we are treated to a personification of Nature:

> You have now as a species had a long innings by reason of your intelligence. It is nearly a million years since first you were knocking stones into shape.
> You thought me moral, you now know me without moral. How can I be moral being, you say, blind necessity, being mechanism. Yet at length I brought you forth, who are moral. Yes, you are the only moral thing in all your world, and therefore the only immoral.
> You thought me intelligent, even wise. You now know me devoid of reason, most of me even of sense. How can I have reason or purpose being pure mechanism? Yet at length I made you, you with your reason. If you think a little you with your reason can know that; you, the only reasoning thing in all your world, and therefore the only mad one.
> You are my child. Do not expect me to love you. How can I love – I who am blind

necessity? I cannot love, neither can I hate. But now that I have brought forth you and your kind, remember you are a new world unto yourselves, a world which contains in virtue of you, love and hate, and reason and madness, the moral and immoral, and good and evil. It is for you to love where love can be felt. That is, to love one another.
Bethink you too that perhaps in knowing me you do but know the instrument of a Purpose, the tool of a Hand too large for your sight as now to compass. Try then to teach your sight to grow.

This is a wonderful imaginative message that gives us insight into the kind of person Sherrington was. It can be understood in different ways, for example Sherrington says: "Nature is like a music to which two friends can listen and both be moved and yet each by a different train of thought."

With his poetic insight Sherrington wins through to an ecstatic optimism:

We traced how, it would seem, we are so fashioned that our world, which is our experience and is one world, is a diune world, a world of outlook and of inlook, of the experienced perceptible and of the experienced imperceptible. This world with all its sweep of content and extent taxes utterance to indicate. Yet it is given us in so far to seize it, and as one coherent harmony. More; it is revealing to us the 'value', as Truth, Charity, Beauty. Surely these are compensation to us for much. And will not this compensation grow; Truth grows; and even as Truth so Beauty. Music as her ear grows finer embraces what once were discords. The mind which began by being one thing has truly – as so often in evolution – gone on to being another thing. Even should mind in the cataclysm of Nature be doomed to disappear and man's mind with it, man will have had his compensation: to have glimpsed a coherent world and himself as item in it. To have heard for a moment a harmony wherein he is a note. And to listen to a harmony is to commune with its Composer?

This paean is a fitting climax to the lecture. But Sherrington remembers his task to give a discourse on Natural Religion. He asks: Has it emotions as other religions? and replies:

Natural Religion has convictions; it must therefore have emotion. Its convictions entertain 'values', and the 'values' constrain emotions. We saw that one of its 'values' is Beauty. Also it knows the sentiment of wonder. Now that Nature is freed from the pseudo-marvels of magic, wonder is for it a truer wonder. Wonder at natural law, to our experience universal and infrangible. Law which has generated in us capacity for inference and reason; whence it is we have them. And there is Truth. Natural Religion along with the great religions holds truth a 'value'. As to it Natural Religion exacts a credibility somewhat other than do they, or, rather, demands another standard of credence. They and it pursue truth, but, for Natural Religion what it holds to be true must be verifiable with an austerity all its own.

He goes on to consider the nature and role of Natural Religion:

If religion has to stir the world, let alone stir man to conflict with the world, the appeal to a Deity which is personal can go far to harness for its purposes the whole dynamism of the psyche. It is equivalent to establishing a 'value' which for its followers resumes all other 'values'. But this source of emotional strength Natural Religion is without, for it sublimes personal Deity to Deity wholly impersonal. In a manner the Θεός of Aristotle is that which it re-approaches.

Granted it can dispense with founding temples and establishing rites, yet it will be incommensurate to its own self-proposed enterprises unless it have passion. Whence then the passion it has? Surely Truth, Beauty, Charity provide passion. The very austerity hedging its acceptance of Truth illustrates the price it puts upon that 'value' and will pay for it. At great cost it would have the truth about Nature – Nature which for it includes man. Its curiosity to know that truth is no mere worship of Reason. Reason it takes for its slave. Reason it says is not a 'value'; it is just a tool for thinking. The aim, the zest, which can employ reason is that which constitutes the 'value'. And that purpose here, is passion to know the 'secrets of Nature', as the old phrase has it.

The final message has great nobility, but we think it may be a message only to an elite. It is too austere and too demanding in its lofty appeal for responsibility. We fear that Sherrington may be optimistic in claiming that ". . . it raises the lowliest human being conjointly with the highest".

Compared with a situation where the human mind beset with its perplexities had higher mind and higher personality than itself to lean on and to seek counsel from, this other situation where it has no appeal and no resort for help to beyond itself, has, we may think, an element of enhanced tragedy and pathos. To set against that, it is a situation which transforms the human spirit's task, almost beyond recognition, to one of loftier responsibility . . . We have, because human, an inalienable prerogative of responsibility which we cannot devolve, no not as once was thought, even upon the stars. We can share it only with each other.

We have chosen to link together with passages of comment and explanation extensive quotations from *Man on His Nature* because we feel that in this book Sherrington 'bared his soul' in a way that did not appear in his letters, which were delightfully and intimately personal, and also that did not grace his conversation, even with those intimate with him until in his latter years of retirement. We at the laboratory were surprised and pleased by his Rede Lecture, which was eagerly read as giving some glimpse of the philosophical thinking he had been developing unbeknown to us. He was very shy about such matters of personal enquiry and belief. He was of course an extrovert in other respects, being a great conversationalist and raconteur about his life experiences, in the sciences and in affairs. But he did not speak about his own poetry or his philosophy. By contrast he was delightful and fascinating in his discussions of poetry and of the philosophers of science from Aristotle to the present time. Thus we can regard *Man on His Nature* as the great source book on Sherrington the human person, who thought and felt deeply on the philosophy of biology and especially on the philosophy of the brain-mind problem.

The great message from the book is Sherrington's indomitable enquiry into the truth about man in Nature, particularly about his evolutionary origin in a mysterious and wonderful process of emergence. As a student of the brain he sees with particular clarity that this emergence has resulted in creatures that not only have bodies with brains, but also 'recognizable minds'. This frank dualism has of course been subjected to the usual rash of criticisms: for example that Sherrington has not defined the dualistic terms, mind and matter (or brain), and so he was confused (Cohen, 1958). That cheap way out is adopted so often by critics when confronted by over-whelming evidence and argument against some cherished belief that is dog-matically held. The excerpts that we have assembled from *'Man on His Nature'* reveal that Sherrington has used the terms: 'brain' and 'recogniz-able mind' consistently and in a manner clear of all ambiguity. However, there is an enigma that Sherrington presents but cannot explain except by an unsatisfying appeal to panpsychism: It is the origin of recognizable mind at an advanced stage of cerebral evolution. The appeal to Mother Nature will not do, as Sherrington so poignantly and wittily states at the end. Sherrington will not countenance any reference to the supernatural. So the enigma remains. For him it is a mystery but not a miracle. Sherrington was in a most dedicated manner following truth as he saw it, and he was deeply concerned that his philosophy of a limited dualism was rejected by most scientists who remained unshaken in their 'religion' of monist-mate-rialism. We can regard this great book as giving his thought, as expressed in the title (cf. p. 256).

In a less controversial field Sherrington reveals his deep feeling for nature, and particularly for animal nature. He was a forerunner of the conservationists. His wonderful imagination gave him vivid insights into life as it was in the urge-to-live and zest-to-live struggles that are basic in the story of creatures eventually clambering to man's estate under the selective influence of great struggles and sufferings. He saw the central nervous system as the most important influence in natural selection and that is certainly true of the last few million years of hominid evolution to *Homo sapiens. Man on His Nature* was criticized not only for its dualism but also for its latent religiosity. As we said at the outset Sherrington was deeply conscious of his audience and of the assigned theme of Natural Religion. He does not indulge in destructive criticisms of revealed religions. They are not for him, but he recognized their great role in the cultural history of man-kind. His sympathy with religion is also shown by his dramatic device of having Fernel act as a frame of reference for the Age of Faith that was superseded by the Age of Science. He came to regard Fernel with empathy and I think even imagined himself to be another Fernel if he had lived in the sixteenth century. Fernel had come to be his *alter ego*. He told me that he envied Fernel his life in an age where it was possible to have an uncompli-cated personal belief system, subscribing without any reservations both to a revealed religion and to a philosophy of nature.

Sherrington was secretive about the Gifford Lectures, as if he feared some critical reaction. In any case he never liked display and was averse to talking about his present activities when they were not immediately concerned with science or affairs. As mentioned in the introduction he actively discouraged any suggestion of a biography. He makes almost no reference to the lectures in his letters at that time. I have a letter from him written on 6 May 1937, when he was staying at the North British Station Hotel in Edinburgh, in which he mentions that he will be there for a further two weeks, but he makes no mention of the lectures he was giving at that time, though we all knew of this! He makes no mention of the lectures in letters to me of 29 May and 4 June. However, I remember a conversation in London, in June 1937 when he told me that he had great admiration for his audience, mostly of clergymen, who had stayed through the whole course despite the fact that he had so little 'comfort' to offer.

In 1951 a second edition of *Man on His Nature* was prepared in a greatly shortened version, 404 pages being reduced to 294. Again it was criticized, for example, by J. Z. Young, because it did not conform with the "established beliefs" of scientific materialism of that time. In February 1952 Sherrington told me that, as he re-read his original 1940 edition, he was greatly disturbed to find that it was so verbose and repetitive, saying with the characteristic twinkle in his eye: "I must have been a garrulous old man when I gave the lectures". This is surely a unique comment from ninety-four years in retrospect of himself in his early eighties. However, we have quoted here from the 1940 edition because we felt that much of value was deleted in his bending to his critics. In particular he tried to delete most of what his critics referred to as "religiosity" (*cf.* Granit, 1966).

In February 1952 he told me that he was deeply disturbed by the inability of most of his scientific friends to appreciate his efforts to build up a scientific philosophy of man. As in so many of his enterprises he was a pioneer far ahead of his time. It is unfortunate that Sherrington did not live to rejoice in the acclaim with which Schrödinger (*Mind and Matter*, 1958) greeted his book with the words: "I cannot convey the grandeur of Sherrington's immortal book by quoting sentences; one has to read it oneself". We three had all been Fellows of Magdalen College Oxford at the same time – 1934 to 1937. Sherrington and Schrödinger were elected in 1936 as Foundation Members of the newly created Pontifical Academy of Sciences. The symposium which I organized for the Academy in 1964 on "Brain and Conscious Experience" was the occasion to commemorate these two great scientists, then deceased, who would have been so attuned to the theme of the conference. The publication in 1966 was dedicated to them conjointly.

Man on His Nature can be compared and contrasted with a more recent philosophical adventure, *Chance and Necessity* by a great biologist, Jacques Monod (1971). Both books are remarkable for their imaginative treatment of biology. There is no finer introduction to the concepts of molecular biology than in Monod's book, but his section on the nervous system is less satisfactory, because of his imperfect knowledge of this field, and his last philosophical chapter is a disaster. There is the severe message that the only authentic knowledge is the message of science. Those who, like Sherrington and myself, recognize the mysterious dualism of man's nature are classed as animists, being relegated to the same abhorrent category as the animist cults of primitive man. Monod rejects all the other values, beauty, goodness, charity, altruism, and acclaims only the austerity of scientific 'truth'. He has eliminated the idolatries of past superstitions so as to impose a new idolatry. This iconoclastic attitude is to be contrasted with the deep and wise humanity of Sherrington that embraces as equals all the values. In the crescendo of his book Sherrington even exalts altruism above truth.

C. Goethe on Nature and on Science

On 4 March 1942 Sherrington delivered the Deneke Lecture at Lady Margaret Hall, Oxford, the theme being "Goethe on Nature and on Science". We can be grateful that this invitation was given to Sherrington in his eighty-fifth year. The lecture explored a theme that he had pondered for many years. As Professor Andrade (1942) has stated so penetratingly, Sherrington was much interested in the strange contrasts exhibited by Goethe:

> We are confronted with the question as to how a man of such mental power, vision and industry as Goethe could devote so much time to the problems of science without leaving any mark in the history of science, without being more, so far as his work on colour is concerned, than a psychological curiosity. Towards a solution of this question, which has been much discussed, especially by German writers, Sherrington's slender booklet contributes more than many ponderous works have done. The author is, of course, peculiarly fitted for this task. Not only is he one of the very greatest scientific figures of modern times, but also he is a poet of extreme sensitiveness, grace and perception, a man of profound knowledge and wide sympathies, a scholar, a linguist and, above all, a man of deep human understanding.

Andrade goes on to state:

> The booklet which is now before us not only helps us to understand Goethe but also, which is just as important, to understand Sherrington. It will bring delight to all his admirers, that is to say, to all who know him or know anything of his work, for it shows the master still writing with all the clear imagery and vivid analysis, with all the generous emotion and keenness of perception which have at all times mitigated the severity of his scientific thought.

The severity of Sherrington's scientific thought is displayed in his criticisms of the extraordinary inability of Goethe, a great humanist, to recognize even the elements of a scientific investigation. Sherrington was himself a student of visual physiology and colour, so he is particularly fitted to examine the pathetic story of Goethe's complete failure to elaborate a tenable theory of colour. Yet the tragedy is that Goethe set more store by his achievement in science than in poetry. Lacking any rational basis for criticism of the Newtonian theory of colour, he had to substitute scurrilous attacks. The lecture is interesting in the light it throws on Sherrington, who in his eighty-fifth year was still an extremely well-informed scholar and a skilful disputant. We can appreciate the way in which Sherrington, a great yet modest scientist and a still more modest poet, speaks about Goethe, a poetic genius who incredibly prided himself much more on his worthless science than on his immortal poetry. Sherrington is merciless on Goethe's pretentious science, especially his extraordinary views on colour.

Goethe was a great observer and generalizer but he failed completely to recognize the nature of the analytical procedures that led Newton to discover the composition of white light. Goethe relied instead on observations of the colours produced by the scattering of light from turbid solutions and on the phenomena of colour produced by contrast. Sherrington wittily presents Goethe's position against Newton:

> To try to analyze light was a shallow blunder. And the manner of the attempt! Through a tiny hole to admit a poverty-stricken thread of light into a darkened room, when by going into the open day any amount of it could be had – no wonder the students laughed and ran off!
> We encounter here in Goethe what seems an almost wilful inability to enter into the physicist's point of view.

He never tested the prisms he was sent by Büttner in order to check Newton's observations,

> ". . . but he did take one look through a prism. To his amazement the white wall at which he gazed through the prism remained white. Colour showed only where something dark edged the white. Colour showed brightest of all on the window frames. Goethe immediately concluded that he had thus discovered the Newtonian account of light to be an error."

So, he indulged in fantasy about the alleged refraction of light, writing: "For here was the citadel of that bewitching princess who in an array of seven colours had befooled the whole world; here lay the grim sophistic dragon threatening everyone who presumed to try his fortune with these illusions".

Sherrington lists and dismisses the four scientific contributions that have been ascribed to Goethe:

That light is *not* resoluble into coloured lights, an error reiterated to his life's end; that the plant is a collection of modified leaves; that the skull is an adapted piece of back-bone – two plausible though superficial conjectures, now, in the fuller light of the cell theory and embryology, set aside; the 'correlation of parts', a clumsy error he misthought a 'law'. Occasion for controversy is therefore past and gone.

Having disposed of Goethe's alleged science on critical scientific grounds Sherrington mellows to a more appreciative attitude. It is here that his lecture is of particular interest in that it illuminates Sherrington as well as Goethe, for they had much in common. In his adoration of Nature Sherrington felt a deep sympathy with Goethe. This passage gives an interesting example of Sherrington's views on Goethe and Nature and also on Science.

Were it not for Goethe's poetry surely it is true to say we should no longer trouble about his science. Such as it was, it is as science not important. Its importance lies in the light it throws on Goethe the poet, and on his conception of Nature. It documents him a poet-pantheist. He thought about Nature over and over. He abounded in originality. His enthusiasm as an observer of Nature was great. But a new fact he met with was apt to send him on a flight of imagination into the unknown. Creative genius in literature, in science his genius longed to create. It could not always abide the waiting for further experiments and more knowledge. Science has to follow experiment where possible, even where the imagined seems extremely probable. Goethe, though devoted to science, had not at root the scientific temperament. He had not, for instance, along with the urge to discovery the sublime detachment of the scientific thinkers.

Of particular interest is the comparison that can be made between Goethe and Sherrington in their views on Nature, for both had a religious regard for Nature, but it was more restrained with Sherrington. With the ascription of poet-pantheist in mind Sherrington comments:

Pantheism always has had an Olympus. So with Goethe, for him his 'Nature' is an Olympian figure. He, a 'visual', visualized her; he saw her a creative Being, coeval with life, a mythical *type* rather than any *character*, dramatic only as a Greek chorus may be dramatic. Goethe was from all evidence a devoted and even an impassioned lover of Nature . . . The perceptible world remained to him a thing of beauty, and the pageant it presented an unfailing delight. He seems sometimes, as we listen to him, to be looking over the shoulder of a creative Being, and to be entranced by watching her amid her work.

Sherrington is much more restrained in his admiration of Nature. His great insight as a biologist gives him a severely realistic attitude.

Nature in many of her aspects is beautiful. Sea, land and sky can have overwhelming beauty; so, too, the world of living things with their forms and colours and movements. To perceive Nature's beauty is perhaps among the loveliest of all human privileges; a quality of peculiar charm because no two of us can enjoy it wholly similarly. All beauty is relative, and for each of us this world is the only world we know. But, beside the lovable, our world has in it also the hateful, the abominable, vice, ugliness, blood-lust and cruelty. To take subhuman nature: the ferret gnawing the earthed rabbit, the wolf pack in pursuit, the leopard at the throat of the deer, and then, the fever-fit of ague, the growing cancer, the whole scheme of destruction from the killer-whale to the ichneumon fly. This and much more, not to speak further of human cruelty and hate. Goethe, the amateur of Nature, must have known these facts, he must have perceived that, in the scheme of Nature, to attack and prey upon others is for the majority of animals, even likest ourselves, their charter of existence.

Nature sows and reaps vast harvests of pain and fear all over our planet, on earth, in sky and sea. Yet turning to Goethe and his rhapsody it would seem unknown to him. It casts no cloud for him, although his great younger contemporary was protesting 'it spoils the singing of the nightingale'. It forms part of that acknowledged problem, the co-existence with us of pain and suffering, physical and mental, animal and human. Yet Goethe says of Nature 'mit allen treibt sie ein freundliches Spiel'. Ein freundliches Spiel! The words seem laden with irony. 'She is too lofty to heed their suffering though they are her own off-spring! To do so would not beseem her'! Strange pride! Goethe's view of Nature remains in this respect an enigma, and it is another view than that of to-day.

Sherrington is moved to portray his own stark realism in introducing further discussion of Goethe's Nature worship.

The living world is, like it or not, a world of natural inequality. Inequality of size is part of that inequality. Upon that field of inequality is sown broadcast the seed of zest-to-life, and not merely broadcast and at certain seasons but in superabundance and always. The price offered? Individual existence. The competition? Internecine. How successful man is biologically is perhaps best answered by remembering that he substantially is the only one of Earth's creatures permitted to die of old age – and not altogether rarely does so. The ocean is more populated then the land, and the naturalist tells us that it is unlikely that any individual life in all the oceans ever dies a natural death. I do not know whether Goethe, with his gift of picturing Nature's problems, guessed – he could not do more than guess – the extent of this competition. He certainly, walking this green planet, and adoring his imagined goddess, observed this universal struggle and endorsed it to a degree that Christianity never has observed it or endorsed it. To him the crown of Nature's god-head was her insatiable 'zest-for-life'. He said, 'Let people serve Him who gives to the beast his fodder, and to man meat and drink as much as he can enjoy. But I worship Him who has infused into the world such a power of production, that, when only the millionth part of it comes out into life, the world swarms with creatures to such a degree that war, pestilence, fire and water cannot prevail against them. This is *my* God!'

It is surprising that Sherrington is so gentle in his comments upon this eulogy of destruction and suffering.

Sherrington finally closes with Goethe's views on God:

In the *Annalen* dating when he was 62, Goethe declares 'with me, a pure, deep, innate and constantly followed conception has been the view that God is inseparably within Nature and Nature inseparable within God, and this idea has been at the basis of my whole existence.' On another of those rare occasions on which he spoke of religion as regards himself, he is reported as saying that the Deity as such was to him inscrutable, but that one aspect of the Deity was not so, Nature.

There is clearly a great gulf between the attitudes of Goethe and Sherrington to Nature. We should recall the quotations from near the end of *Man on His Nature*, (Chap. XII) where Nature is reproaching man for endowing her with all the human qualities, whereas she asserts she is only blind necessity and pure mechanism).

(J.C.E.)

Chapter 8

Books and the Man

Books, old and new, printers and their history, all cast their spell over Sherrington. Raised in a home filled with books – of science, history and poetry – he was addicted all his life to the printed word and to the forms in which it could be presented.

First we shall look briefly at Sherrington's own major publications and then describe his life with books and libraries. "The Integrative Action of the Nervous System", his Silliman Lectures, published in 1906 by the Yale University Press through Charles Scribner's Sons of New York, became a classic almost overnight. The distinguished biologist Robert Yerkes wrote a seven-page review of it, so taken was he by its message. The Yale University Press generously permitted its reprinting in the original form so that every member of the International Congress of Physiology meeting in Oxford in 1947 might be given a copy. A remarkable new foreword of eleven pages was provided by the author, ending, as one might expect, with another clear statement of the "body-mind disparation" (Appendix 11).

While he contributed chapters to textbooks, systems of medicine, memorial volumes, and encyclopaedias, Sherrington's next published volume was, as we have seen, *"Mammalian Physiology, a Course of Practical Exercises"*, published by the Clarendon Press in 1919. Ten years later a second edition was produced with the assistance of E. G. T. Liddell.

A little volume which caught most of his friends by surprise was one of poetry – *The Assaying of Brabantius and Other Verse*, published by the Oxford University Press in 1925. A second and enlarged edition appeared in 1940.

With his young Oxford colleagues in the University Laboratory of Physiology he published in 1932 *Reflex Activity of the Spinal Cord"*, a well-illustrated volume which owed its clarity to the excellent editing of E. G. T. Liddell. It, also, has had a recent re-issue (1972) annotated by D. P. C. Lloyd.

Sherrington's *Selected Writings* were, in 1940, compressed into 532 pages by the editorial skill of his pupil, Derek Denny-Brown, published by Paul Hoeber in New York, and paid for by the guarantors of the British journal *Brain*. It remains a fine testimonial.

The year 1940 saw the Gifford Lectures in print as *Man on His Nature*, published by the Cambridge University Press and by Macmillan in New York. This has been described in the *Sunday Times* of London as ". . . one of the landmarks in the history of man's speculation about his own place in the universe". Reviewers in North America were equally enthusiastic. The earlier chapters were reprinted as *Life's Unfolding* in The Thinker's Library Series in 1943. A second edition, with new preface, appeared in 1951. It was abstracted thereafter by the Readers Digest. In reviewing *Man on His Nature* Professor William Bean called Sherrington "a man of Elizabethan dimensions".

At the end of the war came *The Endeavour of Jean Fernel* (Cambridge University Press, 1946) on which Sherrington had been working for more than twenty years. When it was sent off to the press he felt bereft, and sought solace in the writings of other French scholars. He was reading one of these beside the fire at Eastbourne on 4 March 1952, when the little book slipped quietly from his aged hands.

During the Festival of Britain in 1951 the National Book League arranged a display of the works of one hundred outstanding modern British writers. The selections were made by Rose Macaulay, V. S. Pritchett and C. Day Lewis. Number 77 in the exhibition was *Man on His Nature,* an inscribed copy, together with the writer's portrait, and a photostat of page 301 on which C. S. S. was already making alterations for a revised edition.

The Endeavour of Jean Fernel is a book of great scholarship which brings before us a sixteenth century Paris physician dear to Sherrington's heart. It is not clear how C. S. S. first became interested in Fernel, but as we have already seen he pursued his publications wherever he could find them. Briefly stated, Fernel's protest against the "barbarian" tutors under whom he had suffered caused him to pursue, as a recluse for five years, "humane letters" and mathematics. A quartan fever requiring a long convalescence decided him upon medicine, in which professional course he graduated in 1530. To support himself during those years of study he had been a tutor, and had published three books: *Monalosphaerium* (1527) describing an astrolabe of his own design; *Cosmotheoria* (1528) containing his own measurement of a degree of meridian; and *De Proportionibus* (1528) on the use and theory of fractions. Of these times Fernel was to write descriptively ten years later (as condensed by C. S. S.): "Not to swerve from the path of our forefathers! What if they had never swerved? No, it has been good for philosophy to move into fresh paths; against the voice of the detractor, against the dead weight of tradition, and against the fullness of ripe authority. So shall each age grow its own crop of new authors and new arts".

Again, Sherrington quotes an abridged version of Fernel's view on medicine as a calling:

> Is there a greater blessing vouchsafed to mankind than medicine is? Life is our dearest possession, by which we breathe and enjoy the company of our fellow-beings. Can any calling be worthier than that which preserves and maintains life itself? Is wealth or fortune, in whatever measure, in the last resort, more estimable than is good health? He who succours the sufferer and the sick exercises a knowledge which deserves the admiration and affectionate regard of all men.

We can imagine the pleasure which Sherrington derived from the research and the writing which he lavished upon Jean Fernel. Part II of the biography opens, under the heading "The Earliest Physiology", with a phrase reminiscent of C. S. S. himself: "Fernel became a great figure with the students. They found him a treasury of knowledge, and a voice with a new message. He was devoted to them and his energy was inexhaustible."

Sherrington says ". . . he lived habitually a nineteen-hour day. To warnings against over-taxing himself he would reply, 'fate will give us long enough repose', quoting – true child of the Renaissance – a line from Ovid's Amores". C. S. S. then adds typically in a footnote: "The identification of this source I owe to the kindness of Mr. Henry Deas, Gonville and Caius College".

And so the story proceeds. The sheer scholarship – not to mention the biographical story itself – is overwhelming. Anyone knowing Sherrington's asides over the years must wonder who is actually speaking in some of the Fernel quotations such as this: "Fernel made his 'Anatomy' a concise manual. It was a preface to his account of the working of the body. Anatomy is to physiology, he says, as geography to history, it describes the theatre of events."

Sherrington stresses the fact that Fernel's *Physiology* passed through thirty-one posthumous editions in the ensuing century. His *Pathology* and *Therapeutics* were installments, one might say, of his system of medicine. The early C. S. S. breaks through as he quotes Professor Esmond Long, the well-known historian of pathology, that Fernel ". . . wrote a special pathology which in its organization falls little short of being modern".

It is impossible to accompany Sherrington throughout this sprightly little volume but two quotations may suffice to bring him and his much-beloved Fernel into final focus. The first reads: "Fernel's practice became very large. It left him scant time even for his midday meal. His patients were of diverse rank, attendants at the court, dignitaries, officials, visitors to Paris, and many of the poor. He never neglected the poor. He had started poor himself".

The second summarized Sherrington's quiet nostalgia:

> And so we take our leave of Jean Fernel. His days were taxed, year in and year out, to meet an overwhelming professional practice, and he gave himself to its cares and its exacting routine in no unwilling spirit. But, through all, he was one who never let himself forget that the sick man lay against the great background of living things in general, and the stars and a Deity beyond the stars. He was also one who, amid an age of furious currents of opinion, never relaxed his effort to read Nature without fear or favour, and judge what may be the rightful grounds of the dignity of man. It seems worth while across the centuries, to seek contact with such a one, and, as we do so, the temptation is perhaps to pick out, in the light of today's knowledge, what has proved right in his outlook and to exalt it, that its worth may shine the brighter. But there, I think, he would have been the first to smile and say 'if you value me, do me the favour to render me all in all for what I was. I was right earlier than my time in some things; I was compact of mistakes, too. If I live, let me live in the round and altogether".

From Paris came a four-page letter from Sherrington's friend, Professor Louis Lapicque the neurophysiologist, saying in part:

> Several days ago I received your *Jean Fernel*. What an interesting book! – for everyone, but especially for the Paris physiologists, who are – if I may judge by my own case – terribly ignorant of this background to their science. You have furnished me with wonderful details of our 'Quartier Latin' unknown to me though I have lived in it for sixty years. Your erudition has my admiration and your interest in our country touches me deeply.

Sherrington's readers had come to know Fernel in *Man on His Nature*, but the biographical volume on his hero was a work of such profound erudition that, as Lapicque says, his readers found it utterly staggering. How could a man approaching his ninetieth year produce such a treasure? The answer can only be sought in his long life of classical scholarship, poetic imagination and abiding interest in the history of French civilization. But more than that, it epitomized his thought on life itself, and was his testament.

No account of Sherrington's life with books would be complete without a statement of his gifts to libraries. We have already mentioned those to the Osler Library and to the University of British Columbia. These are dwarfed, however, by the number of incunabula given to the British Museum and of rare medical volumes to the Royal College of Surgeons and to the Royal College of Physicians in London.

Sherrington was "our best benefactor in modern times" according to the British Museum's Keeper of Printed Books, Sir Henry Thomas, writing in 1947. It is impossible to note any but the oldest here, but bibliophiles, and others as well, should know of the princely gifts to the public weal by one man, with only a professorial salary and with no pension (Appendix 12).

In typically generous fashion C. S. S. gave to the British Museum as a tribute to Sir Henry Thomas on his retirement, two Latin translations from the press of Simon de Colines (Paris, 1534): *De Hippocratis et Platonis placitis* and Galen *De Crisibus.*

The files of the Royal College of Surgeons show 113 notes from C. S. S. over the years offering books and important papers to the library. There he used to take one of us (W. C. G.) to tea and to see the Ramón y Cajal papers and volumes which he had deposited there, including some of the great Spaniard's early reprints on the 'boutons terminaux'– and other forms of nerve endings, published even before Sherrington coined the word 'synapse'. It was possible on my return from Spain in the summer of 1936 to add to the Sherrington items the *Trabajos Escogidos* of Ramón y Cajal – a reprinting of the first ten years of his work, the original papers now being totally unobtainable.

The key to Sherrington's selection of the Royal College of Surgeons' Library as recipient of many fine volumes is to be found in a note to the friendly Librarian, William R. LeFanu, written on Osler's birthday, 1947: "When I was young I got so much advantage from the Roy. Coll. of Surgeons Library that it is a pleasure as well as a privilege to attempt to make any return I can, however inadequate".

Already in 1931, C. S. S. had written to the Honorary Librarian, Sir D'Arcy Power: "It greatly enhances the pleasure already given me by acceptance of my small offering as welcome to the College Library. Let me take the opportunity of adding that if you would like them I can send 3 slim 4^{tos} as follows . . .". The same sentiment was expressed by him in 1935: "The library is so excellent and so admirably administered that it is a pleasure to be of any small service to it".

It would be impossible to detail all of these gifts but a few may be mentioned: William Beaumont's gastric classic in the original edition; Von Humboldt on muscle and nerve; *Studies on Paleopathology of Egypt* by Armand Ruffer – his confederate in the anti-diphtheritic drama in 1894; a seventeenth century French volume *L'Art de Saigner* by an anonymous surgeon; *Flora Medica* – on medicinal plants 1829–1830; early works on 'medical electricity' including a rare one by Jean Paul Marat, 1784 – with a note that Charlotte Corday murdered "Citoyen Marat" as C. S. S. designates him; Montanus, published in 1556 in Venice; Quercitamus, 1575, Lyons.

At the age of ninety-two C. S. S. wrote to the R. C. S. Librarian: "I want to thank the Royal College for the Report of Council kindly sent me. I notice from it that the library is interested in the works of Fernel, and I beg to offer for the acceptance of the library the accompanying early editions".

"P. S. The *Fabrica* [of Vesalius] your report extols is spoiled for many of us by the vulgarity of the title illustration. Lieut. Colonel Garrison likened it to 'Barnum advertisements' ".

One other matter affecting the Royal College of Surgeons must be dealt with briefly, i. e., Sherrington's continuing interest in pooling the resources of London's many medical libraries. His statement of his hope for this is well set out in a letter to W. R. LeFanu of 14 November 1938 (Appendix 13).

Once when LeFanu passed to C. S. S. an enquiry from Sir Charles Ballance concerning early publications on dilation of the pupil through stimulation of the sympathetic nervous system, a two-page reply came back. In it C. S. S. showed that a house surgeon at Stafford General Hospital, E. S. Hare, first described the paralytic syndrome in 1838 but died in that year. Johannes Horner however, was given the credit.

To the Royal College of Physicians C. S. S. gave: Raymond Vieussens, *Novum vasorum corporis humani systema,* Amsterdam, 1705; Schelhammer, *De Auditu, Leiden,* 1684; *Acta Medicorum,* Berlin, 1719 and 1720. Erasmus Darwin's *Botanic Garden,* 2nd ed. 1791 with the note

". . . also a small anthology of verse by Charles L. Dana, the neurolog. physician,New York, who gave the Hughlings Jackson Lecture in London in 1927. Mine is the 3rd and enlarged edition, 1922, from a small press run by Dana and his brother at Woodstock – a little country town in Vermont. They call it The Elm Tree Press. As you include in your library scope the verse writings of physicians perhaps you would care to include the verse-selections of physicians?

To the National Institute of Medical Research at Hampstead C. S. S. gave Carl Ludwig's *Arbeiten* and Eckard's *Beiträge.* Sir Walter Fletcher wrote to him:

I think much more of this gift than as a valuable addition to the resources of the Institute Library. I think of it as an act of great personal generosity . . . I think with pleasure also of the indefinable value that your books will always have there, because of their personal association with yourself. I cannot think of them otherwise than as likely to bring good spiritual health to the Institute for long years to come, in some mystical manner of inoculation.

During the second World War Sherrington gave to the National Library of Wales: Diogenes Laertius, *De vita et moribus philosophorum,* Venice, 1490, and *Decem Librorum Moralium Aristotelis tres conversationes,* Paris 1497. His great friend Victor Scholderer was, during the war, at Aberystwyth with the British Museum's collection of 10000 incunabula for safe-keeping. He wrote to C. S. S. as part of a lengthy correspondence: "You are right; to have steady work to do daily is the only thing in these days . . . as you say, it is impossible to believe what is going on [in Paris] is the real France".

It was not only John Fulton who had phenomenal luck in finding rare books in unlikely places. Sir Charles arrived a few minutes early for a meeting of the Trustees of the British Museum one spring day, so spent a few moments looking over the barrows of second-hand books in Great Russell Street. For a shilling he purchased a little French volume and slipped it into his pocket for reading on the train going home after the meeting. On the train he found it to be one of the earliest books printed in Canada: *Règlement de la confrerie de l'adoration perpétuelle du Saint Sacrement et de la bonne mort,* Montreal, 1776. After consulting with Dr. J. A. Gibson of the Prime Minster's office in Ottawa, Sir Charles sent the book to the National Library of Canada.

(W.C.G.)

Chapter 9

Sherrington the Poet

Sherrington as a boy was nourished on good literature in the home of his step-father, Dr. Caleb Rose, Jr. The library and the 'natural history' collections of Dr. Caleb Rose, Sr., were widely known, and Charles' capacity for 'wonder', developed in Ipswich, remained with him all his life. At Queen Elizabeth's School in Ipswich he had the good fortune to come under the tutelage of Thomas Ashe, a promising young poet. The headmaster, Dr. H. A. Holden, was already well known as a classical scholar for his translations.

At the age of nineteen Charles entered the medical school of St. Thomas's Hospital, London. Speaking of those days of 1876 he told a correspondent many years later:

> You ask after verses I am occasionally guilty of! I enclose two reprints from our University magazine – knowing you are a man of discretion and will suppress them. Also two written out – deserving burning more than any heretic – thinking they may beguile you – one describing a little English garden, my mother's, and set down when I was first away from home, and in London lodgings as a first-year student at St. Thomas's Hospital, and a bit homesick for my old country life: – the other 'compodged' for our little boy Carr, now away from home for his first term at school [Shrewsbury]. Carr when at home employs an airgun on the starlings and blackbirds and others of his co-partners in our little garden patch here [16 Grove Park, Liverpool], hence my bath-tub interview with the starling the other morning, as rhymed.

The earlier is presented here under the title *Mus Hortensis* from the second edition of *The Assaying of Brabantius*. It was modified considerably by C. S. S. since its first writing in 1876.

Mus hortensis

To-day, awake with dawn, I saw,
from my high window looking down,
streets empty yet, and scarce a flaw
sullied the blue that coped the town.
I murmured, how will these be changed
by fume and tumult, ere to-night
labour and strife-for-life have ranged

their hours, and toil out-lasted light.
More favoured lives the upland boy,
who feeds from some wild kernel-tree,
whose task is some half-wild employ,
whose herd is costlier housed than he,
but over whom the heavens go wide,
beneath whose feet the spring-time weaves,

whose pathway winds the mountain-side,
or threads the loveliness of leaves.

This rueful heart took flight to reach
a hill-top seventy miles from here,
and a white house where pine and beech
build their green place throughout the year;
its lawn went still undried of dew,
the pigeons crooned their sleepy noise,
and, piped the shrubbery bushes through,
there came the early robin's voice;
a butterfly, bright wings outspread
wide open on the terrace stair,
budged nothing, as if Pan had said
'the foot to harm thee climbs not there'.
The tool-house gable south and east
still sunned its golden apricots;
remembering many an old-time feast
I paced about the happy plots.
Then wading through the deeper grass
that takes the orchard's after-math
I turned to where morn's shadows pass
aslant the ruddy gravel-path,
tip-toeing lest my spaniel's bark
should rend the sacred silence up,
and, no sound coming, to its mark

I filled him fresh his half-dried cup;
and watched the shimmering insect-herds
hunt my wet flowers and mix their grains,
and glimpsed blithe hoppings of the birds
between the silver raspberry canes;
the heavy plums hung purple-blue,
the dark morellos ripe for Dis,
still lapped in westward shadow grew
the great pale stars of clematis;
the garden-roller leaned in peace
its shaft against the jasmined wall,
framed in an opening through the trees
the distance bosomed Bramford Hall;
and west and south and toward the dawn,
as waiting still day's fuller rise,
nine amber window-blinds half-drawn
dimmed the cool rooms for sleeping eyes,
dear sleeping eyes that dreamed perhaps
of me, and drew from memory's place,
forgetful how the months elapse,
some homely vision and my face.

And long could I have led my flock
in that fair place a pasturer
of wandered fancies, but the clock
boomed over towery Westminster.

On going up to Cambridge in 1879 to join his two younger brothers who were already there preparing to study law, Sherrington found his way into Heffer's bookshop where, for a shilling, he bought a first edition of Keats's collected poems.[1] He had already a considerable acquaintance with the work of the poet who had died of tuberculosis at a tragically young age. At school in Ipswich C. S. S. had already put into Latin verse the sonnet of Keats: "On Visiting the Tomb of Burns". Moreover, in the art gallery of the Ipswich museum he had become entranced with a landscape by Charles Bell's pupil, Benjamin Robert Haydon,[2] to whose memory Keats and Wordsworth had each written a sonnet.

We have already referred to the Longfellow paper by C. S. S. which appeared in the Cambridge Review in 1882 (Appendix 1). While he became a great reader of poetry we have no further examples of his own until he arrived at Liverpool as Holt Professor of Physiology in 1895. On the death of George Holt, ship owner and founder of both the chair and the early laboratory of physiology there, C. S. S. wrote:

---

1 Years later he sold it back to Heffer's for £ 100.
2 Teacher of Landseer.

In Memoriam: George Holt of Liverpool

Mother of Ships! not all thy keels that steer
delaying sunset or forestalling dawn,
lessening the watery spaces of the sphere,
not they, nor all thy quays like ramparts drawn
fronting the tideway, nor thy marts where awn
of Egypt's growth soothe Hesperean ear,
where fret wild feet that spurned the prairie lawn,
and fruits lie strewn that crowned the tropic year,

– no, not those wealths thou heap'st upon the shore,
nor all thy triumph above dividing seas,
vouchsafe the glory of thy temple floor
one wreath of bay so beautiful as these
that, while he stayed, with both his hands he bore,
'In Help is Hope' and 'Hope begets Heart's-ease'!

Even two years after his arrival at Liverpool he was still haunted by the stark realities of clinical life which he had experienced at St. Thomas's Hospital, London. His poem of 1897 reflects the concern of a sensitive observer:

St. Thomas's Hospital 1897

Palace of Pain, whose face mocks o'er a flood
rich and impure, the place of state decrees
and council hall of kingdoms bent on good.
There a pale population coughing blood
toil wasted, ulcer burrowed, born of ease
seeks for a little help in its disease.
Thames mirrors thee as it has mirrored trees
and many a happy garden, and healthy wood.
Lo, at thy thousand windows sighs like airs
make the deep curtains move it seems to me,
and white with sunlight still thou art in gloom
grief moans thee through from resonant room to room
so wild at first, but later glad to see
Death reach the pain that wears, and body that bears.

To his former pupil, Harvey Cushing, who had been appointed Professor of Surgery at Harvard he wrote on 9 December 1910:

Your letter speaks of medical men as versifier; it will interest you, therefore, to hear that we have a mutual friend, a 'medicine man' whom we have just discovered to be a real *poet*. Perhaps you know it already. I did not until a month ago, when after spending a weekend with us here, he left us on his departing, a little privately printed and unpublished volume – just printed this year containing some *gems* – poems fit for an anthology of English poems. The medicine man being no other than Henry Head. I am not exaggerating their beauty. Title: 'Songs of La Mouche and Other Verses' – much of it in the manner of Heine.

The "University Magazine" at Liverpool to which C. S. S. referred earlier was the student paper *Sphinx* for which he wrote occasionally. It was in this setting that he first published his poem, "A Transcript from Eucles Comrade of Xenophon", which began: "Then rose the Lydian sun between the hills". This poem appeared in his 1925 volume *The Assaying of Brabantius and Other Verse* as "Cyrus and Panthea" with many changes. Strangely his personal Liverpool copy shows several changes in the lines which did not find their way into the printed volume; e. g.: "Then rose the Asian sun between the hills".

In 1913 Sherrington published in the University of Toronto Monthly a poem "The Bow of the Ship", composed on a trans-Atlantic liner. Carr Sherrington, who came upon it in 1963, told me, "C. S. S. was very fond of it. I think you will like it; it should be republished".

The Bow of the Ship

I am the bow of the ship!
  I fling the foam with my speed,
Like a sea-god's shoulder adrip
  That all things in the high sea heed:
And I was slid from the slip
  By man for man in his need!

From sunrise on to sunset,
  With moon and with no moon,
For him I go and I get,
  And return beseeching no boon,
Content with my bulwarks wet,
  And my strength to restart soon!

Out from the high dock-gate
  To over the ocean rim,
South where the doldrums wait,
  North where the fog-belts swim,
My furrow a white road straight
  Plough'd at behest of him!

Strong men's muscle and brain,
  The toil thereof and the fire,
Spent were on me not in vain;
  I ripen'd to their desire,
From them for joy and for pain
  Is my soul as the son's from the sire!

Later the same year C. S. S. wrote to Cushing in Boston: "I enclose a piece of sea-verse, appropriate perhaps from a seaport physiologist". He was only a seaport physiologist for another two months before he left Liverpool for Oxford – there to swim in the warmer waters of "Parsons' Pleasure" in the altogether, or at "Dames' Delight" properly clad.

The Swimmer

Beyond the bar, mid ocean-vapors brown,
the sun, a murder'd king's cloak'd shield low down
    passes 'neath shadowy spears sloped Zenith high;
the church vane sparkles last in the grey town.

Far out, a swimmer who swims face toward land,
but the ebb drinks him, as it drinks loose sand;
    above his toiling shoulder the slow sky,
and the long surges broadening either hand.

And the last spark dies off the steadfast vane,
the risen vapor thickens into rain,
    close-hooded round by darkening sea & sky,
forsaken, lost, he drifts with his lone pains.

And more the night wind frets the ebb-way race,
curtains of foam swung 'thwart him blind his face;
    now that given ridge, where loud-voiced breakers cry
'the rampart of the ocean', nears apace!

Night, on a world of bursting seas that pour;
and, late, a thing face down on the low shore.
    the dawn draws near; not he will lift his eye;
for him the sun shall smite the vane no more!

Sherrington's move to Oxford in the first week of 1914 brought him into a different world – some colleges being 600 years old. Despite its name, New College had in 1379 incorporated into its grounds the ancient city wall and its defence towers. Across Longwall Street stood Magdalen College, with its beautiful tower and bridge, a deer park and Addison's walk. As Waynflete Professor of Physiology in the University Sherrington was a Fellow of Magdalen. There for the Oxford Magazine he wrote "Spring Term 1914", which appeared in his volume of poems in 1925 as "Oxford" – with its haunting first line.

Oxford

The night is fallen and still thou speakst to me,
what though with one voice sole, with accents many,
Tongued turret and tongued stream, tracked pasture fenny,
and cloister spirit trod, and centuried tree
and, bondsmen loosed in Time's tranquillity,
thy bell dischargèd hours. If wharfage any
thine 'tis where Age shall, nursing late his penny,
smile at long last to hand him Charon's fee.
And now, below, through shadows starr'd, a boat
steals by me laden with singing and young laughter,
and, higher, a wide-flung casement casts afloat
pulses of waltz the which white robes sway after;
vowed Priest of Beauty, these thy shrines among,
thou kneelst with old folk, thou that dancest with young.

This was followed in the same periodical by "Hilary Term 1916", beginning: "Now in the cloister few but old feet roam". In the 1925 volume it was amended.

Now in the cloister few the feet that roam,
ours that must stay, who little can than wait,
exchange our tidings, good, ill, early, late,
and send our 'god-speed' to them past the foam,
the young folk, splashed with death in the trenched
    loam.
Ay, oil the hinges of the ancient gate,
keep burnished bright the goblet's silvern state
against the hour shall hail the soldier home.
You stately tower, from high you saw them go,
and have full many doughty scenes and fair

watched and swung bells above, shattering the air
to honour heroes, you too wait as though
of our poor hearth-bound presence scarcely ware,
you heard from far the filial bugles blow.

With this his war-time poems began, soon to include "To Memory of
R. P. P., Flanders" – to memorialize R. Poulton-Palmer, the brave young
son of Sherrington's colleague, Professor E. B. Poulton, and his wife – one
of the Palmer family long associated with the neighboring city of Reading.

"Admetus Anew" appeared in the Oxford Magazine on 17 November
1916 with the following sub-title: ("This flower of youth, that stands
betwixt us and hell" – Letter from a historian, September, 1916)

When white Alcestis, staying the path of Death
Against her loved's breast, gave her own,
How suffered he who watched above the breath
That ransomed his! for him his new-leased throne
    Stood but a carven stone!

Nor heard he him, the lion-hided, leap
The last ravine that clove the plain;
Only he saw the leaden-lidded sleep
Mask Love's blenched face and marble out its pain;
    He groaned for all his gain.

O heart, my heart, young Love a-dying for thee
That long thy seat endure on high!
What shall it boot, thy length of days to be,
When, *sans* the love-lit zest-enchanted eye,
    Thou yearnest, heart, to die!

To thee, alas, no great-heart Heracles
Shall bring again thy golden day,
Thy day of ere Love died on the frore seas,
A gale-swept song-bird lost, a surge-drowned lay,
    Joy hurricaned away.

Nay, heart, my heart, thou listenest coward lies;
Not love shall sacrifice in vain;
Go, wait thine urn, not lowering thine eyes:
Who knows him dust and counts his toil his gain,
    Life dwarfs for him life's pain.

Thy choice had been for thee the gods had willed
The steep descent and flowerless pit,
Yet, since the task wherefore Love's lip was stilled
Bides thine to do, that Love find guerdon fit,
    Go, crown thy days with it.

In its 30 November 1917 edition the magazine included the following
short poem:

Dream Naïveté on Death

I had passed out upon seas soft as oil,
green with the green of everlasting bronze,
and, as a moon that still the day-tide wans,
faint sailed the sun, a disc of silver foil;
and I was old, so old that the sun's toil
from his beginning was but for the nonce
as beside mine, to beat without response
under cliffs sheer, tiered granite coil on coil.
Then in my dream ensued swift change to me,
as 'twere the mind, shod with some finer fire
than thought, on sharpened peaks, past all the known,
above abysses, felt like a great sea
the wind of realms fair-sphered beyond desire,
and starward shot as earthward a dropped stone.

Another short poem from Sherrington's restless pen graced the Oxford Magazine on 7 March 1919:

Δι, ωςων ην λόγος

In the beginning life, that was from death,
went whirled as flame to scattered sparks asunder,
lonely and many as the stars for wonder,
souls that each one its place imprisoneth;
so, till came speech to use and read lips' breath,
more fine than strings, more passionate than thunder,
bridging the dumb abysses round and under,
that thought reach thought exchanging what mind saith.
And so accomplished, after lapse of time,
dear meed of converse binds life's scattered ones,
with healing of the schism of old prime,
as light rejoins the pulses of old suns;
but ah! each soul finds yet, what though bars broken,
the fairest thoughts lie still beyond thoughts spoken.

When the Oxford University Press published his 67-page volume *The Assaying of Brabantius and Other Verse* many poeple "could not believe it"! One reviewer thought that *Miss* Sherrington had considerable to learn – which caused the retiring President of the Royal Society – and no doubt his friend John Masefield – much merriment.

One of the first to write to C. S. S. thereafter was Walter Morley Fletcher, bibliophile and friend – Secretary to the Medical Research Council:

Dear Sherrington, It was a great delight for me to find your book of poems waiting for me here and I am most grateful to you for your gift. I had long wanted to have some at least of your verses I knew from private rumor you had written, but I had never dared to ask you for them. I shall read this with very great interest, and great pleasure too, I am sure. My chief pleasure though will be in their coming from *you,* and in the friendship you have always so generously given me.

W. B. Hardy (Wesbrook's research supervisor at Cambridge and Carr Sherrington's tutor years later at Caius) wrote from the Athenaeum:

> My dear Sherrington, I have four friends who send me copies of their verse. To three I write such as politeness demands. To you a different acknowledgement is due. I have read your booklet through three times with growing pleasure because it has the real stuff in it ... the real ring and quality is undoubted and I congratulate you on possessing a faculty hitherto unsuspected by me. I am glad to have the book for old association's sake. Thank you for sending it.

The dedications of some of the poems are known. "At Keats' Grave" was dedicated to Geraldine Sharpey-Schafer, the only daughter of Sherrington's great friend, Professor E. A. Sharpey-Schafer. This long and beautiful poem offers considerable insight into Sherrington's life-long preoccupation with Keats, his style, his medical training and his tragic death at such an early age. At the same time the poem gives wings to Sherrington's thoughts on 'words'. How coarse and debased our language has become today as we speak of 'communication', as compared with the almost magical Sherringtonian view of words, as can be seen in the following extracts from his poem on Keats:

Thine was pain; now thine the praise;
dower, they both, of thy slain tongue,
that so led through lovely ways
words and thoughts together clung
themselves singing even unsung.

Words, thy handmaids, under thy spell
shod to follow thy desire
missioned heavenly things to tell,
lapt in music-swayed attire,
shadows moved by thought's leapt fire;

words, raised trumpets blown at morn,
words, foamed sea-capes calling through mist,
words like viol reed and horn
met in mood and half unwist
each by other turned and kissed;

words, deliverance of joy,
words, blithe feet that lift in dance,
flute-throat words of girl and boy
paeaning the Spring's advance,
death not heeding nor mischance;

words sharp-shapen as swords unsheathed,
words calm-lipped as the moon's rim,
words, voiced airs unloosed, breaths breathed
soft as censer-smokes aswim
swathing sacred rafters dim;

words, fleet brooks that rippling tell
April-thoughts to rooted grasses,
or with pause by some brimmed well
halted quiet as a glass is
mirroring day's vault that passes;

words, heaped torrents swol'n with rain,
words, cloud voices league-long blown,
words begotten of human pain
ripened through dark nights of moan;
words like bell-towers sobbing in stone,

passionful more than the brown bird's
fountain'd in June to the night sky;
blazoned sunrises of words
risen anew with a new cry;
words like living looms that ply

still across this day of ours,
weaving fancy's storied woof,
pageants under kingly towers,
or the jolly satyr's hoof
pounding 'neath an acorned roof; . . .

"Never a dirge of roses" was dedicated to John Middleton Murry, a prolific Keats scholar and husband of Katherine Mansfield.

From a teacher in far-off Adelaide, Australia, Sir Charles received an enthusiastic appreciation of his little volume, *The Assaying of Brabantius and Other Verse.* "I have seldom received a present which gave me more delight than your volume of verses; the more so as they came as a complete surprise . . . though I knew your deep interest in poetry.".

The 1925 volume of poetry was dedicated to the foremost clinical neurologist of Britain, Sir Henry Head. He, in turn, wrote to ask if he might dedicate some poetry to C. S. S. In 1940 Professor E. N. da C. Andrade also asked if he might dedicate his volumes of poetry to C. S. S., saying: "I do hope that you will find [in the proofs submitted] enough that you approve to let me use your name in this way". Andrade reported to C. S. S. that

> In reply to Walter de la Mare's letter about your poems, from which I quoted to you, I wrote telling him that you were a great admirer of Hardy and how you had quoted the whole of the poem on the blinded thrush in the concluding chapter of *Man on His Nature.* This morning I have another letter from him in which he says: 'It is curious how sure I felt that Sherrington was a devotee of T. H.'

There remain some untitled and some undated poems. In a large scrapbook kept up by Sherrington's wife, Ethel, there is a brief rhyme in German:

> Gott weiß viel:
> Doch mehr der Herr Professor:
> Gott weiß alles!
> Doch er – alles besser.

Later in the same scrapbook one finds:

> Remember all
> He spoke among you and the man who spoke
> Who never sold the truth to serve the hour,
> Nor paltered with eternal God for power:
> Who let the turbid stream of rumor flow
> Through either babbling world of high or low
> Whose life was work.

Some poetic lines have been found by Carr Sherrington in his father's diaries, and as he says, ". . . the writing in them was miniscule – he took off his glasses to do it. My thought is you might like to have his 1946 one . . . Most of his verses were written lying in a punt on the Cherwell while I did the punting". Of another diary Carr says: "I have come across your name again . . . There are many names in it familiar to you and furthermore it gives evidence of his design of verses. They came to him at odd moments, and were jotted down, improved upon during a train journey or a walk. In short the diary is good evidence of an organized mind and life, for he was then about 84".

Sometime between 1942 and 1943, while in wartime lodgings at Caius College, Cambridge, Sherrington wrote what his son has called ". . . a delightful verse about his mother; I recall her well in silken gown, lace cap and always 'knitting for the boys' ". Then he adds, "C. S. S. was an expert at crochet like his mother".

> Our mother rose from where she sat
> Her needles as she laid them down
> Met lightly, and her silken gown
> Settled; no other move than that.

When he was ninety C. S. S. wrote four short lines on Alexander – whether the Great or the Field Marshall of Tunis, Carr was never sure. The lines could equally well apply to either:

> They say great Alexander with him took
> Across swift rivers and then parching lands
> Over hoar mountains and long burning sands
> The charnel presence of an old blue book.

Another brief quatrain is thought to have been written from Eastbourne in one of his little diaries of which Carr Sherrington said in 1965: "It intrigued me and pleased me that you figure so prominently in these diaries. Few of his students and protegés do – just Penfield and Eccles and one or two others". Carr said these ". . . lines appealed to me immensely":

> It is old letters now that he lives on,
> Dear folded fragments of the past,

> Little I think he cares what chances
> Or if today's noon be his last.

Carr added: "There is little doubt in my mind that these lovely lines expressed his own views of that time, and his thoughts. Equally they are not far from my own thoughts today".

Two days after his ninety-fourth birthday the very arthritic Sir Charles wrote, as a jovial postscript to his letter to Lord Adrian acknowledging congratulations, these four lines:

> Stars! how many there are!
> And this one too!
> So then, I'm in a star;
> And where are you?

(W.C.G.)

Chapter 10

Public Service

While much has been said in the foregoing concerning Sherrington's service on many public bodies, editorial boards and commissions of enquiry, it seems essential to note, in addition, some of the unusual responsibilities which he undertook. While he was not one to ride on to the public stage on a white charger he had his 'lost causes' which he felt he must support.

Although he wrote to various publications on matters of public urgency, he wrote most often to the *British Medical Journal* or the *Lancet* on anti-vivsectionists or on medical educational topics. In one memorable case *(Lancet,* 1894) however, he wisely refused to be drawn into a protracted debate with Victor Horsley, who had suggested that a 'referee' be asked to adjudicate the merits of certain findings on cerebral localization. The problem resolved itself when Horsley died of heat stroke in Mesopotamia in 1915. Sherrington did not publish his paper until 1917, but the personal correspondence preserved in the Wellcome Library still makes interesting reading. No one could impose on Sherrington against his will, and the firmness of his convictions occasionally amazed his academic colleagues.

One of his interests was the Marey Institute in Paris – named after the great physiologist, Étienne Jules Marey, who died in 1904. His 'tambour' is still used in physiological recording today. He was a pioneer in the study of the flight of birds, and it was his book, translated into English under the title *Animal Motion,* which the Wright brothers memorized as schoolboys before embarking on powered flight. In addition Marey was a pioneer in cinematography, and along with Muybridge engaged C. S. S.'s attention in this field. Sherrington was requested by the International Association of Academies to attend the annual meetings of the governing committee of the Marey Institute for several years; he would put off Royal Society meetings in order to do this, so keen was he on French science.

For several generations of life-scientists the Physiological Society of Great Britain has been their academic and professional home thanks to

Sherrington's long and inspired service to it. His reminiscences of the early meetings with much informality and ease of intellectual contact have been transcribed for us by Professor Kenneth Franklin of Oxford.

In 1923 Sherrington received from the Foreign Office the following letter of thanks from the Marquess of Curzon of Kedleston: "His Majesty's Government much appreciate the readiness with which you consented to represent them at the celebrations . . . in France in honour of the centenary of the birth of Louis Pasteur . . . and the dignified manner in which you carried out your mission".

One of Sherrington's early concerns was to develop in Britain research and development laboratories in which answers could be given to major physical and engineering problems facing the country. As President of the Royal Society, he was able to welcome a large number of visitors to the National Physical Laboratory at Teddington, where inspection of the latest experimental aerodynamics research facilities took place. The safe dosage of X rays as well as many admiralty projects were under study in that year. C. S. S. remained interested in this laboratory throughout his life and maintained close personal ties with Sir Joseph Petavel, the director – incidentally an admirer of Sherrington's poetry. In 1928 he welcomed the delegates to the tercentenary celebrations by the Royal College of Physicians of the publication of William Harvey's *De Motu Cordis* (Appendix 9).

When St. Thomas's Hospital and Medical School entered upon a public funding campaign in 1929 Sir Charles undertook the responsibilities of a Vice-President of the Appeal Committee. The Dean of the school wrote very frankly to him: "I hope you will fully understand that under no circumstances was there any desire on the part of the Committee to ask you to become a Vice-President for any financial assistance but purely for the name of Sherrington, for which we at St. Thomas's have the most profound respect". In the same year he spoke at the centenary celebrations of the Zoological Society of London (Appendix 10).

Clearly Sherrington was in demand for many such purposes. In preparing for the Imperial Press Conference of 1931, his friend J. J. Astor asked him to come to the official dinner at the Royal Academy " . . . at which we hope our guests will have an opportunity of meeting representatives of art and literature, and indeed of all the professions".

From Whitehall, in 1934, Prime Minister Stanley Baldwin wrote to C. S. S.:

> On the completion of your second period of service as a member of the Medical Research Council, I wish to take the opportunity of expressing high appreciation of all the help that you have given in that capacity.

The Committee of Privy Council over which I preside are very sensible indeed of their indebtedness for the time and thought which you have given without stint, during these eight years, to this important branch of national work. They would wish cordially to acknowledge this, and I therefore now ask you to accept an assurance of their sincere gratitude.

No doubt, although your formal membership has ended, there will continue to be occasions on which your advice will be of great value, and I am sure that it will then be as willingly given as in the past.

Kenneth Clark, Director of the National Gallery, wrote to C. S. S. in 1934 thanking him for "etched portraits of Mr. and Mrs. Edwards". On another occasion we find Sherrington donating to the National Portrait Gallery the bust of Crome and Crome's palette. With the death of his friend Sir William Bragg, the physicist, Sherrington was asked by Gilbert Murray to fill the vacancy on the Board of Trustees of the British Museum in 1942. It was made clear that it was " . . . the unanimous wish of the Standing Committee that you should allow them to propose your name . . . ". At age eighty-five, this must have set a precedent.

In 1934 the Warden of New College, H. A. L. Fisher, revived the matter of government grants to universities, in a note to C. S. S.:

You may remember that a letter came to me over your signature during the War, when I was at the Board of Education (1917), stating the urgent needs of the University for a Parliamentary grant. The claim which you set out was so strong that I had very little difficulty in convincing the Chancellor of the Exchequer and the Cabinet that Parliament ought to come to the rescue of the two ancient Universities. Nearly 17 years have passed since then, and it occurs to me to ask you whether it might not be opportune that some statement should be given to the Public, in view of the visit of the University Grants Committee next November, of the progress and activities of Oxford Science since it has had the advantage of this aid from the State.

Sherrington's relations with Russian scientists were very warm. He had visited Russia in Czarist days and was considerably embarrassed when asked by the ruling family to select, from an array of treasures, a memento which he would like to take back to England. He chose some chocolate! With Henry Dale he had visited Pavlov's home. At the time of Pavlov's death in 1936 Dale wrote to Sherrington commenting:

It is sad to hear that the great old man Pavlov has gone. I was reminded, on reading of his origin and early history in *The Times* this morning of what you said about the points of similarity between his career and that of Ramón y Cajal. It is strange, indeed, that two great men of such similar humble origins, both making history in the knowledge of the central nervous system from different angles, should each have become a symbolic figure for scientific regeneration, under revolutionary conditions, in his own country.

One of us (W. C. G.) found while on a visit to laboratories in Leningrad and Moscow in 1937 that a letter of introduction from Sherrington opened doors magically. Pavlov's successor, Professor Orbeli, and his wife entertained at Pavlov's farm enjoying honey from Pavlov's bees. We toasted

Sherrington's health, discussed the care of the dogs in winter time, with outdoor "runs" in which the floors were heated, and especially the work of Banting and Best on insulin. Orbeli had taken some of his training in Cambridge and, with his wife, spoke excellent English. He had told the would-be translators of the Oxford School's book *Reflex Activity of the Spinal Cord* that he would help them to prepare a Russian text only on condition that Sir Charles approved.

From 1925 to 1934 Sherrington was a member of the governing body of the Medical Research Council of Great Britain. This organization developed from the provision made by Prime Minister Lloyd George's original legislation which set up the National Health Insurance scheme and allotted "one penny per person" for grants in aid of medical research. This fund in the first year of the scheme approximated £ 57,000 sterling.

The Medical Research Committee as it was then called appointed a skilled and research-trained Cambridge physiologist, Walter Morley Fletcher to be its executive secretary. He forced it to get down to serious business, with fewer "excellent dinners and wit" at the home of Lord Moulton, and more for the future of research. Henry Dale, disheartened, was ready to leave the original committee but when Fletcher was appointed, realized " . . . that the M. R. C. could be pulled out of the mess of jobbery into which it seemed to be sinking".

In 1930 Fletcher wrote to Sir Charles to say that:

> The Medical Research Council yesterday expressed by unanimous vote their desire to submit your name to the Lord President for reappointment . . . I am asked to express the strong desire of all members of the Council that you may be willing to join them again. I hope you will not think it impertinent if I add some personal solicitation on my own behalf as their officer to whom you have always given such ready help.

Sherrington's *credo* for medical progress was best stated when he told his audience at McGill University in Montreal: "Do not, O my brothers, forget research. Science calls us all to it – and the call is from humanity as well".

An account of the recognition given Sherrington by universities, academies and learned societies during his lifetime and posthumously is to be found in Appendix 15.

(W.C.G.)

Chapter 11

The Final Philosophical Messages

In 1947 Sherrington wrote the introduction to the second edition of *The Integrative Action of the Nervous System* (Appendix 11). It was a remarkable survey of his earlier work on reflexes with the addition of a clear distinction between 'habit' and 'reflex'. "Habit arises always in conscious action; reflex behaviour never arises in conscious action. Habit is always acquired behaviour, reflex behaviour is always inherent and innately given. Habit is not to be confounded with reflex action".

Psychologists should take heed of this sharp distinction by the "master of the reflex". The so-called conditioned reflexes are *not* reflexes. Particularly memorable is the wonderfully vivid account of the self!

> Each waking day is a stage dominated for good or ill, in comedy, farce or tragedy, by a *dramatis persona*, the 'self'. And so it will be until the curtain drops. This self is a unity. The continuity of its pressence in time, sometimes hardly broken by sleep, its in-alienable 'interiority' in (sensual) space, its consistency of viewpoint, the privacy of its experience, combine to give it status as a unique existence. Although multiple aspects characterize it, it has self-cohesion. It regards itself as one, others treat it as one. It is addressed as one, by a name to which it answers. The Law and the State schedule it as one. It and they identify it with a body which is considered by it and them to belong to it integrally. In short, unchallenged and unargued conviction assumes it to be one. The logic of grammar endorses this by a pronoun in the singular. All its diversity is merged in oneness.

Finally there is a plea for dualism: "That our being should consist of *two* fundamental elements offers I suppose no greater inherent improbability than that it should rest on one only".

In 1950 at the age of ninety-two Sherrington delivered his final message in a short introduction to a B. B. C. Symposium on the Physical Basis of Mind (Appendix 14). He reaffirms with several examples his belief in dualism and finishes with a very audible chuckle as he recounts in derogatory fashion a story from last century where " . . . the oracular Professor Tyndall, presiding over the British Association at Belfast, told his audience that as the bile is a secretion of the liver, so the mind is a secretion of the brain".

He finishes with the great enigma that remained with him to the end: "Aristotle, 2000 years ago, was asking how is the mind attached to the body. We are asking that question still".

In retrospect we can agree that Schrödinger's eulogism of "Man on his Nature" was richly deserved. It is so because for the first time we are given an attempt to discover how far the resources of the neurosciences can contribute to a solution of the age-old problem of brain and mind. Sherrington modestly recognized that no solution was at hand, but his rigorous exposition led him to the rejection of much philosophical speculation. The main issues of the problem were thus better defined than ever before. He eminently deserves the title "Philosopher of the nervous system" given with remarkable prescience by Asher in 1931.

It is for us to continue in the philosophical field he illuminated. In fact he enjoined me so to do in a most moving appeal on the last occasion we met (February, 1952). He seemed to think his end was near, but I did not expect this to occur nine days later (4 March) from a coronary attack. I hoped for more of those wonderful allocutions. His mind was brilliantly clear and critical as he delivered his last messages to me. I have always regretted that I did not have a concealed tape recorder! For him the greatest adventure and challenge to mankind was to discover what he was and how he came to man's estate in the evolutionary process. There would be no end to this enquiry. To journey is better than to arrive. As a true scientist Sherrington feared arrivals – the claim to have established some incontrovertible truth. Such claims lead to dogmas and superstitions, and are scientific diseases. We quote finally the last sentences of Penfield's admirable offering (1957) to the memory of Sherrington on his centenary:

> He had faith, this old man who was forever young, that success would come to physiology in time, and understanding to scientist and philosopher alike. But he turned from the problem that neither could solve, to see life with the eyes of a poet:
>
> "The night is fallen and still thou speakst to me,
> what though with one voice sole, with accents many,
> tongued turret and tongued stream, tracked pasture fenny
> and cloister spirit trod, and centuried tree."
>
> Nature spoke to him with many tongues and with accents many. He understood her accents and could integrate them in his thinking until he seemed at last to comprehend the meaning of life, the design of the Creator.

(J.C.E. and W.C.G.)

Epilogue

Thus we leave Sir Charles, hoping to have added – not to his lustre which has been so well chronicled by others – but to his wholeness as a human being, full of "busy common sense", a reluctant giant.[1] His great hope was that he could live his life as one who opened rather than closed doors – especially for young people. He left no declamatory doctrine behind him, but rather a body of reproducible knowledge upon which his successors could build. The least dogmatic of men, he held a prescient mirror up to life and living things – a true biologist. His reverence for human life was the keel of his ship; the charts he made of the seas we sail will continue to benefit all men in perpetuity.

The noble philosophy of man that Sherrington delivered in his last great period of creativity offers some much needed illumination in the present dark and troublous times – the clear light from a great spirit. He condemns today's *Homo preadatorius* in all its forms as a regression to an early evolutionary type that has long been superseded by the modern civilizations based on values, that guide living in humane societies. *Homo praedatorius* is an anachronism with the seeds of destruction of all that matters.

Sherrington's great work was accomplished without the competitiveness that threatens the scientific community today. Dedicated scholars can suffer severely from neglect, and with that the standards of scholarship can suffer, too. Success is too often measured by the size of grant support – a grotesque inversion of values. The temptation of the young scientist is to devote his

---

1 C. S. S. wrote of Ferrier (1928) as we might well write of Sherrington. "Slight and erect in figure, genial and alert in bearing, the burden of years long weighed lightly on him. A reflective quietude of voice and manner tended to veil the underlying energy, no less a part of his nature. Shrewd observer, keenly alive to men and things, and not least to aesthetics and to humour, his talk could exert charm, and owed something to a certain piquant directness and penetrative simplicity."

life to the competitive climb of a predaceous man and not to the dedicated and imaginative search for truth.

We trust that the life of Sherrington as here told will be an inspiration and a guide to those searching for the way. We were exceedingly fortunate to know him personally with his modesty, charm, vivacity, good humour and the wonderful range of knowledge on which he could draw with singular aptness. It was an amazing experience to live in daily intimate contact with him. One always associates him with the informality and warmth of the hospitality that Lady Sherrington gave to their home in Oxford. All these remain the rare memories that we treasure throughout our lifetime, memories that become more precious as we learn that such occasions only come once. Sherrington was a scholar and a scientist, an adventurer questing for truth and beauty, and so human a person that his pupils' admiration was transmuted into love.

We have been motivated to write this book by our hope that we may convey some of his essential features to those coming long after this great man. As Liddell so well says: "He had searched long and found much. His kind comes to the world not often in centuries".

(J.C.E. and W.C.G.)

Selected References

The bibliography of Sir Charles Sherrington has been reproduced by Denny-Brown in 1940, Fulton in 1952, Cohen in 1958, so that the authors have felt it unnecessary to repeat its several hundred items here. Throughout the text we have given the standard citations of his work. However, reference must be made to the charming "Memories", read to the Beaumont Club at Yale University and to the Fellows' Society of the Montreal Neurological Institute and the Montreal Physiological Society, in November 1957 – the centenary of Sir Charles' birth – by his son Carr, and privately printed. We have, with the permission of Miss Unity Sherrington, daughter of Carr and Margaret Sherrington, reprinted this lecture as Appendix 17.

As explained in the acknowledgments we have drawn on a large number of personal letters, drafts of speechs and on many printed papers in bringing together what we hope is a warm and faithful portrait of Sir Charles' active life and thought.

There remain, however, a few publications in which the background to our study is amplified, and these we cite hereunder:

Adrian, E. D.: Sensory integration. The Sherrington lectures, p. 20. Liverpool: University Press 1949

Bean, W. B.: Editorial. Curr. Med. Digest. *36,* 363–366 (1969)

Campbell, A. W.: Histological studies on the localization of cerebral function. Cambridge: Cambridge University Press 1905

Cohen, Lord of Birkenhead: Sherrington – physiologist, philosopher and poet, p. 108. Springfield (Ill.): Thomas 1958

Creed, R. S.: Obituary Notice: Sir Charles Scott Sherrington, O. M., G. B. E., F. R. S., 1857–1952. Br. J. Psychol. *44* 1–4 (1953)

Denny Brown, D.: Charles Scott Sherrington. Am. J. Psychol. *65,* 474 (1952)

Denny Brown, D.: The Sherrington school of physiology. J. Neurophysiol. *20,* 543–548 (1957)

Eccles, J. C.: Obituary, Sir Charles Sherrington, O. M., F. R. S., 1857–1952. Br. J. Phil. Sci. *3,* 298–301 (1952)

Eccles, J. C.: Some aspects of Sherrington's contributions to neurophysiology. Notes Records R. Soc. (London) *12,* 216–225 (1957)

Forbes, A.: A Memorial tribute. J. Clin. Neurophysiol. EEG *4*, 213 (1952)

Franklin, K. J.: Francis Joseph Cole, 1872–1959. Biographical memoirs Fellows of the R. Soc. *5*, 37–47 (1957)

Fulton, J. F.: Sir Charles Scott Sherrington, O. M., J. Neurophysiol. *15*, 167–190 (1952)

Fulton, J. F.: Sir Charles Sherrington, Obituary. Lancet *262*, 569 (1952)

Granit, R.: Sir Charles Sherrington: An appreciation. Nature *169*, 688 (1952)

Granit, R.: Charles Scott Sherrington: An Appraisal, p. 188. London: Thomas Nelson 1966

Krige, C. F.: To cure sometimes. A doctor's autobiography. Johannesburg: Da Gama Publishers (no date)

Liddell, E. G. T.: Sir Charles S. Sherrington, 1857–1952. Oxford Magazine *70*, 282–284 (1952)

Liddell, E. G. T.: Sir Charles Sherrington, 1857–1952. Br. Med. Bull. *8*, 379 (1952)

Liddell, E. G. T.: Charles Scott Sherrington, 1857–1952. Obituary Notices of Fellows of the R. Soc. *8*, 241–270 (1952)

Liddell, E. G. T.: The discovery of reflexes. Oxford: Clarendon Press 1960

Moruzzi, G.: Charles Scott Sherrington, 1857–1952. Rivista Sperimentale di Freniatria. *76*, Fasc. 2, 3–6 (1952)

Penfield, W.: Sir Charles Sherrington: An appreciation. Nature *169*, 688 (1952)

Penfield, W.: Sir Charles Sherrington, poet and philosopher. Brain. *80*, 402–410 (1957)

Penfield, W.: Sir Charles Sherrington, O. M., F. R. S.: An appreciation. Notes Records R. Soc. (London) *17*, 163–168 (1962)

Ramón Y Cajal, S.: Recuerdos de mi vida. Translated by Horne Craigie, E. as: Recollections of my life. Cambridge (Mass): M. I. T. Press 1966

Sherrington, C. E. R.: Memories, C. S. S. 1857–1952. Privately printed 1957

Sherrington, C. S.: Obituary notice of Sir David Ferrier. Proc. R. Soc. (London). [Biol.] *103*, viii–xvi (1928)

Swazey, J. P.: Reflexes and motor integration – Sherrington's concept of integrative action, p. 273 Cambridge (Mass.): Harvard University Press 1969

Appendix 1. C. S. Sherrington on Longfellow

From: *The Cambridge Review.* 3 May, 1882

In the short space of three weeks two poets have been snatched from the feast of life they helped to make more beautiful and joyous for us all, poets widely sundered in all other ways yet linked by the bond of poetry in each. Longfellow died on March 24, at Cambridge, Massachusetts; and Dante Gabriel Rossetti on April 9, in Thanet, Kent. Neither of them was born of English parentage; but none could be more English, if dear love of England and a place in the assemblage of those who have made this English tongue the richest treasury of thought that men possess, can make them English.

All lives are forces in the world, have their trajections, and initiate disturbances, which, though untraceable, register the sociology of the planet from their time onward for all ages. Individually most are little forces; but the great men are great forces; their vibrations are ample and intense; and further, are, so to speak, "catching." Napoleon's generals are little Napoleons; Raffaelle's school little Raffaelles. Often, no doubt, the great are more sensitive to the spirit of the age than is the ordinary man, and far more impressionable by its reactions; but preeminently they, more than their fellows, act upon the spirit of the age. Their influence is wide, or deep, or long-continuing: Shakspere's is all of these; Rosseti's certainly the second; Longfellow's perhaps only the first. But how wide his influence is and has been, it is hard to conceive: it is said that 350000 copies of his collected poems had been sold more than a quarter of a century ago. One day, while still comparatively unknown, he was standing in an Evangelical church and heard verses of his own chanted by the congregation. It was only last Christmas that we came across a band of children singing his "Village Blacksmith" to a wild tune of their own in a country lane in Suffolk. He has been literally the poet of the million; and although "fit audience though few" may seem a higher crown of honour, yet to be the people's singer has to the lover of mankind no glory like it. And to be the people's singer, never base, and ever pure in heart, believing in the people's purity, and in the household hearth as in a shrine sacred with chaste loves and duties of comrades, perceiving the pathos of the common-place and sympathising with the everyday–seems to us to have much of priestship and of the holiest in it, and among mortal offices to be nearest the godlike.

Longfellow's style of verse is as far removed from that of the school of "culture" as if a century and not one half of a generation lay between them; but his spirit had much that is one with the priceless element of the most refined modern culture, the enthusiasm of humanity, to which the religion and the philosophy of this day, the Broad Church and the Positivist school, allow so large a scope in our social improvement. His style of verse exactly fitted the people: clear, not too terse; simple, and never strange . . .

Longfellow's verse to us has its chief charm in its "unstrainedness"; its affectation, when it has any, is so slight and apparent that the mind does not stop to pride itself upon power of penetration in perceiving it, and passes it by without interruption of enjoyment, without irritation. It is the easily read affectation of a child – so easy to read that one thinks it but "natural," forgetting the very fact that it is affectation. Will this verse be a living power in the future, as it most assuredly is now? The mechanism of the verse in "Evangeline" is much inferior to that of the "Bothie of Toberna Vuolich," of the "Edith" of Ashe, our Johnian poet. But through all there breathes the same childlike freedom, "so innocent-arch, so cunning-simple." There is no weird line that for a moment seems to open up space and all the worlds; there is nothing to compare with the "Threnody," itself comparable with "Lycidas" and "Adonais"; nothing to set beside the intellectual feasts, the emotional deeps, of "In Memoriam"; those his religion precluded: still less, beside the vast profundities of feeling in the "House of Life." We find nothing in Longfellow to set against the marvellous lyrics of Mr. Swinburne, where everything "suffers a sea-change into something rich and strange:" no wit like Mr. Lowell's, although for a genial humour quite comparable to our Laureate's, turn to the "Spanish Gipsy" and Iagoo's tale in the wigwam in "Hiawatha." Yet despite all this, we believe that the author of "Miles Standish" will long keep a place in the heart of the people. These are stainless pages, wealthy in sunny sketches, in allusions drawn from study of the best of many lands. The love of childhood is as marked, almost as vividly expressed, as Hugo's. And especially "Hyperion" and "Kavanagh" will keep the memory of Longfellow alive in the hearts of his readers: though the Boston transcendental school, the Browning Society at Girton, and bards of the poetry of realism may smile a little contemptuously at admirers of the late Professor of Belles Lettres (hateful phrase) in transatlantic Cambridge. To the poorest child, in whose unpropitious destiny the one thing propitious is the English book he many read, shall the book given be a sealed one? shall the richest casket of human thought be made too difficult for him to open? and he who comes openhanded, even to the lowest, shall not great glory be his from lowest and highest?

Few can now doubt that the North American Republic has entered upon the possession of a political as well as a commercial wealth. Few would have guessed that her advent would be so long deferred. The history of her existence is one long poem. But though the struggles of out-wandering races against nature and against the races they dispossess have generally been rendered vocal by the songs of the conquerors, the early colonists, Puritans and sturdy martyrs they, had little turn for singing . . . Great struggles for great principles usually produce for themselves the genius that shall make them live in story; yet the War of Independence produced at the time no poet – happily for England, let us say. The early editions of Griswold's American Poets are collections of most uninteresting verse, not at all above the ordinary English magazine poetry of the early part of this century, strictly moral always, somewhat lacrymose – hectic, Mr. Rossetti calls it, "with hectic tinge which speaks of the more commonplace, not the more poetically related, forms of consumption." "At bottom nothing but maudlin puerilities, or more or less musical verbiage," says Walt Whitman in his strong way.

But a destiny to civilise a continent made for itself bards at last, Emerson, Whittier, Whitman, Miller, and others. And now, a year later than Bryant's death, Longfellow, eldest of the brotherhood, is dead! Eldest to judge him by his work. For he is nearer akin than Bryant to that class of earlier American writers who, we have said, have little distinctive in them, nothing national; but far removed from these by reason that he is a poet, they poetasters. Bryant is the first American poet, Longfellow is a pre-American poet. Bryant indicates the growth of an American poetry, sprung from New England life and the seed which our great Johnian, the bard of the Cumberland hills, had sown; the health and air of the mountain ("Auf den Bergen ist Freiheit!"), which is the conspicuous element of American poetry, and Emerson has occupied in all its vastness, has been preserved uninterruptedly; Whittier, Emerson, Whitman, Miller, Lowell, Parsons, all possess it. Would that some among our poets had it more? the little breath they have is too often that of a nursery-garden. Poe alone has it not; and his writings are exceptional altogether. The worst part only of him is American, and in his work the higher life of America finds, we would contend, no representation whatever. So far he is not a national poet. Neither is Longfellow. But Poe is not even Anglo-Saxon; Longfellow always is. No one could point to any writing of the latter, even to "Hiawatha," and say with certainty this is not the work of an Englishman; the "Wayside Inn" is an English inn; the "Village Blacksmith" too. As he was fond of saying, Longfellow was a true lover of "old England." Little more than two months before his death the writer of this article received a letter from him, in which he speaks with pleasant recollections of this university and of the kindness shown him by the late Master of Caius. And if he was a true lover of England, surely England in the mass was a true lover of him; his pages must fill a well-known place on the bookshelf of most of us, short though that shelf may be; alas, that there will be no further addition to his store of words that are pleasant to read in the lamplit corner, pleasant to be reminded of by nature in the afternoon fields.

Appendix 2. Extracts from "Marginalia" on Cambridge and London, c. 1880

From: *Science, Medicine and History*. Essays on the evolution of scientific thought and medical practice writen in honour of Charles Singer. Collected and edited by E. Ashworth Underwood. 2 volumes. London: Oxford University Press 1953. (Proofs read and corrected shortly before Sherrington's death on 4 March, 1952)

I was an undergraduate at Cambridge in the opening 80's of last century, and was at Gonville and Caius College. The Master then was the Rev. Dr. Norman Ferrers, whom we saw but little. I sat for the Natural Sciences Tripos. Things were stirring in the Medical School. Langdon-Brown has happily referred to Michael Foster, George Humphry and George Paget as 'the great Triumvirate'. But, for me, an even more appealing triumvirate, in that then small and ramshackle haunt of Physiology, were Gaskell, Langley and Lea, assistants to Foster, and all, like him, belonging to Trinity College. The physiological school was small in numbers but its camaraderie was something unforgettable. After taking an Arts degree I stayed up doing a research with Langley. It was at this time that an elderly visitor looked in one forenoon during the vacation, and I was asked to take him round our very disjointed buildings. We witnessed Langley experimenting on saliva-tion in the cat. The separate nerves were graduately stimulated. Drugs at different dosages injected. The saliva collected from the actual ducts was carefully measured, its digestive power and its amounts recorded. Pieces of the gland preserved for microscopical examination. All was done with a precision and skill which evidently impressed the visitor. Then we went to Gaskell, engaged on his study of the excised tortoise-heart. The beats were recorded graphically and separately from auricle and ventricle; a pile of such tracings fixed and varnished filled a basket near to hand. The visitor, after we left, expressed to me how impressed he was by all this care and skill and exacting enquiry. But he then added that he was surprised and mystified by the problems chosen: such earnestness and care devoted to subjects quite remote from Medicine – salivation in the cat, and the beat of a tortoise's heart! The visitor was a clinician of European repute. All I could say did nothing to shake his conviction that this devoted laboratory work was as regards Medicine sadly beside the mark. The coming years however were not slow to answer this criticism. Langley was discovering what to this day is the fullest picture of secretion as a cell-process. Gaskell was laying the foundation of knowledge of a disease which has become known largely through his work to be the most frequent and deadly of all types affecting the heart. Langdon-Brown rightly styles his work the foundation of 'Modern Cardiology'.

Returning for a moment to Sir George's slightly lame gait, a story went that at the Royal College of Surgeons where the candidates used to wait before a good fire in the large entrance-hall, they witnessed on one occasion the entry of an elderly plainly dressed man who limped. It struck them that this must be a patient on whom they would be examined. They pressed forward, gave him ten shillings, and listened to his account of himself. In the examination room later, they were surprised when the same spare keen-eyed man came forward, this time in the role of examiner. 'No,' he told them, returning the ten shillings, 'we are not going to talk about varicose veins this time.' Sir George never out-stayed his prestige in the Chair, but in some cases the existence of the 'life-tenure' of certain university chairs led at times to quasihumorous situations. At a faculty meeting called to appoint a fresh examiner, the Regius Professor, getting on in years and sadly deaf, presided. Those assembled waited for him to make the first proposal. He did so and to our surprise the name he put forward had passed to the Elysian Fields. A short pause ensued during which a member of the committee seated next to the Regius was heard to whisper to him. The Regius cupped his hand to his ear and regretted that he was a little deaf. Then in a loud stage-whisper the words were repeated, 'Dr. R – is dead sir'. The Regius smiled understandingly in genial reproof: 'Deaf, is he? So am I; but come now, he is not so deaf as all that!'

I imagine that in the training for no other profession does so great a shift of contacts happen so abruptly as for the student of Medicine – or at least did so seventy years ago. The plunge from laboratory life in Cambridge to out-patient work among the poor of a great hospital in London is an experience startling and ineffaceable – an excursion into a strange world. St. Thomas's Hospital dates back to the twelfth century, and is more than coeval with 'Barts'. Its site was for centuries in St. Thomas's Street, the street in which Keats wrote his famous sonnet on Chapman's Homer. It stood opposite Southwark Cathedral, and with Chaucer had seen pilgrims set out for Canterbury from the Tabard Inn near by. Richard Mead, Dr. Johnson's 'Mæcenas', was one of its physicians, and his marble bust is still in its entrance-hall. In the railway age the making of London Bridge terminus displaced the old hospital. In 1870 Queen Victoria opened its new buildings, facing the Houses of Parliament across the tidal Thames. The Germans killed some of its sick and nurses during the late war. Its students are an admixture of London, Oxford and Cambridge. It serves a population which stretches form Bermondsey to Brixton Church, perhaps a million souls. In my student time its 'parish' extended across the river as well – what was then called Regency Street, Millbank, was then the very climax of its poverty. When I was lodged in the 'College House' for A. O. C. duty, I had alongside me on similar duty a Cambridge man, a wrangler, James Niven,[1] and I remember we shared for reading Georges Sand's *Consuelo*. The bell would ring – no telephones then to call us out for a visit. On my first night, the bell rang me and I went down to find a young man waiting to take me to his wife who was in labour. It was Saturday, and after the closing-hour for the public houses – they closed later then than now – but the streets were not yet quiet. We walked west along the Embankment to beyond Doulton's potteries. We entered a doorway and descended a flight of stone steps. Opening a door he ushered me into a basement cellar. It had for window an unglazed opening into the well under a large grid in the pavement. The cellar was roomy and lit by two naked gas flames. My patient lay on a low bed in one corner. This was her second confinement; she was not unduly anxious. The elder child lay asleep across the lap of a neighbour. On the farther side of the cellar were more children, and three adults. I learned that three families tenanted the cellar. My patient had no privacy whatever. Such talk as went on was not noisy, but it was not hushed. It treated my patient as a matter of public interest to the room. I was helped in what I had to do by the husband and a woman evidently known to the room. The husband got hot water, whence I do not know, for there was no grate or fire. Things went well. The neighbour took charge of the last arrival. Before daybreak I prepared to leave. To my astonishment the young husband then

---

[1] James Niven (1851–1925) was later a fellow of Queens' College, Cambridge, and medical officer of health of the City of Manchester until 1922 [Editor].

proposed to see me home – there was no gainsaying him. He insisted on carrying my handbag all the way. Back at the Hospital we parted with a handshake, and I could have cried 'Concitoyen', I admired him so.

There was no other case waiting and I was soon asleep in my little official room. It was ten o'clock in the morning before I woke and my eyes opened on the daily 'poker' party already assembled in the room and at play, with the rattle of pence and the calling of debts. The trivial vulgarity of the scene I woke to contrasted dreadfully with the dignity of the poverty I had glimpsed hardly half a mile distant up the road.

In the late spring of 1914 I had a short trip to Russia, always to be remembered with pleasure. In St. Petersburg, as it was then still called, the Douma was in session, and through the kindness of Sir Bernard Pares, who attended, I met some of its notables. Snow still patched the spacious squares of the city; and the Neva was piled with drifting ice crunching against the bridges. My immediate business was as an organizing secretary of the Société des Académies to prepare for the triennial meeting to be held in St. Petersburg the next year. Our little party from London consisted of three, and the Czar gave us a personal interview at the Summer Palace at Tsarsky-Zelo. But to me the most memorable event of our visit was personal contact with the physiologist Ivan Pavlov. He was overflowing with energy, although an elderly man; he was spare in figure and alert and humorous in manner. He directed three laboratories, and insisted that I should spend a day in going round them with him. I joined him by appointment at ten o'clock in the forenoon, and at five o'clock in the afternoon he still, on encountering a stairway, ran up it rather than walked. He wished me to hear his morning lecture to students; it lasted forty minutes. I could not follow it, my Russian was not adequate, but the discourse was a vivacious affair delivered without a note. His form of address to me was always broken French or German, very rapidly uttered. We drank tea a number of times. He would say 'Tea, tea', pull open a drawer half-full of loose tea, scoop out a handful, throw it into hot water from the samovar, and in little more than a minute we would be drinking the fresh infusion. The laboratory we visited last was in a suburb, and though completely built, not yet completely equipped. A large costly institute, it was lavishly staffed. It was called the 'Tower of Silence', because for the observations its rooms had to be sound-proof. Pavlov had there a number of his trained dogs. We observed their reactions through periscopes. One animal he particularly wished me to see; its training confronted it with a dilemma; its anxiety was pathetic to watch. Remembering my good host's aversion to any mention of the word 'mind' – which his laboratory doctrine excluded – I answered, when he still pressed me for an opinion, that the animal seemed to me in a state of persecution best comparable with that of a Christian martyr. Pavlov was delighted; he laughed and laughed again; he repeated it to others.

When at length the afternoon came to an end, he caught my arm and urged, 'You will dine with us this evening'. I had already promised to dine at the hotel that night with two of the friends with whom I was travelling. 'No, no,' he said, 'bring them to me.' So they came with me. At the invited hour we joined him at his 'apartment' – on the first floor, in a busy street. A maid opened to us, and a moment later Pavlov himself joined us. He helped us with our coats, and made us welcome. Before we left the small lobby he suddenly turned to us and said, 'The police may come to-night. I have not permission for three guests – I have permission for one, but not for three. If they come, they will put to each of you the question, "Why are you here?" The only reply for you to give them is for each of you to say, "I do not know". That is the only reply which precludes all further answer or question'. We broke into a smile. He smiled too and added with a laugh, 'Please remember; that is the right and only reply to make'. The police did not come. Our evening was one of delightful hospitality and entertainment. Mrs. Pavlov was there and a grown-up son and daughter, both of whom spoke English well. A glass case containing butterflies, collected by 'father' when a boy, evoked a number of anecdotes of father's boyhood. We left an hour before midnight. We felt we had been admitted to the hearth of a singularly lovable and simple Russian family.

Appendix 3. Grindelwald in Winter, 1887

From: *The Alpine Journal* 57, 10–14 (1949)

My old friend – perhaps in view of my own formidable seniority I ought to correct that to my younger friend – the Editor, invites me, with his characteristically youthful confidence, to set down for these pages a reminiscence of Grindelwald in winter dating back now more than sixty years. His wish is a command, although I cannot help the misgiving that what he is good enough to find of some interest is really in itself too trivial for this *Journal*. As the Christmas vacation of 1887 drew near and London seemed at its foggiest, a surgical colleague[1] with whom I was in almost daily contact, told me that he and a brother were thinking of going to Switzerland for New Year, and asked 'Would I join them?' 'Yes,' I said, 'although it seems an odd time of year to choose. What place do you propose?' 'Grindelwald,' he said. 'They get a spell of settled weather following Christmas; that is what I hear, but we cannot find anyone who has tried it.' 'Of course Grindelwald will be smothered in snow, but I shall love to come.'

Four days before Christmas, the morning train for Dover found us, a trio, waiting for it on the platform, and waiting as inconspicuously as we could. We had tweed caps with ear-flaps, tweed tunics and knickerbockers, thick woollen stockings and heavy black boots bearing viciously projecting nails. These accoutrements were the more unwelcomely conspicuous because the morning was in fact mild and bright in London, a so-to-say premature harbinger of next year's Spring. As we steamed through Kent the gardens were green and almost gay with blossom. We sped across France, meeting no trace of snow. Basle, still no snow. At Lucerne we got the lake-steamer for Interlaken and found some dozen passengers other than ourselves. They were clearly all of them *commis-voyageurs,* and in the catering line. Our boat stopped everywhere and our travelling companions changed all the way. We got our meal on board, and we thought it a good one. The lake shore was fringed with ice and there was some snow on the roads and sleighs had replaced wheels. Landing at Interlaken we took two sleighs and began to climb the valley-road to Grindelwald. The lake had been blinded in mist, and so was our valley-road. At one place where the road narrowed there hung from overhanging rock the largest icicles I had ever seen – strange and beautiful things, some of them perhaps twelve, or more, feet long. Of the mountain peaks above us, the fog let us see nothing of Jungfrau, and of Wetterhorn and Eiger – not a visible trace.

On the roadway the snow deepened rapidly. A couple of sleighs met us on their way down. Then almost suddenly as we ascended further, the mist thinned and in a matter of minutes we entered sunshine. Wetterhorn and Eiger looked down on us in brilliant beauty, Jungfrau seemed a monument of purity.

A little later, as the light was beginning to fade, we drew up, with a cheerful jangling of bells, at the old Bear Inn. There, expecting us, were its proprietors of that time – the family Boss – represented by Miss Boss and Emil and another brother – was it John? Miss Boss we found a capable

---

[1] Henry Clutton, then an Assistant Surgeon at St. Thomas' Hospital, London; his brother's name was Ralph – Editor.

manager and good business woman as well as host. Two great St. Bernard dogs leaving the log-fire in the hall barked at us and returned to the log-fire. Our rooms awaited us. Bare pine-wood floors, and windows looking out on Wetterhorn. Recent snow clothed the whole landscape. Its spirit seized us at once, and before dusk actually set in we were choosing staves from a collection near the doorway and *luges* from a number left there. It seemed a pity to go indoors, but a bell soon summoned us to supper. We sat down twelve all told at a long pine-wood table, and joined the inn's other guests, all but one of them as English as ourselves. Our doyen, so to say, was Captain Abney, the distinguished photographer. His pockets bulged with lenses and he seemed never tired of trying them out. With him were his daughter and her husband. Then there were Professor Gamgee of Manchester who was an invalid and had had a nervous breakdown, a senior medical student from Barts., and a young Swiss baron, somewhat of a toper. The family Boss usually joined us for supper, occupying one end of the long table; they spoke English easily, and Emil knew London. Emil, we were given to understand, was in the summer time a good mountain guide.

By the time we had finished supper an incredible sky of stars had appeared, and we went outside to look at it. Abney set about actually photographing it, with fantastically prolonged exposures – but he was not well satisfied with his results. We all turned in early, quite ready to do so.

The morning broke gloriously and we soon were out of doors enjoying it. The air felt like a chosen tonic – under an almost cloudless sky – but valley-ward the white mist again hung there. I had walked the road in summer and remembered well how hot and breathless in many places I had found it, though then free of fog. If what I find now is a fair sample of winter Grindelwald, I thought, winter is the right season to come here.

No one else joined our party, though the old inn was not a quarter full. A brand-new relatively huge *annexe* nearby stood closed and empty. How did we put in our time? We were out-of-doors through the whole day, even when it occasionally snowed. There was usually a little fresh snow at some time each night. We had brought skates, and a small piece of ice lay alongside of the inn but was too rough for enjoyable skating; we flooded it several times without improving it. As for skis, they were at that date practically unknown to us and to Switzerland. I fancy tradition tells now they first won their way into Grindelwald from Norway, but at what date I cannot say. In Grindelwald I remember being told in 1889 that skis would not answer because Grindelwald snow was not suitable for them – and I accepted that as a reliable dictum from those who possibly knew. In 1887 we had but that cradle-shaped hobby-horse on runners, the *luge,* not fully

developed at that time. A small one-man sled shod with iron. A number of
these, with a cord attached in front of each, waited patiently at the inn
entrance for use by anyone. What pleasure we got from them! We would
toil up some snow-track half the morning to get the furious fun of a glide
down in less than a twentieth of the time into the village again. The exhil-
aration thus engendered in us, hardworked fog-beridden Londoners, went
to the head. I, for one, found it an irresistible excitement. One afternoon,
however, it gave me a not undeserved scare. Gliding at full-speed down an
ice-bound track on the side of the Faulhorn, on reaching the village street,
finding it empty and a garden gate open just opposite through which the
track plunged further, the temptation was too great for my weak mind.
Instead of stopping, I dashed across and through the gate and found myself
descending a still steeper track through an orchard down toward the Lower
Glacier. About 150 yards ahead I saw descending the same way a figure. I
shouted. Whoever it was had but to step aside into the looser snow – but
some of the village would do this only at the very latest moment. I repeated
the warning cry, *Achtung!* again and again. Still no trace of the expected
response. An impact; I saw a momentary soaring of two legs over my head,
followed by an ominous dull thud on the frozen track behind. I pulled aside
into the soft snow and saw the fallen man lying face upward on the icy path.
I expected tragedy and I had found it. I ran to be of what service I could.
The man I had knocked down still lay motionless on his back and made no
attempt to rise. On my stooping and addressing him he slowly opened his
eyes. Then he said, amicably but indistinctly, 'Good evening.' I felt him all
over. No, not even a scratch. He was contentedly drunk. I helped him up
and saw him on his way and left him finally at his cottage gate.

Christmas was a great event in Grindelwald. The Bear Inn provided a
Christmas tree which was almost a whole tree, and we all helped to load it
with seasonable gifts. Villagers from Grindelwald began to come in on the
afternoon of Christmas Eve, and dancing commenced at once to the accompaniment of a cottage piano and a harp. It then went on continuously, not
merely until midnight but until the *evening* of next day, Christmas Day. The
whole festival culminated in the distribution of presents from the lordly tree
itself, accompanied by intermittent supper from a well-laden table hard by.
Then, by twos and threes and fours the company, well wrapt up and chatter-
ing noisily, began to disperse homeward. Then it was that a conspirator
entered the scene. He laid a wager that he could make the village guests
disgorge their treasured gifts even before they could get them home. We
watched his plot, and truly ludicrous its results were. Most of the company
in order to reach home had to pass the village church and its churchyard.

There with a chalked face, and, beyond that, folded head to foot in a shroudlike sheet, the practical joker hid himself behind the churchyard wall and abided his best opportunity. He waited until the festive homeward throng was at its densest – groups spread right across the road. Then, with an unearthly howl, he showed himself above the churchyard wall, and waved his arms as if a soul in torment. The effect was instantaneous. The whole roadway seemed to answer with one cry. Old and young dropped their parcels and fled terror-stricken. Then our graceless wag climbed over the wall and, picking up a number of the dropped belongings, unsheeted himself and walked back to the Bear Inn to claim his wager.

More snow fell. By Emil's advice, our little party devoted a day to the Faulhorn – a day as it proved of cloudless sunshine. The snow was more than knee-deep in many places, even where we kept to the path. We lingered at the top, because of the view, it was so lovely; as the late afternoon light began to take on sunset tints we watched and stayed to let them grow. Two lakes were in almost full view below us. A scene of indescribable colour developed – the sheet of one lake became violet and that of the other flame-like orange. We could have lingered longer but Emil urged us to start down. As we descended we grew careless of the path and near the village found ourselves wading through untrodden snow deep enough to bury standing hurdles and low gates. However we had but to descend, for all descents led to the village road. Looking back I can remember those sunset lakes still. I remember feeling how little possible it was for the painter to attempt such scenery, and then I recalled some of J. M. Turner's, recently exhibited in Bond Street, lent by Ruskin. They had in my young judgment alone seemed adequate – they were the work of Turner's last years when he revisited Switzerland – the Shakespeare of landscape-painting he seemed to me then, and does so still.

We never took the huge St. Bernard dogs with us on our excursions. I asked why and was told they were intended as watch-dogs for the Inn. Before that was explained to me, I had an experience. One morning getting downstairs earlier than the rest of us, I had gone out for a short walk from the inn-entrance and called the dogs to come with me. They came briskly enough, barking as I thought with the enjoyment. They would rush up the low embankment of cleared snow either side and charge down upon me. They did this more and more frequently and fiercely. Suddenly I appreciated that I was mistaken in supposing this was play on their part. They were hunting and they were hunting in a couple. I had not brought even a stick with me – besides they were as big as calves. I turned, as nonchalantly as I could, in my tracks and talking to them, I hoped, more authoritatively, set my steps back toward the inn, but this did not appease them at all. The inn was out of sight behind a bend of the road. As I made my way I was relieved to hear a voice and the cracking of a heavy whip. The dogs heard too. Emil appeared hastening toward me: 'The dogs can be troublesome' was all he remarked, and we returned together.

The weather remained superb. There was in the courtyard in front of the inn a telescope mounted on a tripod. On turning it toward the mountains one could see *gemsen* on the rock ledges. Emil and a friend from the village went after them once during our stay, but explained that it was the close season. 'However,' he added, 'I am a member of Parliament for this district, and if I start before daybreak no one will say anything!' He could not, he said, take one of us with him. He had his gun and we heard some shots during the day, but seemingly he brought no game back.

Our sixteen days sped far too fast. The weather remained settled until it was time, to our regret, to go down to Interlaken and start homeward. Interlaken itself was still draped patchily in white mist. Our little trip had told us that at some height above the lake the days can be bright and clear and bracing while the lake itself is mist-covered, and lacks sun. On the strength of this experience I spent Christmas and New Year at the Bear again two years later, but the party I found there was much larger, and more cosmopolitan, including some Americans and French; the annexe, however, was still closed. There were still no skis.

It is now sixty years since I was last at Grindelwald, and it is difficult for me even to imagine the changes in the place. Many more hotels I suppose; I hear of a grotto of green transparent ice in the Lower Glacier, and there is a train running up from Interlaken, and crowds of young people with skis. Ah, that I were young still.

As already said, the expressed wishes of Professor Graham Brown I have long regarded as commands. If I now venture, for this once, to flout his Editorial blue-pencil it is because I feel the following incident regarding him too characteristic to be left unrecorded. It should be common property of his friends. My present Editor and myself found ourselves in Zürich some years ago. It was springtime and we went into the fine booksellers there to look round at anything new. Not guessing who my companion was, an attentive attendant drew to our notice a recently published map of a new ascent of Mont Blanc, displaying Graham Brown's conquest of it by a new route. A few days later, from Berne we went on to Nyon-en-Suisse, to call on American friends then living there. Their villa had a strip of lakeside, and our transatlantic hostess took us to it to do the honours of the view across the Lake. There was a fine glimpse of Mont Blanc which she pointed out. 'The highest mountain in all Europe,' she said, 'Had he seen it before?' She added 'There are some who actually climb up it.' 'Even from the wrong side,' I said. 'Poor people', she exclaimed. But Graham Brown never gave himself away; he did not even smile.

C.S.S.

Appendix 4. A Memorial of Ramón y Cajal, 1949

From: Dorothy F. Cannon: *Explorer of the Human Brain. The Life of Santiago Ramón y Cajal.* New York: Henry Schuman, 1949

The subject of this Memoir was, besides much else, a man of outstanding personality. The excellent biographical portrait here furnished of him has brought back to me, vividly, a number of firsthand impressions received half a lifetime ago. Should this Memoir seem perhaps overladen with individual reminiscence, that, whether defect or not, is attributable to the conjunction of an exceptional human character with its unusually successful portrayal by the writer who follows me.

Santiago Ramón y Cajal spent his only visit to England – a visit of some two weeks' duration – as my house-guest. He had been little outside Spain. He was naïvely interested in what he saw of England. He was, for the time being, at a disadvantage conversationally, because he had no English, and what Spanish his hosts possessed did not suffice for more than a few halting sentences. His way out of this difficulty was to employ a sadly imperfect French, which he drove to its utmost limit or beyond. German he did not speak.

His rich voice compelled attention to whatever he said. The memory of that voice reminds me I have a privilege regarding him which, owing to lapse of time, must be becoming rare. My mind's-eye recalls him as he walked and talked and indeed as his outward appearance was, just at that stage of his career when he had recently become, in his own line of science, an international figure. I see him a man perhaps a little below medium height – at least in London – broad-shouldered, spare, and strongly built. Of dark complexion, his olive-skinned face lit by brilliant eyes deep brown in color and of steady gaze. His hair almost black and closely cropped, trespassed low on a wide forehead. The strong face, completely shaven, had mobile, muscular lips. His hands as he sat and talked seemed to ask to be doing something. He was deliberate in his movements, but they were habitually energetic. He did not smoke, not even a cigarette. On being offered, inadvertently twice over, "something to smoke," his reply was a vigorous, "Mais la vie moderne est une chose déjà fort compliquée. Porter du tabac, des allumettes, etc., ça serait de la compliquer encore plus. Merci, non!" His philosophy of life even in little things was never far to seek.

Two days after his arrival, as in the morning we sallied from the house-door into the street, he surprised me by the remark that England's decadence was indeed obvious and that Spain regretted it. I asked him why he thought England decadent. He replied, "Pas de fabriques: pas d'usines." He told me that he had looked for them from the train window as he travelled from Calais, and there were none; and he now found very few in London itself. I said, "In this part of London there are not many, but in London taken as a whole there are many – too many!" I added, "Much business is done in London. Crowds of people come into London every morning for business and leave again in the late afternoon." Feeling that he was still incredulous I asked if he would care to see them. Yes, he would. So next morning by 8:30 we were on London Bridge. The Bridge was flocked with people coming in from the Surrey side and a stream of wheeled traffic along with them. Cajal was deeply impressed; it was difficult to get him away. The next day, at his request, I sent him – I could not go myself – to watch the scene again.

He was strikingly simple in several ways. At dinner one evening whitebait were served. The dish was new to him. He could not be persuaded to eat the tiny fish whole although he saw the rest of us doing so. He persisted in attempting to dissect out the backbone from each one, which was rather a trial to his hostess. We were delighted to find that at meals he would often manage to follow the general drift of talk at table, and that he did not let the language disability deter him from joining in. He would reinforce conversation with a little set speech, a short oration which developed its own peroration. This climax he would emphasize by a final dramatic gesture, for which his left hand had been preparing. That hand had been busily crumbling the bread beside his dinner plate. It would gather the crumbs into a high pyramidal heap and then, to stress his closing words, sweep them with his cupped hand from the table to the carpet, accompanied by a challenging look round, and to the dismay of the maid serving. This may have been a trick of rhetoric acquired at the famous Café Suizo in whose weekly debating club Cajal was, I believe, prominent. Cajal was surprised to find so little café life in London; no outdoor café life at all.

He had more than once mentioned his wish to take from London some gifts for his wife and children, and we lunched at the Army and Navy Stores that he might choose there some things for them. He was amazed at the extent and variety of the store. He spent three hours there but without making a purchase. Each time his fancy dictated a purchase, his Spanish love of a bargain impelled him to open a debate, partly in dumbshow, with the salesman or saleswoman with the object of lowering the price asked! He seemed prepared to devote the whole afternoon to such an attempt. I expect that where he and his wife did their shopping in Madrid, bargaining was still a customary procedure.

This simplicity of Cajal's ways and ideas is mentioned here because it illustrates how singular a mixture he presented of old-time ways and ultra-modern science. There was clearly an element of greatness in him. With peasant-like naïveté as to many of the ordinary conventions of life, there went a scientific enquirer who had transformed with novelty in the space of six short years, and singlehanded, the ancient study of the functional anatomy of the vertebrate nervous system. Is it too much to say of him that he is the greatest anatomist the nervous system has ever known? The subject had long been a favorite with some of the best investigators; previous to Cajal there were discoveries, discoveries which often left the physician more mystified than before, adding mystification without enlightenment. Cajal made it possible even for a tyro to recognize at a glance the direction taken by the nerve-current in the living cell, and in a whole chain of nerve-cells.

He solved at a stroke the great question of the direction of the nerve-currents in their travel through brain and spinal cord. He showed, for instance, that each nerve-path is always a line of one-way traffic only, and that the direction of that traffic is at all times irreversibly the same. The so-called nerve-networks with unfixed direction of travel he swept away. The nerve-circuits are valved, he said, and he was able to point out where the valves lie – namely, where one nerve-cell meets the next one. He insisted that at such a place there is *contact* of one nerve-cell with another, but no *conjunction* of one nerve-cell with another, and he had, of course, support from the old well-known "Wallerian" degeneration, the degeneration always halting at and not transgressing across the surface of meeting of the two cells. The meeting place of the two contacting nerve-cells forms a watershed between two nutritional systems, each system prevailing up to the limit of its own watershed.

Cajal wisely safeguarded his claim to his discoveries by announcing them personally to Mathias Duval in Paris and to Kölliker, the Swiss anatomist in Würzburg. Cajal's demonstration of his facts was arrestingly complete. His new teaching lent itself to explanation by diagram. In a few years it established itself in every up-to-date text-book of neurology and physiology. It is true that an anatomist in Berlin, Waldeyer, published – without consulting Cajal, and somewhat to Cajal's disgust – a conspectus of the Cajal conception, styling it the "neuron" theory. The term, although still current, is now less used than once. Cajal himself clinched his new concepts by illustration with a number of admirable drawings from his own hand in hard black and white. A step amounting to genius, taken by him at an early stage, was his resort to material from the embryo (e. g., the chick) so as to escape the difficulty presented to his metallic methods by the developed myelin-sheath. As evidence of the breadth and sweep of his attitude toward the anatomy of nerve-tracts in general, the following incident, which I give at first hand, is characteristic. I was helping him to choose some microscopic preparations from among those he had brought with him for the illustration of his Croonian Lecture at the Royal Society. He handed me a preparation showing nerve-fibres descending to, and ending in, the spinal cord, and, as he did so, said, "Pyramidal tract." "But," said I, after a hesitation, "isn't this from the chick? Birds have not any pyramidal tract." All he answered was, "Bien; c'est la même chose." My remark, though correct, touched a detail too trivial for him to regard.

A trait very noticeable in him was that in describing what the microscope showed he spoke habitually as though it were a living scene. This was perhaps the more striking because not only were his preparations all dead and fixed, but they were to appearance roughly made and rudely treated – no cover-glass and as many as half a dozen tiny scraps of tissue set in one large blob of balsam and left to dry, the curved and sometimes slightly wrinkled surface of the balsam creating a difficulty for microphotography. He was an accomplished photographer but, so far as I know, he never practiced microphotography. Such scanty illustration as he vouchsafed for the preparations he demonstrated were a few slight, rapid sketches of points taken here and there – depicted, however, by a master's hand.

The intense anthropomorphism of his descriptions of what the preparations showed was at first startling to accept. He treated the microscopic scene as though it were alive and were inhabited by beings which felt and did and hoped and tried even as we do. It was personification of natural forces as unlimited as that of Goethe's *Faust,* Part 2. A nerve-cell by its emergent fibre "groped to find another"! We must, if we would enter adequately into Cajal's thought in this field, suppose his entrance, through his microscope, into a world populated by tiny beings actuated by motives and strivings and satisfactions not very remotely different from our own. He would envisage the sperm-cells as activated by a sort of passionate urge in their rivalry for penetration into the ovum-cell. Listening to him I asked myself how far this capacity for anthropomorphizing might not contribute to his success as an investigator. I never met anyone else in whom it was so marked.

And there is yet another feature of Cajal's scientific verve which reading the accompanying biography has brought to mind insistently; and in it lies an element not without a pathos peculiar to itself. The "Cuban Interlude," so styled in this volume, lays bare to us Cajal's consuming love of country. This patriotism, at once passionate and patient, was at that epoch in Spain submerged in a general flood of contemporary frustration, especially as to all that pertained to distinction and achievement in the realm of natural science. A devastating pessimism reigned in Spain in those years, paralyzing modern Spain's grasp of and competence in science. A comment of Cajal's own countrymen on his early publications ran to the effect: "Who is our Santiago to attempt to teach foreign savants?"

Cajal's own nature was far too strong for such despair. His faith in his country never faltered. His feeling was that if his country's powers had waned, it was for him and his contemporaries to give them renewal. Whence did he draw this inspiration? Not from his father; enough is told us to let us know that, although his father was remarkable and worthy and in a number of respects a forceful character, his struggles had choked out of him all trace of romance. As for Cajal himself, love of and devotion to Spain radiated from him in his daily intercourse. Their utterance did not take the form of fond praise of all Spanish ways of life and modes of thought.

Often his reaction was regret at some defect he detected in Spain as contrasted with elsewhere. At the time when he was in London the "hansom cab" was the London gondola; it provoked from him the quaint comment, "The grey matter grows well under grey skies!" – meaning by "grey matter" the sheet of the brain which anatomy connects with intellect, and by "grey skies" the sky of Britain as contrasted with that of Spain. The picturesque phrase was a favourite with him; it revealed how constantly his mind harped on the intellectual success status of Spain. This solicitude for his country's repute deserves explicit mention here; it was perhaps the most powerful driving-force in the make-up of his whole scientific character. It lifted him altogether above all personal vanity. His science was first and foremost an offering to Spain, a spiritual motive which added to the privilege of knowing the man.

                                                                                    C.S.S.

Appendix 5. Address on Medical Science

From: *The Canadian Journal of Medicine and Surgery.* Vol. XIV, No. 5. Toronto, November 1903

... In nurturing science, I would urge that a community cultivates more than mere utility. And even with regard to mere utility, as the fields of knowledge fall ripe under the ceaseless husbandry of the world's thought, those who would join in the great reaping, and not only glean where others reaped before them, must cultivate for themselves. To do this requires more than the devotion of individuals. It requires the intelligent cooperation of whole groups of individuals. Organized scientific inquiry becomes in advanced countries a conscious aim of the community as a community.

That society may draw due benefit from wells of natural knowledge, three kinds of workers have to stand side by side. First, the investigator, who, pursuing truth, extends discovery, with little or no reference to practical ends. He constitutes the fountain-head of the knowledge that is for distribution. Other hands may reap the harvest, but his sets and rears the seed.

After the investigator comes the teacher. To him it belongs to diffuse the knowledge won. This honorable and difficult task receives its best reward in seeing the small spiritual beginnings of the pupil widen out into the spiritual beginnings of the master. Thirdly, there is the applier of natural knowledge. His part consists in making scientific knowledge directly serve practical needs. It is this work which, to the popular idea, often represents the whole of science, or all of it that is commonly termed "useful." The practical results of this work are often astounding to those ignorant of the steps by which they have been reached. The greatest of these steps, however, is usually the first one, made in the laboratory of the investigator. These three co-workers are co-equal in the priesthood. Science and the applications of science are one growth, united together even as the fruit and the tree. The proper hearthstone round which the community should group these laborers, laboring for a common end, is the University. There the sacred flame of learning is fed from many sides by many hands.

... The bond between Schwann and Pasteur has opened a new perspective, and chemistry and medicine were drawn still tighter by their discoveries concerning those subtle influences named "ferments." Pathology, the study of these processes of the body in disease, even more than physiology, as yet has drawn help from this part of modern chemistry. If the processes of health are in fact the resultant of the due co-operation of ten million little foci of healthy chemical action in the body, the processes of disease are similarly divisible, and have to be traced to the unhealthiness of certain of these minute centres of activity. How extreme is the importance of chemistry to modern medicine no single statement can perhaps emphasize so well as this – that is, I believe, acknowledged on all hands – that in virtue of his chemistry, a chemist, Louis Pasteur, during the latter half of last century, was able to do more to alleviate the diseases of mankind and animals than any single physician of his time.

... I have said enough to remind us how interlocked with science medicine has become. She is applying sciences to her own problems, and they form a vast capital fund from which she can draw wealth. To give instruction in this part of medicine, to turn out men trained in it, is now one of the duties of a medical school. The earnest student has a right to expect such training from his *Alma Mater*. But for it the requirements are importantly different from those that suffice as an introduction to empiric medicine. In the first place, as Pasteur said, we cannot have the fruit without the tree. For scientific medicine the student must, perforce, be thoroughly trained in his sciences before he can really grasp instructions or truly profit from his medical teaching. One of the aims of his instruction in empirical medicine is to teach him to observe for himself, so in his instruction in scientific medicine, one of its aims is to enable him to apply science for himself. How small a fraction of all the realities of medical practice can be met in the few years of preparation of the student in the clinic as he passes through it in his school career. His teacher knows that well, and uses the cases as types whereby the principles of medicine can be fixed as a beginning. The rest must be accomplished by the man himself, as his life's work. The more necessary that the man go forth from his school equipped not only with the present applications of science to disease, but so possessed of the root principles of the sciences adjunct to medicine, that he may grasp and intelligently use the further developments of scientific medicine after he is weaned from his instructors and the school. That is the way to obtain enlightened progress in professional practice. What truer safeguard can a man have, alone it may be, and isolated from the centres of knowledge – what truer safeguard can he have against all the pseudo-scientific quackeries of the day, than some real knowledge of the principles of the sciences, along whose lines the discoveries of medicine must develop?

... The duties of a university do not begin and end with the disciplinary and didactic. Besides schools of instruction, they must be schools of thought. To be this latter, the laboratory must pursue research. Even for the welfare of the class-teaching this is essential. Instructive lectures may be given by men of ability, the whole of whose knowledge is second-hand, but it is doubtful whether the real life of science can be fully felt and communicated by one who has not himself learnt by direct inquiry from nature. Nothing so augments the teacher's power of impressive and incisive teaching of a subject than to have faced problems in it himself as an original enquirer. And, after rudiments have been once fairly acquired, there is for good students no training equal to that given by following even a small research under an experienced leader.

. . . What, then, are finally the uses of these laboratories now opened by your University? They will assist in training men for various honorable callings, especially for that most ancient one of medicine. They will assist, no doubt, also to render life by practical applications of science superficially still more different from what it was only a short generation ago. They will assist to bring home and distribute to your community treasures of knowledge from all quarters of the globe. They will assist – and it is a thought dear to a high-spirited people – themselves to add to the sum total of the treasures of knowledge of the whole human race.

C.S.S.

Appendix 6. Letter to Henry Head re W. H. Gaskell, 1918

Dear Head,
So busied have I been I could not get to your note about Gaskell. He was *always* an inspiration to me and to any work I was able to try. Such inspiration is often subtle and part of its success springs I imagine from its subtlety. One does not like to be driven, but inspiration is *not* driving. My own work began by chance at the wrong end – the cortex – pyramidal degenerations, etc. It was certainly through Gaskell that I very soon felt that. One could not talk with him long without realising that the cord offered a better point to attack physiologically. Also, that the cord was originally and still must essentially be a chain of 'ganglia', as he would say, thinking of invertebrates. The spinal afferent root should show the limits of, and at least part of the make-up of, the metamerism – functional as well as morphological. But when one got on with that, came the stumbling block,

i. e. that in the vertebrate the segments as judged by the skin afferents had overflowed into one another. But at the same time you showed the visceral segmentation and how it had persisted in purer form. I remember how pleased he and I were about your observations and results. He had expected it would be something like that. He had always insisted to me that the bulb-segmentation was more primitive than the spinal. But the bulb lent itself less to laboratory experiment.

Later too, when his own chief interests had passed to the origin of vertebrates, he was still always a bulwark to me about the inhibition of voluntary muscle. To both him and me it always seemed that the taxis of vol. muscles was impossible without inhibition. But we both expected *efferent* inhibitory nerves to them. You remember his vivid interest in Biedermann and the Astacus claw. I used to search for similar things in mammal muscle-nerve. I used to put down – he agreeing – each failure to a swamping of the inhibitory fibres by excitatory mixed in the same efferent nerve. Gradually, in view of one's reflex experiments, it burst upon me that for the vol. muscles, the inhibitories play not on the muscle direct but on the spinal motor cells driving them, and in that sense are all afferent or central. When I told him how things were pointing he came out of his own work, though up to the neck in it then, and went into my story and all its pros and cons, not stinting time for it. Finally he said, yes, of course, here again the somatic part of these segments which is less primitive; visceral muscle inhibition is peripheral, skeletal muscle's inhibition has become central! That gift of sympathetic attention and unselfish switching off from his own problem to a pupil's, was characteristic of his nature. And his transcendant sincerity lent such force to his criticism . . . He personified truth. In a hundred ways I owe him help and inspiration.

I wish that when this war is over some more adequate account of him and his influence may appear; no proper appreciation of him has been given yet.

With kindest remembrances to you both,

Yours ever, C. S. Sherrington

Appendix 7. Osler at Oxford

From: *Centenary Tribute to Osler by Sherrington,* reprinted from the British Medical Journal, Vol. II. July 9, 1949

Osler at Oxford! The impression left upon me is vivid enough, although I feel it far from easy to convey. It had its different sides. My privilege was to join him as a colleague in the teaching when he was still relatively a new-comer to the place. I think he regarded his chair – the Regius Chair of Medicine (attached to Christ Church) – as legitimately to be treated as a sort of sinecure; its very stipend was then rather beggarly, and Osler some-times did not scruple to say so. He looked upon what was expected of him, not, I fancy, as in any ordinary sense a part of the routine teaching of medicine, but rather as a focal point whither to draw together the scattered strands of tradition pertaining to an ancient Faculty, some of them begin-ning to wear thin. I think he felt what was incumbent on him was to main-tain a stately but rather formal professional intercourse, a picturesque cere-monial furbished with tags of scholastic learning, a certain dignity of cus-tom, and the observance of loyalty to certain past ways. In a number of these features Oxford resembled its sister on "reverend" Camus; and Osler was deeply gratified to have as his opposite number Clifford Allbutt, a classical scholar as well as a close friend.

Canadian by birth and upbringing, his ties with the Empire formed a cherished background to his life. The annals of European Medicine were familiar and dear to him, and that his position should link him with Linacre, Sydenham, and Harvey rose, I think, almost daily to his thought. Not that he lived in the past; rather he trod a stage whose scenery was much of it furnished from the past. The very buildings had their fascination for him. Once as I walked alongside him across the open space between the Camera, the Bodleian, and All Souls, he stopped and, looking round, said: "The finest architectural view in Europe."

Love of Rare Books

One of the happinesses he cultivated in Oxford was to serve as showman to parties of transatlantic visitors and to introduce them to his favourite glimp-ses of the University scene – a personally conducted tour, leading finally to lunch at his own house with Lady Osler at the table. The number of guests might be anything up to fifteen or sixteen, and the hostess had little notice of exactly how many there would be. But the babble of conversation was unceasing, and their host seemed able to address them each one intimately – Tom, Jack, Jim, or whatever familiarity dictated. One regular item of their entertainment, laid out for their inspection in a small well-windowed room opposite the "Study," would be some dozen or so choice printed books, each volume open at a selected place. These specimen volumes would include first-rate rarities – a fifteenth-century Aristotle from a Paris press, a Descartes' *Method*, etc.

His library was housed mainly in one large room with open shelves reaching to the ceiling and a couple of turntable bookcases, one of them completely filled with editions of his favourite among all books, Sir Thomas Browne's *Religio Medici*. When he resided at Oxford he was engaged in cataloguing his library on a novel plan – a *Bibliotheca prima*, etc. After Osler's death this catalogue was completed by Dr. William Francis, and issued at the Clarendon Press, at the charge of Lady Osler, in a fine folio volume. The books themselves were bequeathed by him to the McGill University library, Montreal. So far as I know he kept none of his books under lock and key, although he was well aware of the frailty besetting certain book-collectors and could relate instances within his own experience. In the Preface to his monumental catalogue he gives some anecdotes of his own adventures in pursuit of specially desirable volumes. His book-collecting seemed to be a "catching complaint," for I think we may suppose it was started in Harvey Cushing – and in others – by Osler himself. A well-known bookseller in London used to say that he attributed to Osler's influence no small share in the increased antiquarian interest taken in early printed books on both sides of the Atlantic. Osler was certainly a most intriguing devotee of the fashion.

A Special Interest

One of the adjuncts of the Oxford chair exerted quite a special appeal on Osler. In virtue of his tenure of the chair he was Master of an ancient almshouse some ten miles out of Oxford, a picturesque low-roofed cloistered building dating from the foundation of the charity, and enclosing perhaps half an acre of plotted garden. The apartments of the old pensioners themselves faced inwards towards this court. The whole stood in a small village which in itself was old-world, rural, and intersected by little running streams or "freshets" full of watercress grown for the London market. Lady Osler made herself unobtrusively a fairy godmother to these aged dependants. Osler as Master had a couple of rooms under the common roof. I happened to be present when he noticed a sort of strong-box in his bed-chamber there. The key, when inquired for, was not to be found, and Osler, thoroughly intrigued, wired to Chubb's, of London, for an expert to pick the ancient lock. The expert when he came looked at the chest, then, taking a small wooden mallet from his travelling-bag, tapped the sides of the lid and almost at once lifted it. "This chest has not been locked these many years," he said. The box contained deeds, many of them on vellum with seals attached, each seal in its little case fixed to the ribbon belonging to the document. Osler was enchanted. All the way home he could speak of nothing else.

As Consultant

I fancy that his opinion was considerably sought as a consultant during his Oxford years. I was present once when it was – unofficially – appealed to. It interested me to see his manner change at once. It became gravely professional. His voice assumed a deeper tone, his forehead frowned slightly; his lips tightened, his bearing became dramatic and oracular – kindly always, but now dispensing kindness oracularly. His position in Oxford was such that he allowed himself to call on sick people independently of invitation from their doctor. William McDougall, the psychologist, was then in Oxford, and I knew him well. He told me the following. His youngest child, a little maid of 7, was fatally ill. One afternoon Osler called, and after talking with McDougall they both went upstairs to the child's room. Outside her room Osler suddenly stopped and tapped at the bottom of the door. Then, opening it, he stole across to the child's bed with little steps and knees bent to dwarf himself as much as possible, his coat-flaps nearly touching the floor, his face on a level with the child's in bed. The child gazed wonderingly at him. "Mary," Osler said, assuming a small bird-like voice, "I am come to tell you a secret – a nice secret. You are going soon to leave us. You will be leaving on a journey, to a beautiful place, a wonderful place where you will be very, very happy. And all your friends will soon be coming there to join you. I can't stay longer now; I must run off. Good-bye, Mary; God bless you." And he kissed the child gently on the forehead. Then he withdrew as he had come, the little girl watching him wonderingly with a long smile.

Osler's Son

Osler himself had one child, a son, about to enter Christ Church when the first world war broke out. Revere shared some of the tastes of his father, and the pair were in several ways almost like schoolfellows together. The world war had been expected by many, but not by Osler. When it came Osler's parental anxiety was pathetic to see. After a year of delay his son was called up for military training: then, rather more than a year later still, for service abroad. Almost at once (1917) tragedy happened – a chance shell from a far range. The surgeon nearest at hand was the old family friend Harvey Cushing; but there was nothing to be done. To Osler the news was overwhelming. He strove on bravely but hopelessly. The laboratory attendants hearing his step declared it was no longer as it had been. As the year 1919 drew near its close, wintry weather caught him in a hired car far from home in a lonely place towards nightfall, and the car broke down. He and the chauffeur had to pass the night there, and he was chilled through. A day later he arrived home looking ill. He went to bed; bronchopneumonia set in. After some weeks he died, exhausted.

At the funeral service the Cathedral was filled to overflowing – friends attended not only from Oxford but from long distances.

I am not competent even to attempt any judgment of Osler's distinction as a clinician. He had of course a certain position as a man of letters. His literary style was rather obviously formed on his prime favourite, Browne of the *Religio,* without the redundant wealth of classical allusion. One conviction about Osler's influence on his time, of which I am quite sure and to which I would here bear witness, regards the remarkable camaraderie and personal affection which radiated from him. It stood for friendships which were lifelong ties. It was contagious. It propagated itself along his social contacts wherever he moved. His unlocked bookshelves were a part of it. In Baltimore, when he and Cushing occupied adjoining houses, doorways were cut through on each floor to facilitate communication between the households.

Appendix 8. Some Aspects of Animal Mechanism

From: British Association Speech, printed in *The Times*. Thursday 7 September, 1922

It is sometimes said that science lives too much to itself. Once a year it tries to remove that reproach. The British Association meeting is that annual occasion, with its opportunity of talking in wider gatherings about scientific questions and findings. Often the answers are tentative. Commonly questions most difficult are those that can be quite briefly put. Thus, "Is the living organism a machine?" "Is life the running of a mechanism?" The answer cannot certainly be as short as the question. The problem is not the why of the living organism, but the how of its working. It might be thought that it is presented at its simplest in the simplest forms of life. Yet it is in certain aspects more seizable in complex animals than it is in simpler forms.

Mind and Matter

Taking as manifestations of mind those ordinarily received as such, mind does not seem to attach to life, however complex, where there is no nervous system, nor even where that system, though present, is quite scantily developed. Mind becomes more recognizable the more developed the nerve-system. Hence the difficulty of the twilit emergence of mind from no mind, which is repeated even in the individual life history. In the nervous system there is what is termed localization of function which shows mentality, in the usual acceptation of that term, not distributed broadcast throughout the nervous system, but restricted to certain portions of it, among vertebrates to the forebrain, and in higher vertebrates to the relatively newer parts of that forebrain. Its chief, perhaps its sole, seat is a comparatively modern nervous structure superposed on the non-mental and more ancient, other nervous parts. The so-to-say mental portion of the system is placed so that its commerce with the body and the external world occurs only through the archaic non-mental rest of the system. Simple nerve impulses, their summations and interferences, seem the one uniform office of the nerve-system in its non-mental aspect. To pass from a nerve impulse to a psychical event, a sense-impression, percept, or emotion is, as it were, to step from one world to another and incommensurable one. We might expect, then, that at the places of transition from its non-mental to its mental regions the brain would exhibit some striking change of structure. But no; in the mental parts of the brain still nothing but the same old structural elements, set end to end, suggesting the one function of the transmission and collision of nerve impulses. The structural inter-connexions are richer, but that is a merely quantitative change.

I do not want, and do not need, to stress our inability at present to deal with mental actions in terms of nervous actions, or *vice versa*. But facing the relation borne in upon us as existent between them, may we not gain some further appreciation of it by reminding ourselves even briefly of certain points of contact between the two?

One is the so-called expression of the emotions. The mental reaction of an emotion is accompanied by a nervous discharge which is more or less characteristic for each several type of emotion, so that the emotion can be read from its bodily expression. This nervous discharge is involuntary, and can affect organs, such as the heart, which the will cannot reach. Then there is the circumstance that the peculiar ways and tricks of the nervous machinery as revealed to us in the study of pure reflex reactions repeat themselves obviously in the working of the machinery to which mental actions are adjunct. The phenomenon of fatigue is common to both, and imposes similar disabilities on both. Nervous exhaustion and mental exhaustion mingle. Then, as offset against this disability, there exists in both the amenability to habit formation, mere repetition within limits rendering a reaction easier and readier. Then, and akin to this is the oft-remarked trend in both for a reaction to leave behind itself a trace, an engram, a memory, the reflex engram, and the mental memory.

How should inertia and momentum affect non-material relations? Quick though nervous reactions are, there is always easily observed delay between delivery of stimulus and appearance of the nervous end effect. Just the same order of lag and overrun is met in sense reactions. The sensation outlives the light which evoked it, and for longer the stronger the reaction. The times in both are of the same order. Reflex acts commonly predispose to their opposites. So similarly the visual impression of one colour predisposes to that of its opposite.

Features of nervous working resemble over and over again mental. It is mere metaphor when we speak of mental attitudes as well as bodily? Is it mere analogy to liken the warped attitude of the mind in a psycho-neurotic sufferer to the warped attitude of the body constrained by an internal pain? Yet all this similarity does but render more succinct the old enigma as to the nexus between nerve impulse and mental event. Can one say that psychical events are included in the balance-sheet drawn up to prove that the animal mechanism conforms with the first law of thermodynamics? And yet Mr. Barcroft and his fellow-observers, in their recent physiological exploration of life on the Andes at 14,200 ft., noted that as well as their muscles their arithmetic was at a disadvantage there. The low oxygen pressure militated against both. Professor Elliott Smith and Sir Arthur Keith, recasting the shape of the brain from the cranial remains of prehistoric man, can outline for us something of his mentality, using a true and scientific phrenology.

The Seat of the Mind

Could we look quite naively at the question of a seat for the mind within the body, we might perhaps suppose it diffused there. Can we attach any meaning to the fact that it is localized in the nervous system? The nervous system has had the special office from its earliest appearance onward throughout evolutionary history more and more to weld together the body's component parts into one consolidated mechanism reacting as a unity to the changeful world about it. More than any other system it has constructed an individual of unified act and experience. In that system mind, as we know it, has had its origin. The cortex of the forebrain is the seat of mind. From small beginnings it has become steadily a larger and larger feature of the nervous system until in adult man the whole of the rest of the system is relatively dwarfed by it.

The mental attributes of the nervous system are the coping-stone of the construction of the individual. But they do not stop at the individual; they proceed beyond the individual; they integrate from individuals to communities. When we review the distribution of mind within the range of animal forms, we meet with two peaks of development – one in insect life, the other in the vertebrate, with its acme finally in man. In the insect the type of mind is not rational but instinctive, whereas in man there is reason as well as instinct. Yet in both one outcome seems to be the welding of individuals into societies on a scale of organization otherwise unattained. The greatest social animal is man; the powers that make him so are mental.

The living creature is fundamentally a unity. In trying to make the how of an animal existence intelligible to our imperfect knowledge we have to separate its whole into part-aspects and part-mechanisms, but that separation is artificial. Can we suppose a unified entity which is part mechanism and part not? One privilege open to the human intellect is to attempt to comprehend, not leaving out of account any of its properties, the how of the living creature as a whole. The problem is ambitious, but its importance and its reward are all the greater if we seize and we attempt the full width of its scope. In the biological synthesis of the individual it regards mind. It includes examination of man himself as acting under a biological trend and process which is combining individuals into a multi-individual organization, a social organism surely new in the history of the planet. For this biological trend and process is constructing a social organism whose cohesion depends mainly on a property developed so specifically in man as to be, broadly speaking, his alone – namely a mind actuated by instincts, but instrumented with reason. Man, often Nature's rebel, as Sir Ray Lankester has luminously said, can, viewing this great supra-individual process, shape even as individual his course conformably with it, feeling that in this instance to rebel would be to sink lower rather than to continue his own evolution upward.

Appendix 9. Speech at the Reception of the Delegates to the Tercentenary Celebration of William Harvey's "De Motu Cordis"

Royal College of Physicians (London, 1928)

Mr. President, Your Excellencies and Gentlemen,

In William Harvey we call to remembrance one who was Fellow, Censor, Treasurer and, for a day, President Elect, of this College; its benefactor by gift and bequest, and part and parcel for ever of its pride and honour, being a living spring of knowledge. Each year commemorates him in this place by the Oration which bears his name and has its historic and distinguished roll of orators – yourself, Sir, of them.

And now Time in its course completes three and a half centuries since his birth and three from that of his unforgettable book. Wherefore this welcomely representative assembly is met to bear witness to the book and to the man. No book can be its author all in all, yet, in science, no less than in letters the book can be supreme evidence of the man. Harvey's De Motu Cordis embodies not only Harvey's thought but what the hand of Harvey at behest of the thought of Harvey contrived, searched for and found.

At the Renaissance the Spirit of Man turned from an old order, cabined within a rounded scheme of things, to move and inhabit for itself afresh. That new day broke first on Scholarship and Letters. In Science it reset the mechanics of the stars before it bent to the study of terrestrial life. With this latter it adventured first upon the outward forms of organ and of organism. Later it turned to explore in both their inward meaning, the living function itself. For this last step the Renaissance *is* William Harvey.

His picture hangs on the wall yonder. Stripping from it some years we may see him, at two and twenty, hair 'long and curling', eyes 'black and very full of spirit', listening in the steep theatre at Padua to Fabricius, who expounds in Latin the parts displayed below on the anatomy table.

If to us the scene seem remote, being three centuries back, to the young Harvey then and there three centuries seemed little. Aristotle and Galen in living authority were for him as present in that room as was Fabricius speaking. Why therefore so remote to us much then surrounding the young Harvey? The answer comes; Harvey's own work changed the perspective of the whole.

Harvey, pupil and fervent admirer of the masters of antiquity, remained so to the end. But his famous exhortation to others, to search out Nature by experiment, he addressed early to himself. Hence, after Cambridge and Padua, the year of Shakespeare's death finds him as Lumleian Lecturer of this College, teaching from first-hand knowledge the great heresy and the victorious truth that the whole blood as one blood circulates the body in two successive circuits driven thus by a valved muscular pump – no other than that thrice-veiled, age-long mystery the heart!

Harvey for this discovery employed nor means nor appliance other than had been at men's disposal from classical antiquity onward. His triumphing was the triumphing of the new Spirit unaided save by its own freedom. He was the coming of modernity. Yet we must recognize that he was not modern quite all through, for he let ten years pass between his discovery and sending it to press. A slender book it was, most of its reference directed to masters dead nineteen to fifteen centuries before, but in observation its every statement holding to this day! It and its message engendered modern medicine.

A message it was however which had to win its way, and in some quarters did so slowly. Thus, in the College Library here if we turn to the learned Abercromby's *De Pulsus Varietate,* dedicated to Robert Boyle seventy years after Harvey's lectures, we find it opening with the words: *"Nili fontibus meo quidem judicio obscurior pulsus origo est".* But though to David Abercromby in 1685 the origin of the pulse was more obscure than the sources of the Nile, Descartes had already 53 years earlier accepted Harvey's circulation. Harvey, reliant on the truth and on the future though he were, could yet hardly have augured the long train of gifted men who were to extend his work, generation after generation onward, unbrokenly to Einthoven and Starling, so freshly lost to us, and of his own College today, Dale and Lewis, brilliantly extending by discovery his original discovery here in this city, where he lived and taught.

As we follow the pages of the De Motu we cannot but be struck by the self-restraint which pervades Harvey's presentment of his thesis. To supply in forty-nine small pages a refutation of nineteen centuries' tradition of continuous error argues a fine restraint. Yet once, at least, in the book, and self-revealingly, Harvey gave his spirit rein. It is where, relaxing his resolve to forego treating of the Circulation's purpose, he forecasts the supreme uses which must accrue to the blood in virtue of its circulating. In that forecast he breaks out into a passage of such luxury of language that we cannot be far wrong if we divine that its imagery flashes on us another aspect of Harvey, a Harvey other than the Harvey austerely stating proof of a solved problem, a Harvey fired with constructive imagination facing a problem fresh and still to solve; the Harvey who already had asked of the heart valves 'Wherefore?' and they had told him; of the vein-valves, and the heart's motions, and they had told him; the Harvey who on his note-book's cover in red ink wrote as motto: *"Jovis omnia plena"*, "Everything is full of Jove!" This Harvey we may believe was no small part of Harvey the discoverer.

Harvey the discoverer possessed cool judgement. He possessed enthusiasms well. Is it not an enthusiast, and an enthusiast for beauty, who throwing down his Virgil could exclaim in admiration, "The man hath a devil!" One spring of his enthusiasm lay in his philosophy of Nature.

Forerunning at two centuries' distance, and almost word for word, the expressed thought of Claude Bernard, Harvey in his latest writings averred that the very vegetative acts of each item of animal structure "compass results as it were by art, election and foresight." May we not of Harvey himself say in admiration, rephrasing his own phrase, "The man is full of Jove!"

Mr. President, the work of Harvey, the spirit of it no less than the import of it, provides his eulogy and makes superfluous all other. His great discovery, aside from its value as sheer intellect, secured an item of knowledge, than which no other single item has so served to grow, as from a seed, Medicine as we now know it. And it was the reassertion, the rebirth, of the method of experimentation, which wedded to observation has created the medicine – and the surgery – of the civilized world to-day. To engender medicine anew is to engender a whole world of correlated knowledge: and an attendant world of beneficence no less. And Harvey had humor. There is humor when in treating of the respect paid to age and authority he adds the comment, Natura enim nihil antiquius majoribus auctoritatis" Excerpt Anathom. II, p. 242.

The circulation of the blood, the meaning of the heart, the light of a victorious method! May we not affirm that modern scientific medicine does in fact start there. And, that so, we envisage Harvey in his perspective through the ages; Founder of Modern Medicine! He would himself have felt no term can carry richer or lovelier praise from a grateful world.

Appendix 10. Remarks at the Centenary Ceremonies of the Zoological Society (London, 1929)

It is my privilege on behalf of the guests and delegates from England to convey to the Zoological Society of London our united hearty felicitation and good wishes . . .

The kindred Societies throughout the land endorse these sentiments of their elder sister. To how many a child – and man and woman – has it not brought an unforgettable revelation, of living Nature's variety and wealth. Shapes of water and land; shapes sometimes in the delineated page uncouth, but when watched in their native habitat rarely or never so; shapes manifoldly recalling past ages of the Earth. We turn from the tanks to the aviaries and learn how the mute and voiceless Earth changed at the coming of the birds, never to sink back into silence. In the monkey-houses we meet a vociferous population such as might qualify for parliamentary institutions. Mind in the making, epitomized; a very school of psychology. We wonder does animal mind view ourselves across the frontiers as a strange genus, with unaccountably freak ways, disturbing what were else an orderly creation.

But no, we may be sure that within the tanks and enclosures there is little or nothing of such speculation, however naive. There the world is taken for granted. And that contemplative curiosity, which, supreme asset for Science as it is, the Zoological Gardens appetize and feed, is what lifts us above taking the world for granted. Scene upon scene written in the living pages of the Gardens has fascinating interest. Man gets glimpses of his own prehistory. We go to that aqueous fairy-kingdom the aquarium. There in the magical light, gazing at life, poising, fanning or gliding through the water, we almost realize – we seem indeed to remember – how, in literal truth, we all of us were water-babies once.

In these days when he who runs may read modern science has told the citizen that animal life is one great series, and how man "looking before and after" can trace his origin to simpler ancestral forms, not to the gods or angels, but to a prehuman and subhuman animal stage, a stock which itself had in its time, slowly attained to qualities and power, making possible the attainment of man's own present estate. We recognize in that estate a nature which relates us to much we might fain discard, and yet a nature which has been a passport for our further travel upward, and has qualified us to achieve, not only what man in the aggregate has achieved, but what individual man at his best stands for. The Gardens help us to the truth of our own past and hence of our nature. The face images for the mind; and the reflexion in all humility that from some simian grimace there has been evolved with progress of time, the smile of Mona Lisa, is an exhortation to fortify man in his effort to reach higher things and a more highly perfected future. The more we think and observe about our friends, the denizens of the Gardens, the more we feel that if we would understand our own nature we must study theirs . . .

Appendix 11. "Editorial Note" by Professor Samson Wright and "Foreword to 1947 Edition" by Sir Charles Sherrington

From: C. S. Sherrington, *The Integrative Action of the Nervous System.* "New Edition". New York: Cambridge University Press 1947

Editorial Note

Professor Samson Wright

The Integrative Action of the Nervous System was first published in 1906. It was immediately acclaimed as a work of outstanding importance which had refashioned neurophysiology by reason of the wealth of the original experimental observations that it contained, its wide generalizations, its philosophic insight and the stimulus that it gave to subsequent research. It determined in large measure the lines of development of the subject. The book has, however, been out of print for a generation, and it is no longer available – as it should be – to be read by all students of physiology and to be re-read by their teachers and by mature investigators in this field. The Physiological Society felt that it must remedy this unsatisfactory state of affairs, and that it owed a duty to Physiology to bring out a new edition of this work for the benefit of the many who would be inspired by it. Such an action also seemed to be a fitting tribute to the author, who had served not only Physiology, but the Society itself for so long and in so outstanding a manner. Sherrington was for fifty years (1885–1935) an 'ordinary' member of the Society; he became a member nine years after the formation of the Society; he served the Society as its Secretary, member of the Committee, and Editor of its *Journal*. The Society which had notably honoured itself by electing Sherrington to its honorary membership hoped that it might give him pleasure by making one of the works, by which his name will go down to posterity, live once more in the minds of grateful readers. Sherrington readily and generously agreed to the Society's suggestion; I was asked to take charge of the venture. He wrote to me of the proposal that "it is a most generous compliment and I value it accordingly; all that it proposes is very welcome to me". He continued with characteristic modesty: "I have long looked on the book as dead and buried and the suggestion that it has still got a fraction of life is a pleasing thought to me – but whether it has enough to make some resuscitation worth while I must leave to others." The 'others' think the resuscitation very worth-while. The Yale University Press, the owners of the copyright of *The Integrative Action,* with equal generosity transferred their rights in the book to the Physiological Society without cost, on the sole condition that in the new edition the entire text was reprinted – a condition which exactly expressed the Society's wishes . . .

Foreword to 1947 Edition

Sir Charles Sherrington

Let me here tender thanks to the Physiological Society, its Officers and all its Members and quite particularly to Professor Samson Wright, for the present generous compliment paid to my rather elderly book. I comply with pleasure to their request for a foreword to it. Owing to various circumstances, the text of the book has remained exactly as when first published.

This seems a suitable opportunity to deal with some ambiguities which have in course of time arisen.

(*a*)

To describe the action of nerve as integrative is, although true, hardly sufficient for a definition. If the nature of an animal be accepted as being that of a whole presupposed by all its parts, then each and every part of the animal is integrative. This is illustrated strikingly by cancer, the growth of which being outside the integrative plan of the body is destructive both to the normal body and to itself. Our search for a more satisfying definition of nerve has then to ask what is the specific contribution which nerve makes to animal integration. Finger-pointings toward an answer are that nerve in any strict sense of the term is not an element of the plant-world. Nor is it found in unicellular animals, although it is practically universal in the multicellular. In these latter, similarly universal, is an organ of mechanical work, muscle, executant of movements and attitudes, the animal's motor behaviour. This behaviour falls into two divisions. One digestive, excretory, in short visceral; the other inclusive of all which is not merely visceral. This latter behaviour is that of external relation, so called. In it, motor behaviour reaches its highest speeds and precision, nerve attains its greatest and supreme developments.

The volume here reprinted concerns itself predominantly with the type of motor behaviour which is called 'reflex'; it might give the impression that in reflex behaviour it saw the most important and far-reaching of all types of 'nerve' behaviour. That is in fact not so. But reflex action presents certain advantages for physiological description. It can be studied free from complication with the psyche: also free from complication by that type of 'nerve' activity which is called autochthonous (or 'spontaneous') and generates intrinsically arising rhythmic movements, e. g. breathing, etc. But taken in comparison with the great field of behaviour in general, pure reflex action of itself cannot be seen to cover such extensive ground as do the instincts actuated by 'urges' and 'drives'. But the mechanism of these has hardly yet been analysed sufficiently for laboratory treatment. The pure apsychical reflex has a smaller role. Studied in that self-contained animal group, the Vertebrates, behaviour seems to become less and less reflex as the animal individual becomes more and more complexly individuated. The 'spinal' man is more crippled than is the 'spinal' frog.

(b)

A 'reflex' can be diagrammatized as an animal reacting to a cosmical 'field' containing it. Animal and 'field' are of one category, both being comprised within the physicist's term 'energy'. They are machines which interact – a point taken by Descartes. His wheelwork animals geared into the turning universe. Cat, dog, horse, etc. in his view had no thoughts, no ideas; they were trigger-puppets which events in the circumambient universe touched-off into doing what they do. It was a view less strange than might seem from this condensed epitome. But it lets us feel Descartes can never have kept an animal pet. Experiment to-day does, however, put within reach of the observer a puppet-animal which conforms largely with Descartes' assumptions. In the more organized animals of the vertebrate type the shape of the central nerve-organ allows a simple operation to reduce the animal to the Descartes condition. An overlying outgrowth of the central nerve-organ in the head can be removed under anaesthesia, and on the narcosis passing off the animal is found to be a Cartesian puppet: it can execute certain acts but is devoid of mind. That it is devoid of mind may seem a dogmatic statement. Exhaustive tests, however, bear the assertion out. Thoughts, feeling, memory, percepts, conations, etc.; of these no evidence is forthcoming or to be elicited. Yet the animal remains a motor mechanism which can be touched into action in certain ways so as to exhibit pieces of its behaviour.

An outline of the spatial arrangement of nerve illustrates how this comes about. From points within and on the surface of the animal, nerve-threads run to its muscles, but in their course thither are engaged by the central organ and are there relayed; the central organ becoming a sort of switchboard where muscles can be switched on or off. The starting-point of the nerve-thread is not equally responsive to all the various types of the field forces. Each starting-point is armed with a structure, the receptor, which reacts to one specific class of field agency, e. g. one to light, not heat, another to heat, not light. The reaction of the nerve-thread itself is, in all nerve-threads, to generate a repetitive series of brief and minute electric currents which run away from the starting-point and, by relays through the central organ, reach this or that set of muscles determined by the topography of the starting-point concerned. As the play of the 'field' shifts over the animal, different sets of receptors come into and go out of action. The receptors thus analyse the successive situations occurring between animal and field in terms of the selective receptors, and ultimately in terms of the muscles of the limbs, etc. Change in the external situation brings corresponding change in the muscles brought into and released from contraction.

A train of motor acts results therefore from a train of successive external situations.

The movements are not meaningless; they carry each of them an obvious meaning. The scope commonly agrees with some act which the normal animal under like circumstances would do. Thus, the cat set upright (Graham Brown) on a 'floor' moving backward under its feet walks, runs or gallops according to the speed given to the floorway. Again, in the dog a feeble electric current ('electric flea') applied by a minute entomological pin set lightly in the hair-bulb layer of the skin of the shoulder brings the hind paw of that side to the place, and with unsheathed claws the foot performs a rhythmic grooming of the hairy coat there. If the point lie forward at the ear, the foot is directed thither, if far back in the loin the foot goes thither, and similarly at any intermediate spot. The list of such purposive movements is impressive. If a foot tread on a thorn that foot is held up from the ground while the other legs limp away. Milk placed in the mouth is swallowed; acid solution is rejected. Let fall, inverted, the reflex cat alights on its feet. The dog shakes its coat dry after immersion in water. A fly settling on the ear is instantly flung off by the ear. Water entering the ear is thrown out by violent shaking of the head. An exhaustive list would be much larger than that given here. The experiments of Graham Brown and of R. Magnus give excellent examples. But when all is said, if we compare such a list with the range of situations to which the normal cat or dog reacts appropriately, the list is extremely poverty stricken as a conspectus of behaviour. It contains no social reactions. It evidences hunger by restlessness and brisker knee-jerks; but it fails to recognize food as food: it shows no memory, it cannot be trained or learn: it cannot be taught its name. The mindless body reacts with the fatality of a multiple penny-in-the-slot machine to certain stimuli, all of them, as in the case of the penny-in-the-slot machine, physical, and not psychical . . .

(*c*)

We turn to behaviour of a different kind, some say even of a different category of act. The field of the psyche is entered. An old adage has it that to the trodden worm its own trodden self is the world's greater half. That anthropomorphic worm may typify ourselves to us; the 'self' of each of us goes far to epitomize the integration we are now to look at. We can retain the scheme of spatial nervous arrangement we used before, this time, however, not mutilating the central organ, but keeping the animal – the human animal if you will – intact. The receptors at the starting-points of the nerve-thread we find now to be, by conspiracy with a psyche in the central organ, sense-organs. The full panel of the 'five-senses' is in session, and by further collaboration with the psyche, a world of subject and object for the individual is in being. The individual has attained a psychical existence. Phases and moods of mental accrue. Each waking day is a stage dominated for good or ill, in comedy, farce or tragedy, by a *dramatis persona*, the 'self'. And so it will be until the curtain drops. This self is a unity. The continuity of its presence in time, sometimes hardly broken by sleep, its inalienable 'interiority' in (sensual) space, its consistency of view-point, the privacy of its experience, combine to give it status as a unique existence. Although multiple aspects characterize it it has self-cohesion. It regards itself as one, others treat it as one. It is addressed as one, by a name to which it answers. The Law and the State schedule it as one. It and they identify it with a body which is considered by it and them to belong to it integrally. In short, unchallenged and unargued conviction assumes it to be one. The logic of grammar endorses this by a pronoun in the singular. All its diversity is merged in oneness . . .

(*d*)

There remains yet another type of integration which claims consideration, although to saddle it upon nerve may perhaps encounter protest. Integration has been traced at work in two great, and in some respects counterpart, systems of the organism. The physico-chemical (or for short physical) produced a unified machine from what without it would be merely a collocation of commensal organs. The psychical, creates from psychical data a percipient, thinking and endeavouring mental individual. Though our exposition kept these two systems and their integrations apart, they are largely complemental and life brings them co-operatively together at innumerable points. Not that the physical is ever anything but physical, or the psychical anything but psychical. The formal dichotomy of the individual, however, which our description practised for the sake of analysis, results in artefacts such as are not in Nature. Each such is a quasi-organism which does not resemble ourselves, nor does it, *pace* Descartes, resemble dog or cat. For our purpose the two schematic members of the puppet pair which our method segregated require to be integrated together. Not until that is done can we have before us an approximately complete creature of the type we are considering. This integration can be thought of as the last and final integration . . .

This is the body-mind relation[1]; its difficulty lies in its 'how'. As to the utility of the liaison that appears patent enough, namely that the psychical may influence the physical act. In illustration – a simple everyday illustration – a morsel of food in the mouth is subject to the movements of the lips, tongue, cheeks, etc. The conscious self is aware of it, perhaps, acutely – if it is savoury or distasteful. In the former case the self can swallow it, in the latter reject it. If the former, the tongue and fauces push it from the mouth into the grasp of the gullet. That done, our conscious self is aware of the morsel no more, although the morsel is still within the grasp of muscle and nerve and they skilfully deal with it further. The conscious self has, however, lost it and control of it. Even if the morsel be poison the self can no longer directly intervene. That is, the morsel vanishes from an experience at the moment when our choice in regard to it becomes inoperative. The psyche does not persist into conditions which would render it ineffective . . .

When this situation is viewed broadly to-day it reveals a circumstance at first sight strange. We perceive that the immemorial principle of self-conservation is being challenged by a 'new deal'; a novel order of things antagonizes a preceding; a new moral value is appearing over the horizon. The principle of altruism has arisen. A great antinomy is shaping. A behaviour actuated by 'charity' even to the extent of sacrificing one's own self for the sake of another's self. The soldier gives his own life for that of others. This new spirit seems to be largely correlated with the development of man on our planet. Lord Acton had in purpose a History of Liberty. A history of Altruism might be not less worth while. This may be thought to be digressing from physiology, but in fact I do not think it is. St. Augustine's *De Civitate Dei* contains not a little physiology. In so far as physiology involves man as a physiological factor on our planet this great antinomy of which he is the protagonist is not alien to the scope of physiology.

Agreeing that the biological function of the physico-psychical liaison is to enhance the organism's power of disposing of its acts, a further question asks of what service is the physical organism to the psychical? This question is only in part a reciprocal of the other, because only some organisms possess the psychical component. In such as do, however, it is clear that the body-mind liaison provides in a largely physical world the physical means of giving expression to the psychical . . .

---

1 For luminous treatment of this point see W. Russell Brain, *Philosophy* (1946), vol. XXI, p. 134.

Appendix 12. Some Gifts to the British Museum

9 March 1935:

A volume containing two early editions of St. Augustine,

1. De ciuitate Dei, printed by Johannes de Westphalia, Louvain, September, 1488
2. De trinitate, same printer and place, completed Christmas Eve, 1495.

8 June 1935:

1. Gregory IX, Decretals, Speyer, 1492.
2. Boniface VIII, sixth book of the Decretals, Strasburg, 1491 (these two uniform binding).
3. Clement V Constitutions, Strasburg, 1491.
4, 5. Bartolo of Sassoferrato, Super prima (secunda) Digesti novi, Venice, May and April, 1493; and
6. Joannes Antonius de S. Georgio, Super usibus feudorum, Venice, 1498.

13 July 1935:

In addition to the incunabula already reported (c. 5188) thirty-four more selected items, seventeen being incunabula, fifteen of the 16th century, and two of the 17th, including two specimens of early Roman printing, Joannes de Aragonia, Orationes duae, press of Joannes Philippus de Lignamine about 1471.

12 October 1935:

Sir Charles Sherrington, O. M., a further important selection of 21 books, including Arnaldus de Villa Nova, on the art of knowing poisons, and two other medical tracts printed at Milan in 1475, with the arms of Pius VI on the binding; Joannes Bertachinus, Repertorium utriusque juris, Nuremberg, 1483, in 3 vols.; Letters of Phalaris, Milan 1484; and two other incunabula; 10 books of the sixteenth century, especially a fine folio Pontifical, Lyons 1511, which would be the earliest French Pontifical in the Museum (c. 5200).

11 January 1936:

Sir Charles Sherrington, O. M., six printed pieces, equally divided between the fifteenth and sixteenth centuries, including (1) a single leaf, one of several surviving printed on one side only, of an otherwise unknown and therefore supposedly uncompleted edition of the Revelations of St. Bridget of Sweden in the types of Lucas Brandis, Lubeck, about 1478; (2) Bertholdus, Horologium devotionis, Anton Sorg, Augsburg, 1489, in a signed modern Swedish binding; (3) Jean Caron, Opusculum tumultuarium, F. Baligault, Paris, circa 1498; and (4) an edition printed somewhere in Germany of the letter (unrepresented in the Museum) addressed by the Emperor Charles V to the Pope and Cardinals on the occasion of the treaty of peace made between him and the French king, dated Toledo, January, 1526 (c. 5215).

9 May 1936:
Six more interesting books, including three Italian and two German incunabula (the most important being the Bull "Consueverunt Romani Pontifices" of Alexander VI, Rome 1499, Stephan Plannck).

9 October 1937:
Sir Charles Sherrington, O. M., (in succession to other gifts of recent years), twelve volumes, nearly all being printed in France in the first third of the sixteenth century (c. 5277).

9 July 1938:
Sir Charles Sherrington, O. M., seven volumes, one fragmentary, of fifteenth century French printing of rarity and interest, including Joannes Maria Philelphus, Epistolarium Novum, Ulrich Gering, Paris, 1481, the first and very rare edition; Traite de paix entre Louis XI et le duc d'Autriche, Louis Martineau, Paris, 1483; Albertus de Saxonia, Sophismata, etc., Felix Baligault, Paris, 1495; Odo, episcopus Cameracensis, Expositio canonis missae, Gui Marchand, Paris, 1496; Breviarium Tornacense, pars aestiualis, Jean Higman, Paris, 1497, only one perfect copy recorded; and Regula beatissimi patris Benedicti in gallicum sermonem traducta, Geoffrio de Marnef, Paris and Bourges, 1500.

10 December 1938:
1. J. P. de Ferrariis, Practica judicialis, Jacobus Suigus, Venice, 1487, the only book known to have been printed at Venice by this wandering printer;
2. J. Faber Stapulensis (J. Lefevre d'Etaples), Ars moralis [A. Caillaut], Paris, 1494, first edition in a North Italian (?) binding;
3. Modus legendi abbreuiaturas in utroque jure, P. le Dru, Paris, 1495;
4. P. Tataretus, Expositio super Summulis Petri Hispani, for Jean Fabri,

Lyons, 1496; with Fabri's fine device, only known to occur on two books, and hitherto wanting in the Museum;

5. G. Chabutus, Semita diuersarum quattuor viarum, M. Toulouze, Paris 1496 (?) the only known edition, with a fine device, unknown elsewhere;

6. Olivier Maillard, Sermones de aduentu, A. Caillaut, Paris, 1497; very rare first edition of sermons by the most popular French preacher of the day.

8 July 1939:

Sir C. S. Sherrington, O. M. (in continuation of former gifts), four incunabula, three of them law books, viz.: –

1. Aristotle, de virtutibus et vitiis (Ulric Gering: Paris, circa 1480) one of six copies known with the binding label of King Christian VII of Denmark (1766–1808);

2. Vivianus Bononiensis, Casus longi super ff. Veteri et Infortiato (J. Amerbach, Basel, circa 1490), the only early edition of an author unrepresented in the Museum;

3. Martinus de Carraziis, Disputatio in materia legitimationum, U. Scinzenzeler for J. de Legnano, Milan (circa 1495), no 15th century edition of any of this author's works being as yet in the Museum;

4. Nicolaus de Ubaldis, Tractatus de successionibus ab intestato, B. de Vitalibus, 20 June, 1499.

3 August 1940:

Jacobus de Voragine: Passional, oder Leben der Heiligen Winterteil, Augsburg, 1485.

In 1947 he is reported as having given to the British Museum a collection of 56 printed books, mostly printed in the sixteenth century, in France, Italy and Germany, but including two fifteenth century books and five of the seventeenth and twentieth centuries.

Appendix 13. Co-Operative Medical Library Service in London

Broomside, Valley Road, Ipswich, Nov. 14, 1938

My Dear Librarian,

Thank you for the copy of the 'Survey'. I have found much interest in reading it through. Your note with it invites comment from me. Without going into detail, which could only be done properly at considerable space, let me say I am in hearty agreement with the main suggestion, namely fuller cooperation with cognate libraries with which equitable arrangements could be made. It would allow greater devotion of the College library to the particular set of subjects which are peculiarly the Colleges' own – in one word 'Surgery'. By that I would mean Surgery in the fullest sense, including all that the College would understand by the name.

If by collaboration between libraries the College could be relieved from providing a number of the serials and text books, of the non-surgical subjects, it could with a clear conscience devote the money, space, and facilities set free to useful expansion of its collection in subjects more properly especially its own.

That would no doubt affect somewhat a certain fraction of the present clientele of the library. A proportion of its more junior readers would have to go elsewhere. But, as regards the general public and educational interest of these students, their shift would be compensated by an increased convenience afforded by the College library to a more senior class of readers especially concerned with surgery itself in one or other of its aspects. As the Report says the College is now recognized widely as a busy centre of research in experimental surgery. The suggested shift in 'venue' of the library would be in accordance with its recent responsibilities and a boon to its own research worries.

For the College as a step toward cooperation between its library and sister libraries to enter into an 'exchange' arrangement with those libraries would be in accord with a general library 'movement' of today, and doubtless a substantial furtherance of the faculty of surgical study. I fancy it would be of particular value to the provincial medical schools; my experience for what it is worth – leads to me to think some of them not at all well supplied with the literature of surgery. But the 'exchange' scheme would want careful enquiry. The success of the Nat. Central Library in that direction has proved phenomenal. It would be worthwhile perhaps consulting their methods and experience. I believe I am right in thinking that an exchange system of a limited kind is in operation between the 'College libraries' but not Oxford and Cambridge. It involves of course a 'union catalogue' common to the cooperating libraries.

There is much more to be said but this letter is already long. At the moment the main thing I feel is how welcome it is to hear of a step toward that overdue desideratum – some cooperation between the 'medical libraries' in London. London has splendid resources in medical books (I remember how poor, when I was in Berlin, were the medical library collections there as compared with London) but in London the lack of organization between the libraries still sadly impedes the use of its riches. It would be a great step indeed if the College, with its fine library and its public-spirited devotion to surgery and surgical research, would lead the way in cooperation.

I think the 'Survey' a careful report . . . it contains much that is useful to consider.

Yours very truly C. S. Sherrington

W. R. LeFanu, Esq.
Librarian
The Royal College of Surgeons

Appendix 14. Introductory Broadcast for B.B.C. on "The Physical Basis of Mind"

From: The B.B.C. Broadcast Talks *The Physical Basis of Mind*. P. Laslett (ed.). Oxford: Blackwell Scientific Publications Ltd. 1950

[Sir Charles Sherrington's broadcast was prefaced by a short address from Sir Henry Dale, O. M. He introduced him to his audience as 'a veteran of science, still in full mental vigour in his ninety-second year, the greatest physiologist alive to-day. He has been the chief pioneer of the experimental analysis of the central nervous system, and his book *The Integrative Action of the Nervous System* is one of the great classics of physiology and medical science.']

Knowledge of the physical basis of mind is making great strides in these days. Knowledge of the brain is growing, and our theme is almost equivalent to the physiology of the brain. Mind, meaning by that thoughts, memories, feelings, reasoning, and so on, is difficult to bring into the class of physical things. Physiology, a natural science, tends to be silent about all outside the physical. And so the study of the physical basis of mind suffers from falling between two stools.

As a scientific study, it began with observations – that loss of the brain produces loss of mind. But observation of mind is not so straightforward as might be thought. It is not safe even to suppose that mind is universally present in animal life. Most life is, I imagine, mindless, although the behaviour is purposeful. Mind is always an inference from behaviour, and that sometimes is difficult to interpret. It would seem that though there is matter which exists apart from mind, we know of no instance where mind exists apart from matter; that is, if we define 'mind' as we agreed to do.

That the brain is the bodily organ of the mind we have to accept as an established fact. It is perhaps somewhat surprising that the living brain is quite insensitive to handling, or cutting, or even searing with hot iron and so on. The modern surgeon has ascertained that. The most universal agent for provoking activity of nerve is the electric current, but, applied to the living brain, it fails to evoke any obvious effect except in a certain limited area, and there it provokes not 'thoughts,' but limited movements of the body. These movements do not seem 'willed' to the person experiencing them, although he or she perceives them. But the electric current, when applied to the naked human brain, does at times call up 'thoughts.' The experienced brain-surgeon, Professor Wilder Penfield, has examined this effect. He finds that at certain points of the brain surface an electric current will call up to the patient a familiar scene, not always quite the same scene . . .

The physical basis of mind encroaches more and more upon the study of mind, but there remain mental events which seem to lie beyond any physiology of the brain. When I turn my gaze skyward I see the flattened dome of sky and the sun's brilliant disc and a hundred other visible things underneath it. What are the steps which bring this about? A pencil of light from the sun enters the eye and is focused there on the retina. It gives rise to a change, which in turn travels to the nerve-layer at the top of the brain. The whole chain of these events, from the sun to the top of my brain, is physical. Each step is an electrical reaction. But now there succeeds a change wholly unlike any which led up to it, and wholly inexplicable by us. A visual scene presents itself to the mind; I *see* the dome of sky and the sun in it, and a hundred other visual things beside. In fact, I perceive a picture of the world around me. When this visual scene appears I ought, I suppose, to feel startled; but I am too accustomed to feel even surprised.

It is a far cry from an electrical reaction in the brain to suddenly seeing the world around one, with all its distances, its colours and chiaroscuro. Philosophers to-day, I fancy, incline to dividing the world of our experience into two sorts, a material and a spiritual. On the other hand, our scientists, I fancy, lean towards accepting mind itself as a form of energy. I would like to hear Lord Samuel on this. The Victorian era witnessed violent divergences of doctrine upon it. John Stuart Mill protested against those who supposed that, for seeing, the possession of an eye is a necessity. On the other hand, the oracular Professor Tyndall, presiding over the British Association at Belfast, told his audience that as the bile is a secretion of the liver, so the mind is a secretion of the brain.

Aristotle, 2,000 years ago, was asking how is the mind attached to the body. We are asking that question still.

Appendix 15. Honorary Degrees, Fellowships and Memorials

Sherrington is said to have had one of the longest entries ever published in *Who's Who*[1]. However that may be he was honoured by nearly 100 universities and learned societies, with degrees and academic regalia of varying hues, and with honorary memberships and medals. One is intrigued by the fact that honorary membership was conferred on him even by The Burnley and District Medico-Ethical Association in 1905 following his reading to them of an "Original Paper" as their certificate expresses it!

For his eightieth birthday C. S. S. received an illuminated address which was circulated for signatures to his pupils and colleagues around the world. His eighty-fifth birthday was celebrated in many quarters; what pleased him particularly was a letter from Jan Masaryk of the Czech government in

---

1 See Appendix 16.

exile. C. S. S. had known the father, Thomas Masaryk, founder of Czecho-slovakia, in happier times[1].

For his ninetieth birthday on 27 November 1947, *The British Medical Journal* produced a special issue with articles by John Fulton on "Sherrington's impact on neurophysiology", T. Graham Brown on "Sherrington – The Man" and by A. D. Ritchie on "Sherrington as Philosopher". The leading article dealt with his influence on clinical neurology. Dr. F. M. R. Walshe contributed two notable items – an abridged version of his Victor Horsley Lecture of 1946 together with a book review of the second edition of *The Integrative Action of the Nervous System*. Walshe's graceful prose was felt by some to be the highlight of the celebration, in discussing this classic: "In physiology it holds a position similar to that of Newton's *Principia* in physics . . . Here is no medley of *ad hoc* hypotheses but a logical analysis and synthesis bearing the imprint of scientific genius".

Sherrington died quietly in Eastbourne on 4 March 1952 while reading a little French volume by the hearth. Memorial services were held at Gonville and Caius College, Cambridge, on 14 March, and on the following day at Magdalen College, Oxford. The Colleges had their flags at half mast during the ceremonies, which were attended by a very wide variety of friends. At Queen Elizabeth School, Ipswich, a service took place in the Church of St. Mary-le-Tower, following one at St. Margaret, Westminster in the shadow of the Abbey on 20 May 1952.

Obituary notices appeared in nearly every periodical dedicated to the study of the nervous system. In the more general press E. G. T. Liddell, one of Sherrington's successors in the Waynflete Chair at Oxford wrote a very warm and discerning tribute in the Oxford Magazine, 1 May 1952. His summary statement was this: "He knew what questions to ask of Nature and how to ask them". Liddell also wrote a definitive biographical account in the Obituary Notices of the Royal Society (1952).

His long-time Oxford pupil, R. S. Creed, writing in the British Journal of Psychology[2] in February 1953, quoted Sherrington's statement to him: "I am glad to have lived for so long, for I have seen how so much has worked out." C. S. S. was also quoted as saying that his own poems were "Some foot-prints of a lame follower after the Muse". Creed echoed Liddell's sentiments: "He had an uncanny knowledge, partly born of long experi-

---

1 C. S. S. in his 1946–1947 diary wrote: "The contribution of the Czech patriots to the defeat of the Germans was probably greater in proportion to their strength than that of any other people who fought for the United Nations, and the loss of life and the degree of sacrifice probably exceeded, in proportion, that of any country".

2 C. S. S. has served on the editorial advisory panel of the Journal since its beginning in 1904.

ence, of the sort of question to which Nature would vouchsafe an answer, and a wonderful facility in devising the best means for obtaining that answer".

John Eccles, in the British Journal of the Philosophy of Science, on the editorial board of which C. S. S. had served, wrote that Sherrington's great ability was ". . . to find the right and fruitful paths amidst the tangled ideologies that flourish at the onset of a new science". He added: "One can survey his life's effort as the ordered strategy of a campaign" and quoted Sherrington's words, spoken near the end of his Gifford Lectures: ". . . for all I can do [the mental and matter-energy entities] remain refractorily apart. They seem to me disparate; not mutually convertible: untranslatable the one into the other". In the *Journal of Neurophysiology* John Fulton published a touching obituary notice as well as the very useful bibliography of the writing of Sir Charles since his first paper in 1884.

On the centenary of Sherrington's birth Wilder Penfield addressed a meeting of the Canadian Neurological Society under the chairmanship of Professor William Feindel at Saskatoon, on "Sir Charles Sherrington, Poet and Philosopher".

There was no organized effort to commemorate the Sherrington Centenary in Britain in 1957. By good fortune there was in 1957 a Ciba Symposium in London on the Neurological Basis of Behaviour, and this was the occasion to make commemorative remarks and the volume was entitled "Neurological Basis of Behaviour in Commemoration of Charles Scott Sherrington". The President of Magdalen College, Oxford gave a commemorative dinner to which a distinguished group of Sherrington's friends came, as indicated in Figure 7. It was a spendid occasion for enjoying happy remembrances of a great scientist and scholar and a dear friend.

At least four books have been written about the work of C. S. S. – the first being the fourth Sherrington Lecture at the University of Liverpool by Lord Cohen of Birkenhead, published in 1958 under the title *Sherrington – Physiologist, Philosopher and Poet.* The second volume is by Sherrington's pupil, E. G. T. Liddell, *The Discovery of Reflexes,* 1960. In 1966 another pupil, the Nobel Laureate Ragnar Granit of Stockholm wrote *Charles Scott Sherrington – An Appraisal.* The Harvard University Press in 1969 published Judith Swazey's study *Reflexes and Motor Integration. Sherrington's Concept of Integrative Action.*

On the other side of the globe a "Sherrington Room" has been dedicated in the Woodward Biomedical Library of the University of British Columbia. It is a large oak-pannelled room, capable of holding forty students in seminar fashion. It contains most of Sherrington's honorary degree

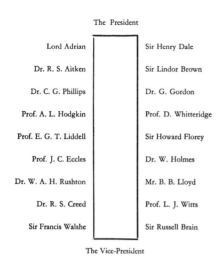

The President

Lord Adrian	Sir Henry Dale
Dr. R. S. Aitken	Sir Lindor Brown
Dr. C. G. Phillips	Dr. G. Gordon
Prof. A. L. Hodgkin	Prof. D. Whitteridge
Prof. E. G. T. Liddell	Sir Howard Florey
Prof. J. C. Eccles	Dr. W. Holmes
Dr. W. A. H. Rushton	Mr. B. B. Lloyd
Dr. R. S. Creed	Prof. L. J. Witts
Sir Francis Walshe	Sir Russell Brain

The Vice-President

Magdalen College

Dinner to celebrate
the centenary of the birth of
Sir Charles Sherrington

Wednesday, 10 July
1957

scrolls, medals, the Eves portrait painted for his family, his court dress, some of his academic hoods, his schoolboy books, watch, and the ice skates which he was wearing when he "fell in" at Sefton Park, Liverpool on a memorable day. But most of all it contains – set around a table made in Ipswich – the ten dining room chairs from Liverpool and Oxford days. To the back of each chair there has been affixed a small brass plate on which are engraved – two names to each chair – the names of some of those who sat on them in his home, at some time past. The names, selected with the help of the Sherrington family, are paired as follows:

Osler – Penfield, Dale – Adrian, Lister – Florey, Fulton – Cushing, Eccles – Denny Brown, Cannon – Forbes, Foster – Hopkins, Wesbrook – Bridges, Río Hortega – Ramón y Cajal, and Rutherford – Bragg.

Nearby is a video-cassette reproducer on which students, faculty and visitors may see the colour television programme on Sherrington made by one of us in co-operation with the Canadian Broadcasting Corporation some years ago along with similar programmes on some of his colleagues such as Wesbrook, Lister, Florey and Osler, and of his predecessors Leonardo da Vinci, Christopher Wren and Willis. A Sherrington Society was established in 1975 under the presidency of Dr. John Smythies, F. R. C. P., with Sir John Eccles, F. R. S. as Honorary President.

238   Appendix 16. Last Entry in "Who's Who", 1952

Much of Sherrington's correspondence has been placed in the Wood-ward Library by Sir Charles' family, together with a few books from his library – not rare books, but well-used little volumes.

Memorial lectures will keep his memory green, but two great classics in the English language will remain as our finest remembrance of him, *The Integrative Action of the Nervous System* and *Man on His Nature*.

Appendix 16. Last Entry in "Who's Who", 1952

Sherrington, Sir Charles Scott, O.M., 1924; G.B.E., cr. 1922: F.R.S.; M.A., M.D., D.SC. (Cantab), F.R.C.P., F.R.C.S.; Hon. D.Sc., Oxford, Paris, Manchester, Strasbourg, Louvain, Upsala, Lyon, Buda Pesth, Athens; LL.D. London, Toronto, Harvard, Dublin, Edinburgh, Montreal, Liver-pool, Brussels, Sheffield, Berne, Birmingham, Wales and Glasgow; late Waynflete Professor of Physiology, Oxford; late Member of Medical Research Council of Privy Council; *b.* 27 Nov. 1857; *m.* 1892, Ethel Mary (*d.* 1933) y.d. of John Ely Wright, Preston Manor, Suffolk; one s. Educ. Caius College, Cambridge, Late Brown Prof. of Pathology, Univ. of Lon-don; Lecturer on Physiology, St. Thomas's Hosp., London; Royal and Copley Medallist and Past-Pres. of the Royal Society; Baly Gold Medallist, Royal Coll. of Physicians; Retzius Gold Medal, Royal Swedish Academy; Hon. Member Royal Irish Academy; Soc. de Neurologie, Paris; associate member of the Institut de France; member Imperial Academy of Medicine, Vienna; Foreign Member of National Academy of Sciences, Washington, French Acad. of Sciences, Real. Academ. d. Scienze, Rome, and of Impe-rial Academy of Sciences, Petrograd; Royal Acad. of Medicine of Belgium and of Madrid; Member of Royal Acad. of Holland, Amsterdam; Royal Acad. of Sweden; Hon. Mem. Royal Danish Academy of Science, Copenhagen; Société de Biologie, Belge; Foreign Mem. Real. Accad. d. Scienze, Bologna; Hon. Fellow of Magdalen Coll., Oxford; Hon. Fellow Caius Coll. Cambridge; Hon. Fellow Roy. Soc. of Edinburgh; Hon Member Physiol. Soc. of America; Soc. Medica di Roma; R. Accadem. di Scienze, Turin. Papal Academy Rome; Anglo-American Secretary, International Congresses of Physiology Liège, Berne, Cambridge, Turin, Brussels, Heidelberg; Vice-Pres. Brit. Child Study Assoc.; Pres. Physiol. Sect. Brit.

Assoc. Cam. 1904; Dunham Lecturer, Harvard, 1927; Lister Oration, Candian Medical Association, Toronto, 1927; Silliman Memorial Lecturer, Yale University, 1904; Page May Memorial Lecturer, University of London, 1910; Croonian Lecturer, Royal College of Physicians, 1913; Member of Board of Trade Committee on Sight Tests, 1910–12; Home Office Committee on Lighting of Factories and Workshops, 1913; War Office Committee on Tetanus, 1916–17; Scientific Com. of the Central Board of Control, Alcohol, 1916–17; Professor of Physiology, Univ. of Liverpool, 1895–1913; Fullerian Professor of Physiology, Royal Institution of Great Britain, 1914–17; late Chairman, Industrial Fatigue Research Board, 1918; Nobel Laureate for Medicine, 1932; Gifford Lecturer, University of Edinburgh, 1936–38; a Trustee, British Museum. *Publications:* The Integrative Action of the Nervous System; Mammalian Physiology, 1916; School Hygiene (part author) 1913; papers to the Royal and other scientific societies, especially on the brain and nervous system; Selected Writings, 1939; Assaying of Brabantius, and other Verse, 2nd. ed. 1940; Man on his Nature: the Gifford Lectures, Edinburgh, 1940, 4th ed. 1946; The Endeavour of Jean Fernel, 1946. *Address:* Gonville and Caius College, Cambridge. *Club:* Athenaeum.

Appendix 17. Memories by C.E.R. Sherrington

From: *Charles Scott Sherrinton (1857–1952).* Memories by C. E. R. Sherrington. A pamphlet for private circulation, printed in 1957

These "Memories" were delivered as the Beaumont Lecture (Yale University) on 15 November 1957.

They were also read at McGill University to the Fellows' Society of the Montreal Neurological Institute and the Montreal Physiological Society on November 1st, 1957.

Foreword

Autumn, 1957

My father was averse to the idea that any extensive biography should be written about him. He had read many biographies and liked but few of them. His thoughts were that any achievements he could lay claim to would, in themselves, form some monument to his long working life – to him his work was in itself a pleasure rather than a toil.

Others truly qualified have set out in scientific proceedings and journals the story of his researches and their contributions to physiology, to neurology and to other branches of the natural sciences. Yet, many years ago, he handed me certain letters which he prized, including one quoted in this monograph from Longfellow. It is my thought that his wish would have been that some human story should be designed, after his death, which would tell in light-hearted vein – for good story-telling was one of his attributes even to the end – of the influences and events which affected his life and guided his thoughts. The centenary of his birth would seem an appropriate time to unfold this story.

Many have asked for it, and now, with all homage, I present it.

C. E. R. Sherrington

CHARLES SCOTT SHERRINGTON

On March 30th, 1908, there was a sale of drawings and pictures in London, at Christie's, and many of them came from the home of Mrs. Caleb Rose of Ipswich – she died in May 1907 at the age of 89. Mrs. Rose, the widow of Dr. Caleb Rose, had been previously the wife of James Norton Sherrington of The Hall, Caister, near Norwich, and she was the greatly beloved mother of Charles Scott Sherrington.

Looking back over exactly half a century I can place the Christie sale as the turning point of my father's life; it meant for him that the home he had loved so much was gone forever and, from that time onwards, the outlook was concentrated on the future not on the past, except for those unutterably happy memories which remained vivid to him until the very end, for he spoke to me of them with some yearning the evening before his death.

Thus his life can be divided almost equally into the two periods 1857–1908 and 1908–1952. Memories of the home at Edgehill House, Ipswich, still stand out clearly in my own mind and, since its influences were so strong on my father's career, a few words may not be out of place.

The family went regularly to London and, as was the wont of those days, stayed in rooms; thus it happened that my father was born in Islington – he never remembered the address but recalled that on later visits with his younger brothers it was a house near where the North London Railway trains from Broad Street pass on their way to Willesden and Kew over a high viaduct.

Brought up at Ipswich, the great influence on his life was his step-father, Dr. Rose, whose own son – by an earlier marriage – was Edward Rose who became a dramatist of note and was at one time dramatic critic of the 'Sunday Times'. It was the happiest of families, there being two younger brothers – William Staunton Sherrington who became a barrister and took a leading part in Masonry, and George Stuart Sherrington who was an athlete of no mean distinction – he was long connected with the Corinthians. Neither of these brothers married and both died before my father.

The three boys all went to Ipswich School where the great classical scholar H. A. Holden was the then headmaster; he imbued in my father a knowledge and love of the classics which was never destined to be lost. At that time his brother, W. S. Sherrington, was regarded as the brilliant one of the trio, winning many school prizes and a scholarship to St. John's College, Cambridge.

An even greater influence on Charles Sherrington at that time was Thomas Ashe, an assistant master at the school. He was a poet of considerable distinction who published several books of poems, probably the most notable being 'Songs of a Year' in 1888. It was Ashe who fired my father with ideas of foreign travel, for Ashe at an early age travelled widely and they kept in touch until 1880 at least. It is my understanding that Ashe died quite young but his influence lasted for many decades, for Sherrington's love of poetry, literature and books may be traced to him and it continued until my father's death in 1952; towards the close, it became, one realised, his first and last love.

If these early interests were strong there was also no lack of athletic activity; Charles Sherrington played soccer for his school and later for Ipswich Town, but he was outshone as an athlete by his youngest brother, G. S. Sherrington, who later went up to Trinity College, Cambridge, gained it is believed a double Blue, and was almost 'sent down' for bathing in Trinity fountain on a Sunday morning. He finally became a solicitor in London.

It was probably due to Dr. Rose, whom my father adored as much as be adored his mother, that he determined on a medical career and left Ipswich to train at St. Thomas's, where he played rugger for the hospital. His plan to go to Cambridge had fallen through, owing to a severe financial blow the family had suffered through the failure of a bank in East Anglia; thus, after a short period at St. Thomas's, he went to Edinburgh University as a medical student for a while, until the financial situation improved, when he entered Gonville and Caius College, Cambridge, where he was a contemporary of his two brothers, W. S. Sherrington at John's and G. S. Sherrington at Trinity. His days at Edinburgh never appealed to him and he spoke little of that period, but he once showed me his old rooms near the 'Royal

Mile' and for a time he roomed in Portobello. Poverty was probably the cause of his Edinburgh difficulties, for he had given up what share there was of help from the family for the sake of his two younger brothers. Those who knew him in after life are not likely to dispute this interpretation of a bleak but brief period.

Cambridge revived his spirit and morale; he rowed for Caius and played rugger for the college, whilst even earlier he had ventured to Switzerland with other medical students, thus becoming one of the earliest British winter visitors to Grindelwald, the main sports then being tobogganing and lugeing. Cycling on the 'bone-shakers' of the seventies was a favourite sport of the Sherrington boys and their contemporaries at Ipswich School; devoid of brakes these bicycles could only negotiate a steep hill by expert footwork, bad for any shoe or boot, the alternative was to trust one's luck in the nearest bank!

It is almost impossible to assess influences, but my own memories of Edgehill House at Ipswich lead me to the following appraisement. In that happiest of family homes there lay a treasure store of pictures, since Dr. Sherrington had been a personal friend of J. B. Crome, David Cox and the Girlings; besides the pictures, including sketches by Landseer, there was the palette of 'Old Crome' and his bust, which my father later presented to the National Portrait Gallery. The house was literally full of pictures – on chairs, on tables – for there was no room to hang them – Cotmans, Cromes, Coxs, some of which now grace the art gallery in Norwich Castle. There were endless collections – fossils, shells, coins, stones, minerals and the like – for it was the age of collections, but there were endless books too, on architecture, archaeology, medicine, the classics and painting. Over the years many painters and engravers spent hours of leisure there – to quote but one, Edwin Landseer. A fine portrait of Mrs. Rose by W. R. Symonds in 1902 reveals her as still a lovely lady at 84.

From Holden came the urge to classics, from Ashe the urge to literature, foreign languages and travel, from Dr. Rose the knowledge of medicine, architecture and archaeology. Yet withal there was healthy amateur athleticism of that day – football, bicycling, wherrying on the Broads, swimming at Felixstowe or rowing on the Gipping.

I draw this picture, incomplete though it be, for it explains the limitless interests of the subject of this monograph. When he started out on life's career, hard though it was for many years, he was not ill-equipped to deal with the problems he would face in terms of knowledge in many spheres nor in terms of health as an athlete.

Cambridge

It was probably the financial problem which led to Charles Sherrington's arrival in Cambridge in October 1879 as a non-collegiate student, but the following year was to find him at Gonville and Caius College. A letter from his mother had congratulated him on the results of his 'Little Go'.

The influences of Thomas Ashe remained strong at this period and the study of medicine by no means occupied all his time. Poetry and painting and the study of printing were his second, if not his first, interest and one of the verses sent from Cambridge, England, to Longfellow at the close of 1881, describing a rural incident, brought forth a delightful reply from the poet in Cambridge, Massachusetts, dated January 10th, 1882. It was probably signed – and the signature is quite firm – during the poet's last illness. The letter refers to a visit to Caius in the summer of 1868 and how he remembered its 'Gate of Honour' and "its amiable and excellent Master Dr. Guest who had a mania for building".

The search for old books and poetry in the early '80s was rewarded by the find of a first edition of Keats at Heffers bookshop. This was acquired for sixpence – it had a fly-leaf missing. Half a century later the little Keats was sold back to Heffers for about £ 100.

It must have been unusual for a student even in those times to pass medical exams prior to studying at Edinburgh and Cambridge, but it is recorded that my father entered St. Thomas's Hospital, London, in September, 1876, as a perpetual pupil and passed his Primary Examination for the Membership of the Royal College of Surgeons in April 1878. The cup he acquired as a member of the St. Thomas's 1st XV at Rugby football in 1879 still bears witness to this fact. This would seem to prove that his time at Edinburgh as a student was short-lived.

Wanderings abroad in search of medical experience, books, architecture and to improve his languages filled his vacations. Sometimes they nearly ended in disaster as when, penniless in Bordeaux at the end of a visit to France, he worked his way back to England on a wine boat from the Gironde. As he once expressed it, there was plenty of wine, much cork (from Spain) and even more work.

It is for others, for I am in no way qualified, to trace out the years when science and physiology began to shape the career which was to prove his destiny: it has been admirably recounted by D. Denny-Brown, E. G. T. Liddell, J. F. Fulton and R. S. Creed. What this little outline does attempt to do, however inadequately, is to explain the influences on his life, those signposts on the road that everyone meets, and the chances by which one takes the path to the left or to the right – for usually there is no turning back.

Fortunately some letters of those years have been preserved and certain of them provide clues as to how his mind was working in his rooms on Hills Road – his address in 1881. In parenthesis one may comment on the care with which he preserved the letters which he valued and saw the value of not, in mere monetary terms, but in their future historical interest, or their useful guidance to him – his loving letters from his mother, the excellent advice he received from Ashe, or from those who were the leaders of the time in medicine and the natural sciences. All the more is this surprising to those who remember his study, a welter of correspondence, pamphlets and books, that made the household task of dusting impossible. In contrast, any envelope brought by the postman which was considered to contain an income tax demand or a bill was promptly consigned to the wastepaper basket! Thus a family duty was to unearth such unopened letters each morning and study their grim contents – that was my mother's daily task.

The life at Caius he always looked back upon with pleasure though work was hard, involving duties at Addenbrooke's Hospital, some of which were not easy. Bicycling enabled him to know most of the surrounding country and to go home regularly; sailing on the Broads brought him into contact with J. S. Austen, then at Emmanuel I believe. Together they once hired a boat at Ramsgate and were nearly drowned through running ashore on the Goodwin Sands. J. S. Austen later became a powerful force in the City of London with many interests in transport and railways in South America, as a colleague of Lord St. Davids. When in college the rooms he loved best were those in the 'Gate of Virtue', where early in 1888 he became engaged to Ethel Wright of Preston Manor, near Lavenham; their marriage by the Dean of Caius in 1891 can be said to have linked East and West Suffolk. Over the years each considered the other half of the county very inferior!

Of the influence of my father's life, in those Cambridge days, of Michael Foster, Langley and Gaskell, others have told in some detail, but one of his own letters to Ipswich, headed Corpus Buildings, Cambridge – there is no year – describes amusingly his life with a Mr. Wherry, whose housekeeper "a Hebe quite beyond praise who provided a neat little dinner of three courses and cheese at 7 and an excellent breakfast at 8". Mr. Wherry, a widower, was a surgeon specialising on the eye, and had married a Miss Albinia Lucy Cust, a hospital nurse; everything in the house from music to sketches, recipes and mixtures for colds was labelled A. L. C.

Langley and Michael Foster are mentioned in this letter.

He joined, as a Demonstrator, Professor (later Sir) George Humphry in the Anatomy Laboratory in 1883 and this led to a visit to Strasbourg to work with Goltz. My father never forgot this picture of Alsace, then being rapidly Germanised, as an occupied country. Many years later his honorary degree from Strasbourg gave him particular happiness. An outbreak of cholera in Spain took him there, with C. S. Roy of Cambridge and J. Graham Brown of Edinburgh in 1885. The Baedeker he used has some interesting notes and the trio, engaged on inoculating the inhabitants, met with a rough reception at Toledo, where the Consul – a Scotsman – rescued them from a volley of stones. On their return collectively chose a truly Scottish present in gratitude to Consul McPherson and Roy was deputed to despatch it. After his death the beautiful ram's horn, with a cairngorm and replete with the tools to handle snuff, was discovered in his laboratory. Mrs. Roy-Batty, as she then was – a sister of Lady Thompson of Trinity – presented it to me on my marriage, in memory of the Spanish saga of 1885.

The following year, 1886, found him in Italy, again on cholera work, and at Venice he ran out of funds: discovering that he could practice medicine there he carried on his work for a time by such activities. The days in Italy developed his love of painting, architecture and early printing. In contrast, Berlin, where he later worked with Virchow, was devoid of similar interests, though visits to the Reichstag proved illuminating in that he was made to realise the impotence of opposition to Bismarck, whose appearances he described as reminding him of a cuckoo set high in a cuckoo clock. The door opened, Bismarck appeared, read his speech without looking up and on conclusion folded his papers and disappeared, not even troubling to hear the comments on his speech.

The year 1887 marked his election as a Fellow of Gonville and Caius College and his appointment as a Lecturer in Systematic Physiology at St. Thomas's Hospital; he was then thirty.

London

An amusing letter from Sherrington to his stepfather, though not dated with the year, probably can be ascribed to this period; it describes his rooms at 69 Lambeth Palace Road. "It is a pleasure to live in a place where the cabman says 'thank you' for a 2/- fare from Liverpool Street. I have never done so before." He concludes with the remarks that he felt as comfortable as his step-brother Teddy (Edward Rose) appeared to be in 'Varna' and, significantly, the rooms were over an instrument maker's shop. Expert worker as he was with precision instruments himself, this must have been an added attraction.

It was in 1891 that he was appointed Brown Professor of Pathology at the University of London, which meant that he succeeded Sir Victor Horsley at the Brown Institution – so closely associated with the development of veterinary science. The Brown appointment on March 10th, 1891, made marriage possible, as a letter, still extant, from his mother to his fiancée, reveals.

They were married on August 27th and the honeymoon was spent abroad. The Reverend Hewitt, whom I can well remember as an old and distinguished-looking man, who had officiated with the Dean of Caius at the wedding at Preston St. Mary, welcomed them to Alassio where he had a villa, and the passport – dated 25th August, 1891, No. 49969 – was signed 'Salisbury'. It cost sixpence and should have carried the 'Signature of the Bearer', but my father forgot that, and no one seems to have questioned his omission!

His writing, and in part my mother's, tells of each day's events – 'Genoa (very hot, no letter from bankers).' They called on Angelo Mosso and went with him by boat to Baveno. My mother records: "C. in bad temper because of a cold" and he wrote "Ethel had heavy lunch of blackberries" – a proof that honeymoons change not over the centuries. The Michael Fosters joined them for a time and there are some comments on the Gotthard, thus, frontier formalities in those brave days demanded no formalities and no mention. A money draft for £ 30 addressed to Genoa never reached them 'ere their return and, unendorsed, to this day it remains a model of calligraphy.

The London home was 27 St. George's Square, a district of which my mother was fond since she had known Westminster well in her school days, Sundays being often spent at the house, in Little College Street, of one of the senior masters at Westminster School.

Ramon y Cajal was a guest at St. George's Square and caused some embarrassment since, before leaving the house after breakfast he had locked his room, his lantern slides being arranged all over the floor for a lecture that evening. My mother wondered why all the neighbours were gesticulating and pointing to the house. She went to find out – in true Spanish style all the bedclothes of her guest were draped from the balcony. Nothing could be done until Ramon y Cajal returned, key in pocket.

It was during the London period that my young cousin, G. V. Sturgeon, fell desperately ill with diphtheria at Ashcombe, near Lewes, in Sussex. My father's advice was sought and he travelled down the next morning from Victoria to Lewes, with vaccine hurriedly prepared. He was met there by the local doctor: in a dogcart my uncle drove them to Ashcombe, the vaccine was administered to the little boy that same morning. This story of the early use of vaccine for diphtheria has been recorded fully but may well be the subject of brief mention.

The London days were, to the best of my knowledge, happy ones and an incident not, I believe, hitherto metioned was the trials made with silk parachutes on Sunday mornings from the tower which adjoins the main buildings of St. Thomas's Hospital. They always impressed my mother, perhaps because she recalled the view on a clear summer day from the top of that tower – a view over London north, west, south and east, from Hampstead Heath to the North Downs.

Football days were long over, but there were opportunities, at weekends, for bicycling, tennis, sculling and golf, judging from the letters written in 1894. There were also many visits abroad, most of them involving attendances at Physiological Congresses, as at Liége in 1892 and Berne in 1895, but there were also winter sports holidays at Grindelwald and summer bicycling rambles in Normandy, Touraine and Anjou. Paris was often included because he loved its 'Rive Gauche', where he had lived and worked, once seeing Pasteur perform an operation.

Many interesting evenings had been spent at the home in Hampstead of his step-brother Edward Rose, who had achieved considerable success with his dramatisation of "The Prisoner of Zenda". My mother enjoyed meeting the literary circle which gathered there, including Bernard Shaw and, of course, Anthony Hope; there were also painters and engravers of distinction, including Edwin Edwards. Thus were the links with Ipswich days and the Norfolk School preserved.

A presentation at Oxford in July 1895 to my father, and also to my mother who was then doing much of his secretarial work, occasioned much happiness – a reception was given by the Burdon-Sandersons. There was a tinge of regret that so few were present from Cambridge, for which there was apparently a reason. The occasion, doubtless connected with his work as Anglo-American Secretary, International Congresses of Physiology, merits mention, since it was my father's first official link with Oxford and heralded, in days to come, many memorable years there, as well as the connection with Magdalen of which he was so proud and spoke so often when he had recorded four-score years and ten.

In the summer of 1895 came the appointment as professor at the University of Liverpool – then University College. With Sherrington's essential background of London, East Anglia and the southern counties one might have expected some evidences of regret at taking up an appointment, in spite of the promotion it offered, in a northern industrial city. All the contemporary evidence is to the contrary, however, and his description of the new home, the city of Liverpool – as it then was – written in October 1895, is one of his more entrancing letters. Incidentally it reveals one reason for his success – to wit his ability to find hapiness wherever he found himself and in whatever company. It matched his humility to which there were so many tributes at the time of his death fifty-seven years later.

Liverpool

Curiously, writing to his mother in October 1895 from Grove Park, Liverpool, he described the house as in many ways like his devoted home at Edgehill, Ipswich. The french windows opening into the garden, the branching stairway and the like; also he found the town more like Ipswich than London with "the distances small, and the traffic countrified, and the shops too". He records that his new colleagues were "cordial and friendly in the extreme and some of them strike one as remarkably nice". It is a significant letter for it goes on to state that the days are bright and sunny here in comparison with London, "I feel so cheered to be out in the country as compared with London, that I believe I shall soon be doing good work here, much better than I ever did in London, the sky of which unstrung me to a degree I hardly realised before we settled here".

His first impressions of Liverpool, and they changed little in the succeeding years, stand out in strong contrast to those of Harvey Cushing who came to spend a month there with Sherrington in 1901. One may read Cushing's reactions in John Fulton's admirable life of Harvey Cushing.

The British Association held its 1897 meeting in Canada and the diary, which I still possess, tells of the Atlantic crossing on the Allan Liner 'Parisian' – the journey to Victoria, B.C., and back and the return on the Dominion vessel 'Vancouver' to Moville. Rat Portage was reached on August 28th and Ipswich reached from Dublin at 9 p. m. on September 30th. Lord Lister was a member of the party as were Professor Farmer, Dr. Gaskell, Dr. Bower, Dr. McAllister, Sir John Evans, Dr. Adami, Professor Bowdich, Professor Poulton, Professor Rücker (co-secretary of the Royal Society), and Lord Kelvin, who seems to have made a disappointing speech at Banff in the Rockies.

My mother records that ginger beer on top of Mount Royal in 1897 was very poor: my father, after having a duel with a Czech professor about the bath at the Grand Union Hotel, Ottawa, "where Grand Duchesses were in waiting", nearly finished his career at Vancouver when the wooden barrier at the end of the corridor on the seventh floor of the hotel, then being extended, dropped to the ground when he leaned on it. It was only lodged, not fixed; gripped by my mother, he remarked "The sign of a new country with great possibilities".

The life at Liverpool was brightened not only by the friendship shown him by many of his colleagues but also by the great kindness of many important figures in the shipping world of those days. Although, perhaps, invidious to select examples, specific mention may be made of the Booths, the Holts, the Brocklebanks, the Bowrings, the Glynns, Sir William Johnston and Mr. John Rankin. In other spheres there were the Sings, the Reynolds, the Gaskells and Sir William Forwood. Brought up on austere lines, many were great patrons of the arts and music and their knowledge of the world, through their shipping and merchant interests, made them authorities on many subjects and frequently delightful conversationalists. To move in those circles, as was essential, on an academic salary proved an agreeable task – though not free from anxiety – but the sincere friendship of these great Merseyside families made life easier than it would otherwise have been.

Meetings and other work required journeys to London weekly, if not more often. The 8 a.m. up and the 5.55 p.m. back from Euston provided an excellent non-stop journey to Edgehill, invariably on time and with breakfast and dinner en route – in fact one could stay in the diner all the journey. Much business was done on these trains and an instance of Liverpool kindness and generosity to my father may be exemplified by one of these journeys. Sitting with Sir William Johnston for dinner – and Sir William always insisted on being host – at a table for two, a special arrangement on the 5.55 p.m., my father's host asked about his work and expressed a wish to help, if he could, in some small way. "Was there anything that the Physiological Laboratory wanted?" Sherrington turned quickly over in his mind those things he badly needed and finally explained a small precision instrument that would be a great help. Johnston was interested, asked the price, and, on being told that it should not exceed £100, pulled out his cheque book – towards the end of the journey – and wrote the cheque, handed it to my father who put it in his wallet and expressed his warm gratitude as the train came to a stop at Edge Hill, Liverpool. The next morning on looking at the cheque he discovered that his laboratory had been donated not £100 but a sum of many times that amount.

In 1903 he received the Hon. Degree of LL.D. at Toronto University, delivering the dedicatory address at the opening of the new medical buildings. He sailed on the 'New England' – a Dominion Line vessel – on September 16th, stayed with Macallum at Toronto, delivered an address at Chicago University – a city he greatly admired – and returned by the 'Cedric' from New York. Before sailing he lunched by chance at the Savile Club with Dr. (later Sir William) Osler, who was sailing on the 16th also, but by the 'Oceanic'. Less than two years later Osler was an Oxford resident and only six years later my father was within an ace of becoming resident in Canada or in New York City.

The year 1904 was a busy one since he was President that year of the Physiological Section of the British Association, the meeting being at Cambridge, while the same year he delivered the ninth Silliman lectures at Yale – going on to Johns Hopkins and the University of Pennsylvania. On this journey his wife accompanied him and the happy memories of Yale, Boston, New York, Baltimore, Philadelphia and Washington always remained vivid to them both, high-pointed by good friendships formed, or renewed – Arthur T. Hadley, Harvey Cushing and Osler to select but a few.

With Liverpool, then the main British bridgehead for the States, no month went by without American or Canadian visitors in transit staying at 16 Grove Park. To me their arrival gave great joy, for they had that happy knack of treating a child as a reasonable being and an equal; special friends were Alex Forbes, who was accompanied by his charming bride, meeting at our home his brother, Cameron Forbes, on his way back from the Far East, and Harvey Cushing. Others I recall were Jacques Loeb and Dr. Roaf of Toronto, whose son was working with my father, and F. R. Miller also from Canada. Truth to tell, Canada had stolen Sherrington's heart – he had revelled in the days at Ipperwash Bay or Muskoka when staying with the Macallums. Long stakes he cut at that time, intending to convert them into walking sticks, still provide a memory of Ontario. Thus, there came a day when, having received an offer of a professorship at Toronto, after considerable cogitation he accepted and duly posted the acceptance on a Friday night. Second thoughts by the Sunday morning determined him to stay in Liverpool – he spent most of that Sunday at the General Post Office recovering the letter which was awaiting the next sailing to Canada.

It was, then, by an extremely narrow margin that I did not automatically become a Canadian citizen; it was some twelve years later that I landed there as a settler, called by the opportunities which opened in a New World. Another offer came from Columbia at the end of 1908 over the signature of Nicholas Murray Butler. My father found many attractions in the proposal but he felt that in due course, in honour bound, he would have to take up American citizenship and he hesitated, finally replying in the negative, though he was ever grateful to Columbia for that chance. It was a long letter, as was the wont of the President of Columbia, beautifully expressed and remains, full of interest, as an heirloom. Fortune's wheel turns curiously – it was fourteen years later that his son was appointed to the staff of another American University – Cornell.

In February 1907 my father had to attend meetings in the Netherlands and Germany and, choosing the Parkeston-Hook of Holland route with its then through carriage from Liverpool Central, booked to arrive in Amsterdam on the 21st. It was my tenth birthday and he regretted being absent, but fortune smiled and the first engagement on the Continent was delayed for two days. On the evening of the 21st we learned of the wreck of the 'Berlin' with heavy loss of life.

Two accidents befell him in 1908: skating at Christmas under the Iron Bridge in Sefton Park the ice gave way and, though the depth of water was not great, the predicament, with thin ice adjoining, was not a pleasant one since other skaters were out of sight. The effects of immersion were temporary, but the other accident affected him for the rest of his life; it was also due to skating, but of the roller variety – then a popular sport: he fell on the rink in Renshaw Street with his left arm stretched out. The arm mended but slowly and, later, arthritis developed, all the more serious as he was left-handed – forty years later this developed into a crippling stage.

In 1913 the Waynflete Professorship of Physiology at Oxford, with a Fellowship at Magdalen, was offered to him and in this instance there was but little hesitation. He was then nearing sixty and the age of retirement was looming ahead but he felt that he could yet accomplish. Events proved his judgement to be right and at Oxford there was no retiring age – and no pension.

Glancing back in perspective, the years at Liverpool were, I believe, the happiest in his life, and my mother's too, but such a comparison is perhaps invalid for how can one compare superlatives? He loved Oxford and Magdalen dearly, but the events of 1914 were no passing clouds – they heralded more than four decades of world disaster, unsettlement and international stress. This period prior to 1914 was of comparative peace and stability though Sherrington, knowing Germany so intimately, foretold with some exactitude what was to come; by many he was regarded as an alarmist.

Saturday mornings were always spent at the laboratory and, customarily, Sunday mornings too, but Saturday afternoons and occasionally a whole week-end was enjoyed in sculling on the Dee, golf at Hoylake, bicycling into Shropshire, Cheshire or North Lancashire, or on expeditions to Haddon Fall, a ramble over Frodsham hills or a long tramp on the shore from Formby to Southport.

The Philharmonic concerts at Liverpool and the Richter concerts at Manchester gave great enjoyment and were social events of those days, as was the beginning of the Liverpool Repertory Company; the poems – later to be published in "The Assaying of Brabantius" – were mostly written in Liverpool days, where he rejoiced in the comradeship of Walter Raleigh – later they were destined to re-unite at Oxford.

Liverpool was at times tough, as was witnessed by the strike scenes of 1911: my father always walked to the laboratory by way of the streets behind Smithdown Road. One winter's evening in deep snow coming home with a visiting professor from Sheffield an icy snowball, from a side street, removed his hat at great speed and left an ugly cut on his forehead but, leaving his friend with surprising speed, he caught the marauder within some fifty yards and, having rolled him in the snow, returned to explain that it reminded him delightfully of his Cambridge days. I recall his return home battered but unbent, whilst Macdonald retailed what he had witnessed. On returning from Glasgow one night after acting as visiting examiner, and with the fees – then paid in cash – in his pocket, he was attacked in an oil-lighted non-corridor compartment between Preston and Liverpool (Exchange). It was an unpleasant incident and he never knew how his assailant had judged his momentary wealth.

Summer vacations permitted the continuation of rambles abroad 'en bicyclette'. From Maintenon a postcard I still retain rejoiced me at $5^1/_2$, for on it was the following doggerel, scribbled in the Jardin du Chateau, which I never could visit myself until fifty years later: –

"In this old garden with moat for warden,
Madame de Maintenon, cheeks pink and paint on 'em,
Sat and eat toffee and sipped black coffee,
In her beautiful bonnet fresh roses upon it which much
nicer to wear is than a bonnet from Paris."
(August 25th, 1902)

To his wife in these years at Liverpool, Sherrington owed much for, in addition to looking after his papers, involving what one would today call secretarial duties, her knowledge of languages, particularly French, was more than that of an amateur. She was accomplished in French long before they were married and, throughout Liverpool days, one day per week was given to French conversation. Music, literature, architecture and travel appealed to her immensely and she found herself at home in every walk of life, whether as an organist in her village church or hostess on the most formal of occasions. She possessed that happy attribute of showing interest in, and some knowledge of, most subjects under discussion and even more in the people, whoever they might be, whom she met.

Oxford

Though the years at London and Liverpool had brought to him many distinctions, Honorary Degrees at Universities and Membership of many learned societies, it was in his Oxford days that he received the highest honours that a country, and indeed the world, can accord to a scientist for his researches. He liked to think that they were offered to him as a man as well as for the work he had accomplished, for they demonstrated that he was much beloved by many in whose hands lay their bestowal. He accepted them in a spirit of humility, as was appropriate to one who had entered Caius with little but his brains to help him as he passed through the Gate of Humility.

More than once on receiving some honour he would exclaim "there must be some mistake, this is not intended for me, it is 'X' who should have received this". There is only one honour which, being suggested, he felt unable to accept for financial and other reasons, and he had to reply in the negative to the then President of the Board of Education. In the years came the Presidency of the Royal Society, the Knight Grand Cross of the British Empire, the Order of Merit and the Nobel Prize. All these he delighted in, as did his friends who were legion, but these tributes did not affect his modesty.

The Oxford that he came to he already knew well, having spent summer vacations there – as he had also, as a lover of Shakespeare, at Stratford-on-Avon. By bicycle he knew well the surrounding territory, its lovely villages and their churches; he knew each college quad intimately and could announce each detail of its architecture. Oxford in 1913 had only just lost its horse-trams in the 'High' and in Banbury Road and its horse-buses in Woodstock Road, but Morris was beginning to change that scene.

Oxford he loved and came to love even more, though some of its social and formal life he found a trifle rigid and inhuman. In the Osler home however, there was a refreshing and stimulating refuge from formality. War came soon after his new home had been established in north Oxford, adjoining the Cher on which he could indulge in canoeing and punting. Much of his writing was done on the river.

The year of his appointment at Magdalen involved a visit to the Physiological Congress at St. Petersburg. Berlin lay on the outwards journey, with a three-hours' customs hold-up on the Russian border (not on his account), and a return via Moscow and Warsaw. A lunch on the invitation of the Tsar at Tsarskoé Sélo provided memories: he remembered the menu when over ninety and quoted it correctly, not knowing that a copy was still extant. The Tsar asked Sherrington news of the former's cousin and finally my father had to admit that he had not met him recently! The Russian host at this luncheon, on May 3rd, 1913, in his welcome, to which my father had to reply, stated that it was the Tsar's wish that each guest should carry away a souvenir from his table. Desperately Sherrington looked around the table, which was loaded with candelabra and silver, but finally his eye lighted on packets of chocolate with photographs of the Tsar, Tsarina and the Tsarevitch – he suggested that the guests would like these. Today, in 1957, that chocolate in its silver paper with photographs of the Royal Family of Russia still exists, stale, but a record of what was and will never return.

Long an admirer of Russia, he dined with Pavlov, being warned by his host not to be surprised if police arrived during dinner, since it was not permitted to have two guests to dinner in a private home. The police did not, in fact, arrive, but on the way by special train to Tsarskoé Sélo, guards swung on to the train from both sides simultaneously, examining each compartment for hidden arms.

Bereft of undergraduates and with but few assistants in 1914–1915 he became involved in much Government work – the problem of gas masks, industrial fatigue and the like. In the summer of 1915 he disappeared on a bicycle, presumably for a holiday, leaving no address: a collar stud, which was lost and could not be replaced, disclosed his whereabouts. He was a bench-worker 'incognito' at a munitions plant in Birmingham. His shift time, 7 a. m.–6 p. m., did not permit any visit to a shop to obtain a collar stud. His great interest in industrial fatigue – he was Chairman of the Industrial Fatigue Board in 1918 – had determined him to study fatigue 'in situ', on the pay he earned, and this period he afterwards described as one of the most useful in his life, even if it did necessitate crossing Birmingham on his bicycle in the early hours of the morning. He was then nearly 60.

His first visit abroad after the Armistice was to Paris in November 1918. It was not without incident as a trap-door in the R.F.C. plane flew open beside my father's seat during the Channel crossing – no accident ensued. In 1919 he was one of the British delegates to the celebrations in honour of the centenary of Pasteur's birth; a problem arose owing to the adamant refusal of the Foreign Office in London to provide a wreath to lay on Pasteur's grave. This difficulty was overcome by the British Ambassador in Paris being asked to do his best – the best consisted in providing a wreath which could hardly be delivered to the delegates who were staying at the Grand Hotel and which certainly dwarfed all other floral tributes to Pasteur! Return from Paris was made via Bruxelles, with a meeting of the Belgian Academy of Sciences.

It was during his Presidency of the Royal Society, 1920–1925, that some concern was felt at the possibility of "The Times" becoming a party political journal and a committee was set up to determine the future continuity of "The Times" as a national institution. As President of the Royal Society he served on this committee and took keen pleasure in the satisfactory results which followed its deliberations and decisions.

A visitor who was especially appreciative of being shown round the laboratories in Oxford in 1921 was the Prince of Siam, his letter of thanks to Sherrington was beautifully worded. The kindly comments he received on the publication of his verses "The Assaying of Brabantius and other Poems", gave him as much pleasure as scientific success: the letters from Thomas Hardy, Edmund Gosse, Henry Head and Charles Richet were especially prized.

An activity at Oxford to which he gave of his best was the Rhodes scheme, though his links with Canada, Australia, New Zealand, South Africa and the United States were not limited to undergraduates coming to Oxford from those countries as Rhodes scholars: Sunday afternoon and evening was open house at his home, which was often referred to as 'Chadland'; there must be many scattered in four continents who recall Lady Sherrington's welcome and her grace as a hostess. Her long illness, and finally her death in 1933, clouded the days when Sir Charles, as he then was, received an Honorary Degree at Upsala and a few weeks later the Nobel award, with E. D. Adrian (now Lord Adrian), at Stockholm. To cross the North Sea four times within a month in November/December at the age of seventy-six is evidence of his stamina.

The year 1934 witnessed the completion of his eight years of service on the Medical Research Council: a warm letter of thanks from Stanley Baldwin records the event. Wisdom prevailed in regard to his retirement from the Waynflete professorship in 1935, but his ties with Magdalen held firm in an Honorary Fellowship, and those ties he greatly cherished as he did the generosity of the College on his retirement.

Life at Oxford for over twenty years he had enjoyed immensely, though at the time he was President of the Royal Society with almost daily visits to London – on many occasions two visits in one day – it was no sinecure. His contacts at Magdalen and other Colleges, his friendships with those most knowledgeable in the arts, as well as the sciences – Robert Bridges as an example – preserved his zest for life and conversation and, thus, there was a wrench to leave a city where kindness had been shown him from every side and where kindred thoughts and kindred interests were shared with his friends and they were legion.

Ipswich Again: Cambridge: Eastbourne

The choice of Ipswich for the years of retirement was not unnatural. For him it held so many happy memories and, after a short, unsuccessfull experiment in a small house, he acquired 'Broomside', adjoining Broom Hill – now the property of Ipswich Town. Broom Hill had belonged to Brooks Hall, where school friends had lived; thus did he return to haunts of youthful days and boyhood escapades.

The main task facing him was the preparation of the Gifford lectures for Edinburgh University – these later became the book "Man on His Nature" which will long remain a monument, not only to his working life, but to the thoughts he held towards the culmination of that life, and also his choice of words to express those thoughts. There were other activities too, such as Governor of his old school and service for Ipswich town in an advisory capacity, touching on museums, its health services and so forth. Indeed the days were no idle ones at 'Broomside' and, on completion of the Gifford lectures, he turned to another work – the life of "Jean Fernel" – a book which, when published, has charmed many at home and abroad by its account of the early days of medicine in Paris. His love of Paris and its 'Rive Gauche' stands out clearly in the pages of this book, enjoyed as they have been by many Frenchman too.

His work as a Trustee of the British Museum brought him many interests and some new friends: to him it was a labour of love and he was never happier in those years than in searching for rare and early books which, if he could obtain them, he presented to the British Museum or some other library. Amongst the libraries which benefited from this activity was that of the University of Wales. The large number of letters extant of thanks from national libraries bear witness to his energy and generosity in this sphere.

His days were much brightened by the letters, and the visits, he received from those who had worked with him in earlier years and whose interests were wide and akin to his own. Alex Forbes, Wilder Penfield and John Fulton were prominent amongst transatlantic residents – those nearer home would provide an overlong list.

The second World-War shattered rudely his dreams of peaceful retirement and in 1940, after heavy damage by aerial attack on adjoining property, he was advised to move from Ipswich in view of his more than four score years. An interlude with his brother in North London involved even more nights in air raid shelters, and it was A. V. Hill, who, to the relief of his family, persuaded him to reside temporarily in Cambridge, where he had so many friends and manifold interests. The Bull Hotel in Kings Parade proved but a short-lived refuge – it was requisitioned at short notice and he found himself homeless, though his Honorary Fellowship of Caius permitted him use of the College on the kind invitation of the Fellows.

From the predicament in which he now found himself he was rescued by the Master of the College and Mrs. Cameron, for although there were no rooms available or, indeed suitable, for anyone of that great age in the College, the Master offered him accommodation in his own home – the Lodge. It was more than a generous and kindly gesture, it was generosity 'in extremis', and, if Sherrington's work since he had first entered Caius in 1880, had brought some honour and lustre to the College, the College repaid now in a hundred ways the reflected honours from his achievments. The charm of the Lodge with its courteous hostess, the long discussions with the Master, the free and easy conversation with the Fellows, the use of the Senior Common Room and the Library made his closing years, in surroundings hallowed by memories, as delightful as they could be. Men of over eighty are apt to be dictatorial and invariably have foibles of their own; Cambridge is no stranger to such problems but one feels that at times the Master and the Fellows of Gonville and Caius College must have possessed souls of ineffable patience.

The crippling onslaught of fibrositis demanded treatment at a nursing home – run by nuns – and at Droitwich, but there was no permanent cure – transfer to Espérance, again a Catholic establishment, at Eastbourne seemed the best course to adopt. Words come not easily to express adequately the care with which he was attended by the Sisters. Although not a Roman Catholic many of his family had been, one being a Mother Superior in a convent in Whitechapel, others of the family had long been resident in Spain. In the Oxford days the Pope had named him as a British member of the Pontifical Academy of Sciences and he had formed an admiration for the Roman Catholic Church, but he was no catholic and there was little call for the Sisters to show him the great kindness they did.

His last years were spent in a quiet house not far from the shore at Eastbourne; many came to visit him and as long as he could walk he enjoyed his contacts with Eastbourne School, the masters and some of the boys, who, surprisingly, seemed to enjoy being with a nonogenarian and bringing their problems of life to him.

He once when ninety expressed some shame that he was not still earning as much as he was spending. A distinguished French scientist who visited him found, to his surprise, that his French was still fluent, and, as we left the house, exclaimed with awe 'c'est un homme' – a tribute my father would have enjoyed.

Deafness grew and, for a period, his eyes gave trouble but remarkably repaired themselves – fibrositis finally held him to his rooms. Conversation to the end was like his earlier self – discussion usually turned to books, literature and painting, architecture and hence to travel. He talked much of his mother and early Ipswich days, and those memories were still concise but of more modern days vagueness rapidly increased. So often he complained that he had lived too long and was being a nuisance to so many people, but so long as the wealth of experience and history remained clear his reminiscences were still fascinating. On the evening of March 3rd, 1952, we discussed, for I was leaving the next week for America, the visit to Canada in 1897 and he described the flowers he had then found in the Rockies. Twenty-four hours later the paper he was reading was heard to drop from his hands: the world had lost one who had toiled long to increase its health and happiness but had equally enjoyed that toiling.

After his death, on the table by his chair, there was found a poem which had never been published. It had been written to his mother for her birthday – October 14th, 1893. Here it is: –

Thee, mother, in dead hours of night
when stars are out o'er thee and me
and on thy roof their holy light
my thoughts encompass utterly.

Day thou hast filled so full with love
then ended, sleep has loosed thy lids
and those brown eyes they float above
lie blind with peace, as Nature bids;

or haply dreaming work in dream
some gentle service love designs
some patient good that wrought with gleam
and quiet joy of face, outshines

upon the heavy-hearted ones
like dawn to eyes that fever-left
turn windowward and know the sun's
kind light again. O far bereft

my passion makes me near; I see
thy hands upon the coverlet
that were tonight enclasped for me
and nightly in old days were set

upon my forehead yielding calm
before the prayer at thy knees made
was uttered and the little psalm
and, last, Goodnight, God bless you! said.

At the end of these verses, in pencil in her handwriting, were the words "Never was there a Mother so blessed with sons". Thus was the ending like the beginning.

"Ab initio ad finem"

Index

---

* C. S. Sherrington('s).

Karl R. Popper
Penn, Great Britain

John C. Eccles
Contra, Switzerland

The Self
and Its Brain

66 figures. XVI, 597 pages. 1977
Cloth DM 39,–; US $ 19.50; £ 9.40
ISBN 3-540-08307-3
Available from your bookseller

Contents:
Materialism Transcendens Itself. The Worlds 1, 2 and 3.
Materialism Criticized. Some Remarks on the Self.
Historical Comments on the Mind-Body-Problem.
Summary. – The Cerebral Cortex. Conscious Perception. Voluntary Movement. The Language Centres
of the Human Brain. Global Lesions of the Human
Cerebrum. Circumscribed Cerebral Lesions. – The
Self-Conscious Mind and the Brain. Concious
Memory: The Cerebral Processes Concerned in
Storage and Retrieval. – Dialogues.

In Part I, Popper discusses the philosophical issue
between dualist or even pluralist interactionism on the
one side, and materialism and parallelism on the other.
There is also a historical review of these issues.

In Part II, Eccles examines the mind from the neurological standpoint: the structure of the brain and its
functional performance under normal as well as abnormal circumstances, for example when lesions
(especially those surgically induced) are present. The
result is a radical and intriguing hypothesis on the
interaction between mental events and detailed neurological occurrences in the cerebral cortex.

Part III, based on twelve recorded conversations,
reflects the exciting exchange between the authors as
they attempt to come to terms with their conflicting
opinions. This part preserves the intimate quality of the
dialogues, and shows how some of the authors' viewpoints changed in the course of these daily discussions.

Springer
International

Prices are subject to change without notice

John C. Eccles

Facing Reality

Philosophical Adventures by a Brain Scientist

36 figures. XI, 210 pages. 1970
DM 25,–; US $ 11.00
(Heidelberg Science Library, Volume 13)
ISBN 3-540-90014-4

Contents:
Introduction: Man, Brain and Science. – The
Neuronal Machinery of the Brain. – Synaptic
Mechanisms Possibly Concerned in Learning
and Memory. – The Experiencing Self. – The
Brain and the Unity of Conscious Experi-
ence. – Evolution and the Conscious Self. –
The Understanding of Nature. – Man, Free-
dom and Creativity. – The Necessity of Free-
dom for the Free Flowering of Science. – The
Brain and the Soul. – Education and the World
of Objective Knowledge. – Epilogue. –
References.

From the reviews:
"This book is an account of the views of a brain
scientist of world renown on the lifelong interplay between the conscious self and the
external world. It is based on various lectures
and papers written over the last few years,
including some unpublished material…
The reality of which he speaks in the title of his
book is above all the reality of self awareness
and death awareness. These two are at the heart
of many present discontents, and as a brain
scientist Sir John Eccles is distressed that the
problems should so often nowadays be treated
with irrationality and not with reason. Sir John
has often broken a lance with the philosophers
and has read widely. This is a deeply interesting book."
Durrant's British Medical Journal

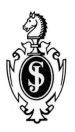

Springer-Verlag
Berlin
Heidelberg
New York

John C. Eccles

The Human Mystery

The GIFFORD Lectures
University of Edinburgh 1977–1978

1979. 89 figures. XVI, 255 pages
Cloth DM 34,–; US $ 18.70
ISBN 3-540-09016-9

Contents:
The Theme of Natural Theology: How the
Challenge Will be Met. – Origin and Evolution
of the Universe. – Planetary System and Planet
Earth. – Origin of Life and Biological
Evolution. – Human Evolution: The Story
of Cerebral Development. – Cultural Evolu-
tion With Language and Values: The Human
Person. – From the General to the Particular:
The Creation of a Self. – Structure of the Neo-
cortex; Conscious Perception. – Learning and
Memory. – The Mind-Brain Problem: Experi-
mental Evidence and Hypothesis.

Sir John Eccles, 1963 Nobel Prize winner and
Distinguished Professor Emeritus of the University of New York, ponders what he calls,
"the great and mysterious problems" presently
beyond science and which "may be, in part,
forever beyond science." In this series of
GIFFORD Lectures which he presented at the
University of Edinburgh in February/March
1978, Sir John addresses problems, such as the
origin of the Universe in the "Big Bang," the
origin of life, the manner in which biological
evolution was constrained to lead eventually
to Homo sapiens, and finally to the origin of
each individual conscious self.

The last three lectures are on the human brain
and the brain-mind problem. The most recent
concepts on the structure and function of the
brain are shown to lead to hypotheses of brain-
mind interaction in perception, in memory, in
voluntary action and in the manifestation of
self-consciousness.

Within this almost infinetely wide range of
enquiry these lectures should serve to uncover
many extraordinary contingencies on the way
to the origin of each one of us a consciously
experiencing being.

Prices are subject to change without notice